MANUAL OF
EMERGENCY AIRWAY
MANAGEMENT
FOURTH EDITION

Editor-in-Chief

Ron M. Walls, MD
Chair, Department of Emergency Medicine
Brigham and Women's Hospital
Professor of Medicine
Division of Emergency Medicine
Harvard Medical School
Boston, Massachusetts

Senior Editor

Michael F. Murphy, MD
Professor and Chair
Department of Anesthesiology and Pain Medicine
University of Alberta
Edmonton, Alberta, Canada

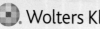 Wolters Kluwer | Lippincott Williams & Wilkins
Health

Philadelphia · Baltimore · New York · London
Buenos Aires · Hong Kong · Sydney · Tokyo

Senior Acquisitions Editor: Frances DeStefano
Product Director: Julia Seto
Production Manager: Bridgett Dougherty
Senior Manufacturing Manager: Benjamin Rivera
Senior Marketing Manager: Kimberly Schonberger
Design Coordinator: Stephen Druding
Production Service: S4Carlisle Publishing Services

Library of Congress Cataloging-in-Publication Data

Manual of emergency airway management / editors, Ron Walls, Michael Murphy. — 4th ed.
     p. ; cm.
  Includes bibliographical references and index.
  ISBN 978-1-4511-4491-8 (alk. paper)
  I. Walls, Ron M. II. Murphy, Michael F. (Michael Francis), 1954-
  [DNLM: 1. Airway Obstruction—therapy—Handbooks. 2. Emergency Treatment—Handbooks. 3. Intubation, Intratracheal—Handbooks. WF 39]

616.2'00425—dc23
2011045971

Care has been taken to confirm the accuracy of the information presented and to describe generally accepted practices. However, the authors, editors, and publisher are not responsible for errors or omissions or for any consequences from application of the information in this book and make no warranty, expressed or implied, with respect to the currency, completeness, or accuracy of the contents of the publication. Application of the information in a particular situation remains the professional responsibility of the practitioner.

The authors, editors, and publisher have exerted every effort to ensure that drug selection and dosage set forth in this text are in accordance with current recommendations and practice at the time of publication. However, in view of ongoing research, changes in government regulations, and the constant flow of information relating to drug therapy and drug reactions, the reader is urged to check the package insert for each drug for any change in indications and dosage and for added warnings and precautions. This is particularly important when the recommended agent is a new or infrequently employed drug.

Some drugs and medical devices presented in the publication have Food and Drug Administration (FDA) clearance for limited use in restricted research settings. It is the responsibility of the health care provider to ascertain the FDA status of each drug or device planned for use in their clinical practice.

To purchase additional copies of this book, call our customer service department at (800) 638-3030 or fax orders to (301) 223-2320. International customers should call (301) 223-2300.
Visit Lippincott Williams & Wilkins on the Internet: at LWW.com. Lippincott Williams & Wilkins customer service representatives are available from 8:30 am to 6 pm, EST.

10 9 8 7 6 5 4 3 2 1

Dedication

This book is dedicated to those dauntless providers who work around the clock and around the globe, in hospital, in the field, and in the air, accepting the responsibility to provide timely, effective airway management to save lives often in the face of overwhelming challenge and without expectation of recognition or reward.

PREFACE TO THE FOURTH EDITION

Here, we proudly present the fourth edition of the manual, with complete reorganization of the content, rich new material, and a broader pool of highly talented contributors, who teach with us in The Difficult Airway Course: Emergency™. The creation of a new edition is much more than just an opportunity to update what has become a very authoritative and useful book. Equally importantly, this book has become our "thinking spot"; the place we go to quietly ponder, evaluate, and create. This is an important retreat every four years from our immersion in the practice and teaching of airway management. For, although we sedulously follow new developments in airway management, and scrupulously and continuously parse the literature, it is only when we are planning a new edition of the manual that we withdraw from our other activities and actively discuss (and debate) what we consider to be the key developments in the evolution of airway management. It is these discussions that lead to dramatic alterations in our content and recommendations from edition to edition. In the second edition, we added extensive discussion of rigid fiberoptic instruments (intubating fiberoptic stylets) and for the first time dedicated a chapter to video laryngoscopy, then an emerging technology with great promise. The algorithms, which have been modified for every edition, were freshened, and we developed more chapters on special clinical circumstances. From the second to third edition, we reconsidered some "entrenched" wisdom, and abandoned it. The Sellick maneuver, long a staple of rapid sequence intubation, no longer was recommended, based on our analysis that the potential for harm was at least as great as the potential for good. Similarly, we revisited our pretreatment drugs and our widely used and familiar mnemonic, LOAD. De-fasciculation and atropine pre-treatment for children failed to make the cut, leaving us only with lidocaine and fentanyl, in a new ABC mnemonic. The lighted stylet, eclipsed by similar fiberoptic devices of much greater utility, was on the chopping block as well, but in the end, we included it, but in a de-emphasized role. Again, the algorithms, especially the difficult airway algorithm, were updated, and new devices were added in such numbers as to cause a reorganization of the material in that section of the book. So, here we are with the fourth edition, the most significant revision of the book in its history. We have completely reorganized the chapters into more cohesive sections, beginning with the cognitive and anatomical bases for airway management, moving into oxygen delivery, then basic airway management (which includes extra-glottic devices), tracheal intubation, pharmacology and techniques (RSI, formerly Chapter 3, now is Chapter 19), pediatrics, EMS, and special airway considerations. We again have modified the difficult airway algorithm, the result of thinking at length about the "forced to act" situation, when the provider recognizes a difficult airway, but the patient is deteriorating so rapidly that immediate action is required, despite the anticipated (or dreaded) difficulty. All sections of the book are updated, none so richly as the discussion of the various video laryngoscopes; a transformative technology, incubated in Jack Pacey's impromptu laboratory in Burnaby, British Columbia over a decade ago, signaling the inevitable demise of direct laryngoscopy. As always, when we put a book to bed, we feel immense satisfaction, tempered by the reality that we have but captured the moment, and the near future of a rapidly evolving field. We are comforted by Terry Steele's vision in helping us create Airway World, a vibrant on-line resource that allows us to continually update and educate our community of colleagues, whether regarding a new device or drug, best techniques, or breaking research. Just as this manual is our interpretation of the knowledge and skill set necessary for emergency airway management, Airway World (www.airwayworld.com) is our hedge against the future, our opportunity to keep you up to date, confident, and informed.

As always, we are grateful for the opportunity to contribute, humbled by the enormity of the challenges faced by our colleagues in emergency airway management, and energized by the prospect of helping, in our small way, to save more lives.

Ron M. Walls, MD   Michael F. Murphy, MD
Boston, MA   Edmonton, Alberta

ACKNOWLEDGMENTS

Nothing of value grows without foundation. My career and contributions have been possible only because of the enormous strength, love, and support of my wife, Barbara, and my children, Andrew, Blake, and Alexa, who have imbued me both with the passion to reach for the sky and the good sense to always keep at least one foot on the ground. I am grateful also to the national faculty of our airway courses, and the innumerable emergency medicine residents and faculty whose self-lessness, commitment, dedication, and prowess inspire me to continue questioning, challenging, learning, and teaching.

Ron M. Walls, MD
Boston, MA
December 2011

I dedicate this book to the faculty of the Airway Courses we teach, the authors of the book chapters we edit, and the endless debate among us regarding airway management in the interest of our patient's lives. No work of this significance could be possible without the support and encouragement of my family: my partner, Deb, and my children, Amanda, Ryan, and Teddy.

Michael Murphy, MD
Edmonton, AB
December 2011

CONTRIBUTORS

Jennifer L. Avegno, MD

Assistant Professor
Section of Emergency Medicine
Louisiana State University Health Sciences
    Center – New Orleans
New Orleans, Louisiana

Aaron E. Bair, MD

Associate Professor
Emergency Medicine
University of California, Davis School
    of Medicine
Sacramento, California

Diane M. Birnbaumer, MD

Professor
Department of Medicine
David Geffen School of Medicine at UCLA
Associate Program Director
Department of Emergency Medicine
Harbor-UCLA Medical Center
Torrance, California

Kerry B. Broderick, BSN, MD

Associate Professor
Department of Emergency Medicine
University of Colorado at Denver
Attending Physician
Department of Emergency Medicine
Denver Health Medical Center
Denver, Colorado

Calvin A. Brown, III, MD

Assistant Professor of Medicine
Division of Emergency Medicine
Harvard Medical School
Attending Physician and Student Program
    Director
Department of Emergency Medicine
Brigham and Women's Hospital
Boston, MA

Stephen Bush, MA (Oxon), MBBS

Clinical Director, Urgent Care
Emergency Department
Leeds Teaching Hospitals Trust
Consultant in Emergency Medicine
Emergency Department
St James's University Hospital
Leeds, United Kingdom

Steven C. Carleton, MD, PhD

Professor
Department of Emergency Medicine
University of Cincinnati College of Medicine
Attending Physician
Center for Emergency Care
University Hospital
Cincinnati, Ohio

David A. Caro, MD

Associate Professor & Residency Director
Department of Emergency Medicine
University of Florida College of
    Medicine – Jacksonville
Jacksonville, Florida

Peter M.C. DeBlieux, MD

Professor of Clinical Medicine
Emergency Medicine
Louisiana State University Health Science
    Center
Clinical Professor of Surgery
Tulane University School of Medicine
New Orleans, Louisiana

Valerie A. Dobiesz, MD, MPH

Professor
Department of Emergency Medicine
University of Illinois
    College of Medicine
Associate Residency Director
Department of Emergency Medicine

University of Illinois Medical Center
at Chicago
Chicago, Illinois

Jan L. Eichel, CFRN, BA, EMT-P

Director of Clinical Operations
West Michigan Air Care
Kalamazoo, Michigan
Midwest Regional Course Director
The Difficult Airway Course: EMS
Airway Authority Education
Scotts, Michigan

Frederick H. Ellinger, Jr., EMT-P

Flight Paramedic
Mid-Atlantic MedEvac
Hahnemann University Hospital
Philadelphia, Pennsylvania

Abbie L. Erickson, PharmD

Clinical Pharmacist
Department of Pharmacy
Northwestern Memorial Hospital
Chicago, Illinois

Kevin M. Franklin, BS

Flight Nurse
West Michigan Air Care
Research Coordinator
Department of Emergency Medicine
Michigan State University – Kalamazoo Center
for Medical Studies
Kalamazoo, Michigan

Michael A. Gibbs, MD

Professor of Emergency Medicine
UNC School of Medicine - Charlotte Campus
Chair
Department of Emergency Medicine
Carolinas Medical Center
Charlotte, NC

Steven A. Godwin, MD, FACEP

Professor and Chair
Department of Emergency Medicine
University of Florida College
of Medicine – Jacksonville
Assistant Dean, Simulation Education
University of Florida College
of Medicine – Jacksonville
Jacksonville, Florida

Michael G. Gonzalez, MD

Chief
Department of Emergency Medicine
Landstuhl Regional Medical Center
Landstuhl, Germany
Deputy Director
Critical Care Air Transport Teams
United States Air Forces – Europe
Ramstein Air Base, Germany

Alan C. Heffner, MD

Assistant Clinical Professor
University of North Carolina School
of Medicine
Director, Medical Intensive Care Unit
Director of ECMO Services
Pulmonary and Critical Care Consultants
Department of Internal Medicine
Department of Emergency Medicine
Carolinas Medical Center
Charlotte, North Carolina

Andy S. Jagoda, MD

Professor and Chair
Department of Emergency Medicine
Mount Sinai School of Medicine
Mount Sinai Hospital
New York, New York

Erik G. Laurin, MD

Associate Professor
Department of Emergency Medicine
University of California, Davis
Sacramento, California

Robert C. Luten, MD

Professor
Department of Emergency Medicine
Department of Pediatrics
University of Florida School of Medicine
Jacksonville, Florida

Nathan W. Mick, MD

Assistant Professor
Department of Emergency Medicine
Tufts University School of Medicine
Director of Pediatric Emergency Medicine
Director of Clinical Operations
Department of Emergency Medicine
Maine Medical Center
Portland, Maine

Michael F. Murphy, MD

Professor and Chair
Department of Anesthesiology and Pain
   Medicine
University of Alberta
Zone Clinical Chief
Department of Anesthesia
Edmonton Zone
Edmonton, Alberta, Canada

Joshua Nagler, MD

Assistant Professor
Department of Pediatrics
Harvard Medical School
Attending Physician
Division of Emergency Medicine
Children's Hospital Boston
Boston, Massachusetts

Patrick A. Nee, FRCP, FRCS, FCEM, FFICM

Consultant
Emergency and Critical Care Medicine
Whiston Hospital
Merseyside, United Kingdom
Visiting Professor of Emergency Medicine
Liverpool John Moores University
Liverpool, United Kingdom

Bret P. Nelson, MD

Associate Professor
Department of Emergency Medicine
Mount Sinai School of Medicine
New York, New York

Robert F. Reardon, MD

Associate Professor
Department of Emergency Medicine
University of Minnesota
Faculty Physician
Department of Emergency Medicine
Hennepin County Medical Center
Minneapolis, Minnesota

John C. Sakles, MD

Professor
Department of Emergency Medicine
University of Arizona College of Medicine
Attending Physician
Department of Emergency Medicine
University Medical Center
Tucson, Arizona

Mary Beth Skarote, NREMT-P

Program Manager
Disaster Medical Services
North Carolina Office of EMS
Raleigh, North Carolina

Julie A. Slick, MD

Assistant Professor
Department of Clinical Medicine
LSU Health Sciences Center
New Orleans, Louisiana

Katren R. Tyler, MD

Associate Professor and Associate Residency
   Director
Department of Emergency Medicine
University of California Davis School
   of Medicine
Attending Physician
Department of Emergency Medicine
University of California Davis Medical Center
Sacramento, California

Robert J. Vissers, MD, FACEP

Chief
Department of Emergency Medicine
Legacy Emanuel Medical Center
Adjunct Associate Professor
Department of Emergency Medicine
Oregon Health Sciences University
Portland, Oregon

Ron M. Walls, MD

Professor of Medicine
Division of Emergency Medicine
Harvard Medical School
Chair
Department of Emergency Medicine
Brigham and Women's Hospital
Boston, Massachusetts

Richard D. Zane, MD

Professor and Chair
Department of Emergency Medicine
University of Colorado
   School of Medicine
University of Colorado Hospital
Denver, Colorado

CONTENTS

SECTION IV. Tracheal Intubation

SECTION V. Pharmacology and Techniques of Airway Management

SECTION VI. Pediatric Airway Management

SECTION VII. EMS Airway Management

SECTION VIII. Special Clinical Circumstances

1

The Decision to Intubate

Ron M. Walls

Timely, effective airway management in an emergency can mean the difference between life and death, or between ability and disability. As such, airway management is the single most important skill of the emergency physician, and emergency airway management is one of the defining domains of the specialty of emergency medicine. Anesthesia providers, hospitalists, and intensivists often are called upon as the primary responders to airway emergencies arising in hospital inpatient units. Paramedics and critical care transport personnel are responsible for the out-of-hospital airway. Regardless of specialty or locus of care, these practitioners must maintain the cognitive base and technical skill set required for swift, decisive airway management, which is often required without warning and in suboptimal circumstances.

The emergence of new technology, principally the various methods of video laryngoscopy, is changing the fundamental approach to airway decision-making, particularly with respect to difficult intubation. Nevertheless, emergency airway management, whether in the emergency department (ED) or elsewhere in the hospital or prehospital setting, still comprises a series of complex actions:

- Rapidly assess the patient's need for intubation and the urgency of the situation.
- Determine the best method of airway management.
- Decide whether pharmacologic agents are indicated, which to use, in what order, and in what doses.
- Construct a plan in the event that the primary method is unsuccessful; recognize when the planned airway intervention has failed, and quickly and effectively execute the alternative (rescue) technique.

Physicians responsible for emergency airway management must be proficient with the techniques and medications used for rapid sequence intubation, the preferred method for most emergency intubations. The entire repertoire of airway skills must be mastered, including bag-mask ventilation, conventional and video laryngoscopy, flexible endoscopy, the use of extraglottic airway devices, adjunctive techniques such as use of an endotracheal tube introducer (ETI, EI; also known as the gum elastic bougie), and surgical airway techniques (e.g., cricothyrotomy).

This chapter focuses on the decision to intubate. Subsequent chapters describe airway management decision-making, methods of ensuring oxygenation, techniques and devices for airway management, the pharmacology of airway management, and considerations for certain special clinical circumstances, including the prehospital environment and care of pediatric patients.

INDICATIONS FOR INTUBATION

The decision to intubate is based on three fundamental clinical assessments:

1. Is there a failure of airway maintenance or protection?
2. Is there a failure of ventilation or oxygenation?
3. What is the anticipated clinical course?

The results of these three evaluations will lead to a correct decision to intubate or not to intubate in virtually all conceivable cases.

A. *Is there a failure of airway maintenance or protection?*
A patent airway is essential for adequate oxygenation and ventilation, and protection of the airway against aspiration of gastric contents is vital. The conscious, alert patient uses the musculature of the upper airway and various protective reflexes to maintain a patent airway and to protect against the aspiration of foreign substances, gastric contents, or secretions. The ability of the patient to phonate with a clear, unobstructed voice is strong evidence of both airway patency and protection. In the severely ill or injured patient, such airway maintenance and protection mechanisms are often attenuated or lost. If the spontaneously breathing patient is

not able to maintain a patent airway, an artificial airway may be established by the insertion of an oropharyngeal airway or a nasopharyngeal airway. Although such airway devices may restore a patent airway, they do not provide any protection against aspiration. As a general rule, any patient who requires the establishment of a patent airway also requires protection of that airway, and the use of an oropharyngeal or nasopharyngeal airway should be considered a temporizing measure, pending establishment of a definitive airway: placement of an appropriate (cuffed for adults and uncuffed for small children) endotracheal tube in the trachea.

A patient who is seemingly able to maintain a patent airway and adequate gas exchange cannot be assumed to be able to protect the airway against the aspiration of gastric contents, which carries a significantly increased risk of morbidity and mortality. It has been widely taught that the gag reflex is a reliable method of evaluating airway protective reflexes. In fact, this concept has never been subjected to adequate scientific scrutiny, and the absence of a gag reflex is neither sensitive nor specific as an indicator of loss of airway protective reflexes. The presence of a gag reflex has similarly not been demonstrated to ensure the presence of airway protection. In addition, testing the gag reflex in a supine, obtunded patient may result in vomiting and possible aspiration. Accordingly, the gag reflex is of no clinical value when assessing the need for intubation and should not be used for this purpose.

The assessment of spontaneous or volitional swallowing is probably a better assessment of the patient's ability to protect the airway than is the presence or absence of a gag reflex. Swallowing is a complex reflex that requires the patient to sense the presence of material in the posterior oropharynx and then to execute a series of intricate and coordinated muscular actions to direct the secretions down past a closed airway into the esophagus. The finding of pooled secretions in the patient's posterior oropharynx indicates a potential failure of these protective mechanisms, hence a failure of airway protection. In the absence of an immediately reversible condition, such as opioid overdose or reversible cardiac dysrhythmia, prompt intubation is indicated for any patient who is unable to maintain and protect the airway. A common clinical error is to assume that spontaneous breathing is proof that the ability to protect the airway is preserved. Although spontaneous ventilation may be adequate, the patient may be sufficiently obtunded to be at serious risk of aspiration.

B. *Is there a failure of ventilation or oxygenation?*
Stated simply, "gas exchange" is adequate to sustain vital organ function. If the patient is unable to ventilate adequately, or if adequate oxygenation cannot be achieved despite the use of supplemental oxygen, then intubation is indicated. In such cases, the intubation is performed to facilitate ventilation and oxygenation rather than to establish or protect the airway. An example is the patient with status asthmaticus, for whom bronchospasm and fatigue lead to ventilatory failure and hypoxemia, heralding respiratory arrest and death. Airway intervention is indicated when it is determined that the patient will not respond sufficiently to treatment to reverse the cascading events leading to respiratory arrest. Similarly, although the patient with severe acute respiratory distress syndrome may be maintaining and protecting the airway, he or she may have progressive oxygenation failure and supervening fatigue that can be managed only with tracheal intubation and positive-pressure ventilation. Unless ventilatory or oxygenation failure is resulting from a rapidly reversible cause, such as opioid overdose, intubation is required.

C. *What is the anticipated clinical course?*
Most patients who require emergency intubation have one or more of the previously discussed indications: failure of airway maintenance, airway protection, oxygenation, or ventilation. However, there is a large and important group for whom intubation is indicated, even though none of these four fundamental failures is present at the time of evaluation. These are the patients whose conditions, and airways, are predicted to deteriorate, either because of dynamic and progressive changes related to the presenting condition or because the work of breathing will become overwhelming in the face of catastrophic illness or injury. For example, consider the patient who presents with a stab wound to the midzone of the anterior neck and a visible hematoma. At the time of presentation, the patient may have perfectly adequate airway maintenance and protection and be ventilating and oxygenating well. The hematoma, however, provides clear evidence of significant vascular injury. Ongoing bleeding may be clinically

occult because the blood often tracks down the tissue planes of the neck (e.g., prevertebral space) rather than demonstrating visible expansion of the hematoma. Furthermore, the anatomical distortion caused by the enlarging internal hematoma may well thwart a variety of airway management techniques that would have been successful if undertaken earlier. The patient inexorably progresses from awake and alert with a patent airway to a state in which the airway becomes obstructed, often quite suddenly, and the anatomy is so distorted that airway management is difficult or impossible.

Analogous considerations apply to the polytrauma patient who presents with hypotension and multiple severe injuries, such as chest trauma. Although this patient initially maintains and protects his airway, and ventilation and oxygenation are adequate, intubation is indicated as part of the management of the constellation of injuries (i.e., as part of the overall management of the patient). The reason for the intubation of such patients becomes clear when one examines the anticipated clinical course of this patient. The hypotension mandates fluid resuscitation and evaluation for the source of the blood loss, including likely abdominal CT scan. Pelvic fractures, if unstable, require immobilization and likely embolization of bleeding vessels. Long bone fractures often require operative intervention. Chest tubes may be required to treat hemopneumothorax or in preparation for positive-pressure ventilation during surgery. Combative behavior confounds efforts to maintain spine precautions and requires pharmacologic restraint and evaluation by head CT scan. Throughout all of this, the patient's shock state causes inadequate tissue perfusion and increasing metabolic debt. This debt significantly affects the muscles of respiration, and progressive respiratory fatigue and failure often supervene. With the patient's ultimate destination certain to be the operating room or the ICU, and the need for complex and potentially painful procedures and diagnostic evaluations, which may require extended periods of time outside the resuscitation suite, this patient is best served by early intubation. In addition, intubation improves tissue oxygenation during shock and helps reduce the increasing metabolic debt burden.

Sometimes, the anticipated clinical course may be such that intubation is mandated because the patient will be exposed to a period of increased risk. For example, the patient with multiple injuries who appears relatively stable might be appropriately managed without intubation while geographically located in the ED. However, if that same patient requires CT scans, angiography, or any other prolonged diagnostic procedure, it may be more appropriate to intubate the patient before allowing him or her to leave the ED so that an airway crisis will not ensue in the radiology suite, where recognition may be delayed and response may not be optimal. Similarly, if such a patient is to be transferred from one hospital to another, airway management may be indicated on the basis of the increased risk to the patient during that transfer.

Not every trauma patient or every patient with a serious medical disorder requires intubation. However, in general, it is better to err on the side of caution by performing an intubation that might not, in retrospect, have been required, than to delay intubation, thus exposing the patient to a potentially disastrous deterioration.

APPROACH TO THE PATIENT

When evaluating a patient for emergency airway management, the first assessment should be of the patency and adequacy of the airway. In many cases, the adequacy of the airway is confirmed by having the patient speak. Ask questions such as "What is your name?" or "Do you know where you are?" The responses provide information about both the airway and the patient's neurologic status. A normal voice (as opposed to a muffled or distorted voice), the ability to inhale and exhale in the modulated manner required for speech, and the ability to comprehend the question and follow instructions are strong evidence of adequate upper airway function. Although such an evaluation should not be taken as proof that the upper airway is definitively secure, it is strongly suggestive that the airway is adequate *for the time being*. More importantly, the inability of the patient to phonate properly, inability to swallow secretions, or the presence of stridor, dyspnea, or altered mental status

---

BOX 1-1. Four Key Signs of Upper Airway Obstruction

- Muffled or "Hot Potato" voice (as though the patient is speaking with a mouthful of hot food)
- Inability to swallow secretions, either because of pain or obstruction
- Stridor
- Dyspnea

The first two signs do not necessarily herald imminent total upper airway obstruction; stridor, if new or progressive, usually does, and dyspnea also is a compelling symptom.

---

precluding responses to the questions should prompt a detailed assessment of the adequacy of the airway and ventilation (see Box 1-1). After assessing verbal response to questions, conduct a more detailed examination of the mouth and oropharynx. Examine the mouth for bleeding, swelling of the tongue or uvula, abnormalities of the oropharynx (e.g., peritonsillar abscess), or any other abnormalities that might interfere with the unimpeded passage of air through the mouth and oropharynx. Examine the mandible and central face for integrity. Examination of the anterior neck requires both visual inspection for deformity, asymmetry, or abnormality and palpation of the anterior neck, including the larynx and trachea. During palpation, assess carefully for the presence of subcutaneous air. This is identified by a crackling feeling on compression of the cutaneous tissues of the neck, much as if a sheet of wrinkled tissue paper were lying immediately beneath the skin. The presence of subcutaneous air indicates disruption of an air-filled passage, often the airway itself, especially in the setting of blunt or penetrating chest or neck trauma. Subcutaneous air in the neck also can be caused by pulmonary injury, esophageal rupture, or, rarely, gas-forming infection. Although these latter two conditions are not immediately threatening to the airway, patients may nevertheless rapidly deteriorate, requiring subsequent airway management. In the setting of blunt anterior neck trauma, assess the larynx for pain on motion. Move the larynx from side to side, assessing for "laryngeal crepitus," indicating normal contact of the airway with the airfilled upper esophagus. Absence of crepitus may be caused by edema between the larynx and the upper esophagus.

After inspecting and palpating the upper airway, note the respiratory pattern of the patient. The presence of inspiratory stridor, however slight, indicates some degree of upper airway obstruction. Lower airway obstruction, occurring beyond the level of the glottis, more often produces expiratory stridor. The volume and pitch of stridor are related to the velocity and turbulence of the ventilatory airflow. Most often, stridor is audible without a stethoscope. Auscultation of the neck with a stethoscope can reveal subauditory stridor that may also indicate potential airway compromise. Stridor is a late sign, especially in adult patients, who have large diameter airways, and significant airway compromise may develop before any sign of stridor is evident. When evaluating the respiratory pattern, observe the chest through several respiratory cycles. Symmetrical, concordant chest movement is the expected finding. In cases where there is significant injury, paradoxical movement of a flail segment of the chest may be observed. If spinal cord injury has impaired intercostal muscle functioning, diaphragmatic breathing may be present. In this form of breathing, there is little movement of the chest wall, and inspiration is evidenced by apparent increase in abdominal volume caused by descent of the diaphragm. Auscultate the chest to assess the adequacy of air exchange. Decreased breath sounds indicated pneumothorax, hemothorax, pleural effusion, or other pulmonary pathology.

The assessment of ventilation and oxygenation is a clinical one. Arterial blood gas determination provides little additional information as to whether intubation is necessary and may be misleading. The clinical impression of the patient's mentation, degree of fatigue, and severity of concomitant injuries or conditions is more important than isolated or even serial determinations of arterial oxygen or carbon dioxide (CO_2) tension. Oxygen saturation is monitored continuously by pulse oximetry, so arterial blood gases rarely are indicated for the purpose of determining arterial oxygen tension. In certain circumstances, oxygen saturation monitoring is unreliable because of poor peripheral perfusion, and arterial blood gases may then be required to assess oxygenation or to provide a correlation with pulse oximetry measurements. Continuous capnography (see Chapter 8) may be used to assess changes in the patient's ability to ventilate adequately, and the measurement of arterial CO_2 tension contributes little additional useful information, although often a single arterial blood gas measurement is used to provide a correlation baseline with end-tidal CO_2 readings. In patients with obstructive lung disease, such as asthma or chronic obstructive pulmonary disease, intubation may be required in the face of relatively low CO_2 tensions if the patient is becoming fatigued. Other times, extremely high CO_2 tensions may be managed successfully without intubation if the patient is showing clinical signs of improvement (e.g., increased alertness, improving speech, and less fatigue).

Finally, after assessment of the upper airway and the patient's ventilatory status, including pulse oximetry, capnography (if used), and mentation, consider the patient's anticipated clinical course. If the patient's condition is such that intubation is inevitable and a series of interventions is required, early intubation is preferable. Similarly, if the patient has a condition that is at risk of worsening over time, especially if it is likely to compromise the airway itself, early airway management is indicated. The same consideration applies to patients who require interfacility transfer by air or ground or a prolonged procedure in an area with diminished resuscitation capability. Intubation before transfer is preferable to a difficult, uncontrolled intubation in an austere environment after the condition has worsened. In all circumstances, the decision to intubate should be given precedence. If doubt exists as to whether the patient requires intubation, err on the side of intubating the patient. It is preferable to intubate the patient and ensure the integrity of the airway than to leave the patient without a secure airway and have a preventable crisis occur.

EVIDENCE

- **Is the gag reflex a useful indicator of the need to intubate?** Although it persists, inexplicably, in clinical practice, the gag reflex largely has disappeared from research evaluations, except with respect to whether it relates to the development of aspiration in overdose patients.[1] In a study of 111 patients requiring neurologic observation in the ED, Moulton et al.[2] found no correlation between the Glasgow Coma Scale (GCS) and the presence or absence of a gag reflex. The gag reflex was noted to be variably present across the range of GCS from 6 to 15, independent of the patient's perceived need for intubation.[2] The gag reflex is not involved in laryngeal closure or protection of the airway. Bleach[3] found an absent gag reflex in 27% of fully conscious patients who had undergone speech therapy and videofluoroscopy to assess for possible aspiration after neurologic events. There was no correlation between aspiration and the presence (or absence) of the gag reflex.[3] Davies et al.[4] studied 140 healthy adults, half of whom were elderly, and found that 37% lacked any gag reflex. Chan et al.[5] studied 414 patients with acute poisoning and noted absence of the gag reflex to be only 70% sensitive in identifying patients who required intubation. In one small study, all patients who required intubation had an absent gag reflex; however, the use of a GCS score of 8 or less outperformed the gag reflex, and evaluation of the gag reflex added nothing to the assessment of the GCS score alone.[5]

REFERENCES

1. Elzadi-Mood N, Saghaei M, Alfred S, et al. Comparative evaluation of Glasgow Coma Score and gag reflex in predicting aspiration pneumonitis in acute poisoning. *J Crit Care*. 2009;24:470.e9–470. e15. Epub 2009 Jan 17.

2. Moulton C, Pennycook A, Makower A. Relation between the Glasgow Coma Scale and the gag reflex. *BMJ*. 1991;303:1240–1241.

3. Bleach N. The gag reflex and aspiration: a retrospective analysis of 120 patients assessed by video-fluoroscopy. *Clin Otolaryngol*. 1993;18:303–307.

4. Davies AE, Kidd D, Stone SP, et al. Pharyngeal sensation and gag reflex in healthy subjects. *Lancet*. 1995;345:487–488.

5. Chan B, Gaudry P, Grattan-Smith TE, et al. The use of Glasgow Coma Score in poisoning. *J Emerg Med*. 1993;11:579–582.

2

Identification of the Difficult and Failed Airway

Ron M. Walls • Michael F. Murphy

DEFINITION OF THE DIFFICULT AND FAILED AIRWAY

Although both difficult and failed airways are discussed in this chapter, the two concepts are distinct. A difficult airway is one for which a preintubation examination identifies attributes that are likely to make laryngoscopy, intubation, bag-mask ventilation (BMV), the use of an extraglottic device (EGD; e.g., Combitube and laryngeal mask airway [LMA]), or surgical airway management more difficult than would be the case in an ordinary patient without those attributes. Identification of a difficult airway is a key component of the approach to airway management for any patient and is a key branch point on the main airway algorithm (see Chapter 3). The key reason for this is that, in general, one should not administer a neuromuscular blocking medication to a patient unless one has a measure of certainty that oxygenation can be maintained if laryngoscopy and intubation fail. Accordingly, if a difficult airway is identified, the difficult airway algorithm is used.

A failed airway situation occurs when a provider has embarked on a certain course of airway management (e.g., rapid sequence intubation [RSI]) and has identified that intubation by that method is not going to succeed, requiring the immediate initiation of a rescue sequence (the failed airway algorithm, see Chapter 3). Certainly, in retrospect, a failed airway can be called a difficult airway because it has proven to be difficult or impossible to intubate, but the terms "failed airway" and "difficult airway" must be kept distinct because they represent different situations, require different approaches, and arise at different points in the airway management sequence. One way of thinking about this is that the difficult airway is something one anticipates and plans for; the failed airway is something one experiences.

Airways that are difficult to manage are fairly common in emergency practice, with some estimates being as high as 20% of all emergency intubations. However, the incidence of overall intubation failure is quite low, generally approximately 1% or less. Intubation failure can occur in a setting where the patient can be oxygenated by an alternative method, such as by BMV or using an EGD, or in a setting where the patient neither can be intubated nor oxygenated. The true incidence of the "*can't* intubate, *can't* oxygenate" (CICO) situation is unknown in emergency intubations but is estimated to represent between 1 in 5,000 and 1 in 20,000 operating room intubations.

This chapter explores the concepts of the failed and the difficult airway in the setting of emergency intubation. Recognizing the difficult airway in advance and executing an appropriate and thoughtful plan, guided by the difficult airway algorithm (see Chapter 3) will minimize the likelihood that airway management will fail. Furthermore, recognizing the failed airway promptly allows use of the failed airway algorithm to guide selection of a rescue approach.

THE FAILED AIRWAY

A failed airway exists when any of the following conditions is met:

1. Failure to maintain acceptable oxygen saturation during or after one or more failed laryngoscopic attempts (CICO) *or*
2. Three failed attempts at orotracheal intubation by an experienced intubator, even when oxygen saturation can be maintained *or*
3. The single "best attempt" at intubation fails in the "Forced to Act" situation (see below).

Clinically, the failed airway presents itself in two ways, dictating the urgency created by the situation:

1. **Can't** *Intubate*, **Can't** *Oxygenate:* There is not sufficient time to evaluate or attempt a series of rescue options, and the airway must be secured immediately because of an inability to maintain oxygen saturation by BMV or with an EGD.
2. **Can't** Intubate, **Can** Oxygenate: There is time to evaluate and execute various options because the patient is oxygenated.

The most important way to avoid airway management failure is to identify in advance those patients for whom difficulty can be anticipated with intubation, BMV, insertion of an EGD, or cricothyrotomy. In the "Forced to Act" scenario, airway difficulty is apparent, but the clinical conditions (e.g., combative, hypoxic, and deteriorating patient) force the operator's hand, requiring administration of RSI drugs in an attempt to create the best possible circumstances for tracheal intubation, with immediate progression to failed airway management if that one best attempt is not successful (see Chapter 3).

THE DIFFICULT AIRWAY

The emergency airway algorithms are discussed in Chapter 3. According to the main emergency airway management algorithm, RSI is the method of choice for any non-crash airway when airway management difficulty is not anticipated. This requires a reliable and reproducible method for identifying the difficult airway. This evaluation must be expeditious, easy to remember, and complete.

In clinical practice, the difficult airway has four dimensions:

1. Difficult laryngoscopy
2. Difficult BMV
3. Difficult EGD
4. Difficult cricothyrotomy

A distinct evaluation is required for difficult laryngoscopy, difficult BMV, difficult EGD, and difficult surgical airway management, and each evaluation must be applied to each patient before airway management is undertaken (Fig. 2-1).

Difficult Laryngoscopy: LEMON

The concept of difficult laryngoscopy and intubation is inextricably linked to poor glottic view; the less adequate the glottic view, the more challenging the intubation. This concept, developed during an era when almost all intubations were done by direct laryngoscopy, appears to hold true even in the era of video laryngoscopy. Almost all research relating certain patient characteristics

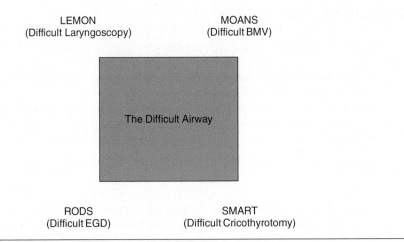

Figure 2-1 ● Difficult Airway Box. Note that the *four corners* represent the four dimensions of difficulty.

to difficult or impossible intubation is based on studies of direct laryngoscopy. It is not possible to determine, based on current information, whether these same characteristics predict difficult video laryngoscopy, and, if so, to what degree. Video laryngoscopy almost invariably produces an excellent glottic view, independently of the need to align the various airway axes, as must occur during direct laryngoscopy (see Chapters 12 and 13.) Difficult laryngoscopy and intubation are uncommon, even rare, when certain video laryngoscopes are used. It follows that evidence-based guidelines for prediction of difficult video laryngoscopy may be challenging, or even impossible, to develop. Pending further information, however, we recommend performing a difficult laryngoscopy assessment, using the LEMON mnemonic, on all patients for whom intubation is planned.

Cormack and Lehane introduced the most widely used system of categorizing the degree of visualization of the larynx during laryngoscopy, in which an ideal laryngoscopic view is designated grade 1 and the worst possible view grade 4 (Fig. 2-2). Cormack–Lehane (C–L) view grade 3 (epiglottis only visible) and grade 4 (no glottic structures at all visible) are highly correlated with difficult or failed intubation. C–L grade 1 (visualization of virtually the entire glottic aperture) and grade 2 (visualization of the posterior portion of the cords or the arytenoids) are not typically associated with difficult intubation. The C–L grading system does not differentiate precisely the degree to which the laryngeal aperture is visible during laryngoscopy: a grade 2 view may reveal little of the vocal cords, or none at all if only the arytenoids are visible. This has led some authors to propose a 2a/2b system, wherein a 2a shows any portion of the cords and a 2b shows only the arytenoids. Grade 2b accounts for only about 20% of grade 2 views. However, when a grade 2b view occurs, two-thirds of patients are difficult to intubate, whereas only about 4% of patients with grade 2a views are characterized as difficult intubations. A grade 1 view reveals virtually the entire glottis and is associated with almost universal intubation success.

Despite scores of clinical studies, no evidence to date reliably identifies which patient attributes predict successful laryngoscopy and intubation and which predict failure. Lists of anatomical features, radiologic findings, and complex scoring systems have been explored with only limited success. In the absence of a proven and validated system that is capable of predicting intubation difficulty with 100% sensitivity and specificity, it is important to develop an approach that will enable a clinician to quickly and simply identify those patients who *might* be difficult to intubate so an appropriate plan can be made using the difficult airway algorithm. In other words, when asking the question, "Does this patient's airway warrant using the difficult airway algorithm, or is it appropriate and safe to proceed directly to RSI?" we value sensitivity (i.e., identifying all those

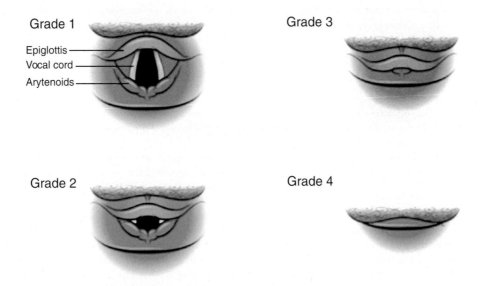

Figure 2-2 ● C–L laryngeal view grade system.

who might be difficult) more than specificity (i.e., always being correct when identifying a patient as difficult).

The mnemonic LEMON is a useful guide to identify as many of the risks as possible as quickly and reliably as possible to meet the demands of an emergency situation. The elements of the mnemonic are assembled from an analysis of the difficult airway prediction instruments in the anesthesia, emergency medicine, and critical care literature. The mnemonic, developed for The Difficult Airway Course™ and the first edition of this book, has been externally validated and has been adopted as a recommended airway assessment tool in Advanced Trauma Life Support (ATLS). The mnemonic is as follows:

L—*Look externally:* Although a gestalt of difficult intubation is not particularly sensitive (meaning that many difficult airways are not readily apparent externally), it is quite specific, meaning that if the airway looks difficult, it probably is. Most of the litany of physical features associated with difficult laryngoscopy and intubation (e.g., small mandible, large tongue, large teeth, and short neck) are accounted for by the remaining elements of LEMON and so do not need to be specifically recalled or sought, which can be a difficult memory challenge in a critical situation. The external look specified here is for the "feeling" that the airway will be difficult. This feeling may be driven by a specific finding, such as external evidence of lower facial disruption and bleeding that might make intubation difficult, or it might be the ill-defined composite impression of the patient, such as the obese, agitated patient with a short neck and small mouth, whose airway appears formidable even before any formal evaluation (the rest of the LEMON attributes) is undertaken. This "gestalt" of the patient is influenced by patient attributes, the setting, and clinician expertise and experience, and likely is as valid for video laryngoscopy as for direct laryngoscopy.

E—*Evaluate 3-3-2:* This step is an amalgamation of the much-studied geometric considerations that relate mouth opening and the size of the mandible to the position of the larynx in the neck in terms of likelihood of successful visualization of the glottis by direct laryngoscopy. This concept originally was identified with "thyromental distance," but has become more sophisticated over time. The thyromental distance is the hypotenuse of a right triangle, the two legs being the anteroposterior dimension of the mandibular space, and the interval between the chin–neck junction (roughly the position of the hyoid bone indicating the posterior limit of the tongue) and the top of the larynx, indicated by the thyroid notch. The 3-3-2 evaluation is derived from studies of the geometrical requirements for successful direct laryngoscopy, that is, the ability of the operator to create a direct line of sight from outside the mouth to the glottis. It is not known whether it has any value in predicting difficult video laryngoscopy, for which no straight line of sight is required. The premises of the 3-3-2 evaluation are as follows:

- The mouth must open adequately to permit visualization past the tongue when both the laryngoscope blade and the endotracheal tube are within the oral cavity.
- The mandible must be of sufficient size (length) to allow the tongue to be displaced fully into the submandibular space.
- The glottis must be located a sufficient distance caudad to the base of the tongue that a direct line of sight can be created from outside the mouth to the vocal cords as the tongue is displaced inferiorly into the submandibular space.

The first "3," therefore, assesses mouth opening. A normal patient can open his or her mouth sufficiently to accommodate three of his or her own fingers between the upper and lower incisors (Fig. 2-3A). The second "3" evaluates the length of the mandibular space by ensuring the patient's ability to accommodate three of his or her own fingers between the tip of the mentum and chin–neck junction (hyoid bone) (Fig. 2-3B). The "2" assesses the position of the glottis in relation to the base of the tongue. The space between the chin–neck junction

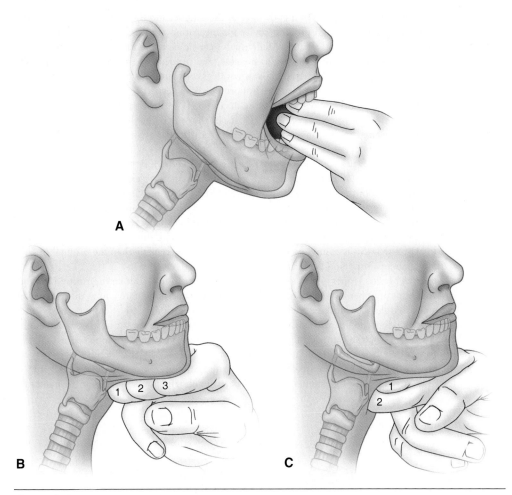

Figure 2-3 ● **A:** The first 3 of the 3-3-2 rule. **B:** The second 3 of the 3-3-2 rule. **C:** The 2 of the 3-3-2 rule.

(hyoid bone) and the thyroid notch should accommodate two of the patient's fingers (Fig. 2-3C). Thus, in the 3-3-2 rule, the first 3 assesses the adequacy of oral access, and the second 3 addresses the dimensions of the mandibular space to accommodate the tongue on laryngoscopy. The ability to accommodate significantly more than or less than three fingers is associated with greater degrees of difficulty in visualizing the larynx at laryngoscopy: the former because the length of the oral axis is elongated and the latter because the mandibular space may be too small to accommodate the tongue, requiring it to remain in the oral cavity or move posteriorly, obscuring the view of the glottis. Encroachment on the submandibular space by infiltrative conditions (e.g., Ludwig angina) is identified during this evaluation. The final 2 identifies the location of the larynx in relation to the base of the tongue. If significantly more than two fingers are accommodated, meaning the larynx is distant from the base of the tongue, it may be difficult to reach or visualize the glottis on direct laryngoscopy. Fewer than two fingers may mean that the larynx is tucked up under the base of the tongue and may be difficult to expose. This condition is often imprecisely called "anterior larynx."

M—*Mallampati score:* Mallampati determined that the degree to which the posterior oropharyngeal structures are visible when the mouth is fully open and the tongue is extruded reflects the

relationships among mouth opening, the size of the tongue, and the size of the oral pharynx, which defines access through the oral cavity for intubation, and that these relationships are associated with intubation difficulty. Mallampati's classic assessment requires that the patient sit upright, open the mouth as widely as possible, and protrude the tongue as far as possible without phonating. Figure 2-4 depicts how the scale is constructed. Class I and class II patients have low intubation failure rates, so the importance with respect to the decision whether to use neuromuscular blockade rests with those in classes III and IV, particularly class IV where intubation failure rates may exceed 10%. By itself, the scale is neither sensitive nor specific; however, when used in conjunction with the other difficult airway assessments, it provides valuable information about access to the glottis through the oral cavity. In the emergency situation, it frequently is not possible to have the patient sit up or to follow instructions. Therefore, often only a crude Mallampati measure is possible, obtained by examining the supine, obtunded patient's mouth with a tongue blade and light, or by using a lighted laryngoscope blade as a tongue depressor to gain an appreciation of how much mouth opening is present (at least in the preparalyzed state) and the relationship between the size of the tongue and that of the oral cavity. Although not validated in the supine position using this approach, there is no reason to expect that the assessment would be significantly less reliable than the original method with the patient sitting and performing the maneuver actively.

O—*Obstruction/obesity:* Upper airway obstruction is a marker for difficult laryngoscopy. The four cardinal signs of upper airway obstruction are muffled voice (hot potato voice), difficulty swallowing secretions (because of either pain or obstruction), stridor, and a sensation of dyspnea. The first two signs do not ordinarily herald imminent total upper airway obstruction in adults, but critical obstruction is much more imminent when the sensation of dyspnea occurs. Stridor is a particularly ominous sign. The presence of stridor is generally considered to indicate that the airway has been reduced to <50% of its normal calibre, or to a diameter of 4.5 mm or less. The management of patients with upper airway obstruction is discussed in Chapter 34.

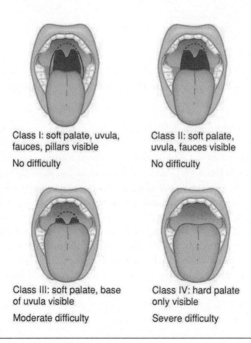

Class I: soft palate, uvula, fauces, pillars visible

No difficulty

Class II: soft palate, uvula, fauces visible

No difficulty

Class III: soft palate, base of uvula visible

Moderate difficulty

Class IV: hard palate only visible

Severe difficulty

Figure 2-4 ● The Mallampati Scale. In class I, the oropharynx, tonsillar pillars, and entire uvula are visible. In class II, the pillars are not visible. In class III, only a minimal portion of the oropharyngeal wall is visible, and in class IV, the tongue is pressed against the hard palate.

Although it is controversial whether obesity per se is an independent marker for difficult laryngoscopy or whether obesity simply is associated with various difficult airway attributes, such as high Mallampati score or failure of teh 3-3-2 rule, obese patients frequently have poor glottic views by direct or video laryngoscopy, and obesity, in itself, should be considered to portend difficult laryngoscopy.

N—*Neck mobility:* The ability to position the head and neck is one of the key factors in achieving the best possible view of the larynx by direct laryngoscopy. Cervical spine immobilization for trauma, by itself, may not create a degree of difficulty that ultimately leads one to avoid RSI after applying the thought processes of the difficult airway algorithm. However, cervical spine immobilization will make intubation more difficult and will compound the effects of other identified difficult airway markers. In addition, intrinsic cervical spine immobility, such as in cases of ankylosing spondylitis or rheumatoid arthritis, can make intubation by direct laryngoscopy extremely difficult or impossible and should be considered as a much more serious issue than the ubiquitous cervical collar (which mandates inline manual immobilization). Video laryngoscopy requires much less (or no) head extension, and provides a glottic view superior to that by direct laryngoscopy when head extension or neck flexion is restricted. Other devices, such as the Airtraq or the Shikani optical stylet, also may require less cervical spine movement than direct laryngoscopy.

Difficult BMV: MOANS

Chapter 9 highlights the importance of BMV in airway management, particularly as a rescue maneuver when orotracheal intubation has failed. If the airway manager is uncertain that neuromuscular blockade–facilitated orotracheal intubation (RSI) will be successful, he or she must be confident that BMV is possible, oxygenation using an EGD is possible, or, at the very least, a cricothyrotomy can rapidly be performed.

The validated indicators of difficult BMV from various clinical studies can be easily recalled for rapid use in the emergency setting by using the mnemonic MOANS.

M—*Mask seal/male sex/Mallampati:* Bushy beards, blood or debris on the face, or a disruption of lower facial continuity are the most common examples of conditions that may make an adequate mask seal difficult. Some experts recommend smearing a substance, such as KY jelly, on the beard as a remedy to this problem, although this action may simply make a bad situation worse in that the entire face may become too slippery to hold the mask in place. Both male sex and a Mallampati class 3 or 4 (see earlier) airway appear also to be independent predictors of difficult BMV.

O—*Obesity/obstruction:* Patients who are obese (body mass index >26 kg per m²) are often difficult to ventilate adequately by bag and mask. Women in third-trimester gestation are also a prototype for this problem because of their increased body mass, and the resistance to diaphragmatic excursion caused by the gravid uterus. Pregnant or obese patients also desaturate more quickly, making the bag ventilation difficulty of even greater import (see Chapters 36 and 39). The difficulty bagging the obese patient is not caused solely by the weight of the chest and abdominal walls and the resistance by the abdominal contents to diaphragmatic excursion. Obese patients also have redundant tissues, creating resistance to airflow in the upper airway. Similarly, obstruction caused by angioedema, Ludwig angina, upper airway abscesses (e.g., peritonsillar), epiglottitis, and other similar conditions will make BMV more difficult. In general, soft tissue lesions (e.g., angioedema, croup, and epiglottis) are amenable to bag and mask rescue if obstruction occurs, but not with 100% certainty. Similarly, laryngospasm can usually be overcome with good bag and mask technique. In contrast, firm, immobile lesions such as hematomas, cancers, and foreign bodies are less amenable to rescue by BMV, which is unlikely to provide adequate ventilation or oxygenation if total obstruction arises in this context.

A—*Age:* Age older than 55 to 57 years is associated with a higher risk of difficult BMV, perhaps because of a loss of muscle and tissue tone in the upper airway. The age is not a precise cutoff, and some judgment can be applied with respect to whether the patient has relatively elastic (young) or inelastic (aged) tissue.

N—*No teeth:* An adequate mask seal may be difficult in the edentulous patient because the face may not adequately support the mask. An option is to leave dentures (if available) in situ for BMV and remove them for intubation. Alternatively, gauze dressings may be inserted into the cheek areas through the mouth to puff them out in an attempt to improve the seal.

S—*Stiff/snoring:* This refers to patients whose lungs and thoraces are resistant to ventilation and require high-ventilation pressures. These patients are primarily those with reactive airways disease with medium and small airways obstruction (asthma and chronic obstructive pulmonary disease [COPD]) and those with pulmonary edema, acute respiratory distress syndrome (ARDS), advanced pneumonia, or any other condition that reduces pulmonary compliance or increases airway resistance to BMV. Also, a history of snoring (or of sleep apnea) predicts more difficult BMV. This risk factor may not be detectable in the setting of an emergency intubation, though, as it requires historical information.

Difficult EGD: RODS

In the emergency setting, extraglottic airway devices have emerged as credible first line devices for ventilation and oxygenation, instead of the traditional bag and mask; as alternatives to tracheal intubation in some patient circumstances (especially out of hospital), and as valuable airway rescue devices.

Studies have identified factors that predict difficulty in placing an EGD and providing adequate gas exchange. These can be assessed using the mnemonic RODS.

R—*Restricted mouth opening:* Adequate mouth opening is required for insertion of the EGD. This requirement varies, depending on the particular EGD to be used.

O—*Obstruction/obesity:* If there is upper airway obstruction in the pharynx, at the level of the larynx or glottis, or below the vocal cords, an EGD may be impossible to insert or seat properly and will not bypass the obstruction to achieve ventilation and oxygenation. Obesity creates two challenges to oxygenation using an EGD. First, redundant tissues in the pharynx may make placement and seating of the device more difficult. Usually, this is not a significant problem. More importantly, obese patients require higher ventilation pressures, largely because of the weight of the chest wall and abdominal contents. The former causes resistance to ventilation by increasing the pressures required to expand the chest, and the latter causes resistance to ventilation by increasing the pressures required to cause the diaphragm to descend. Depending on the EGD chosen, and positioning of the patient (it is better to attempt ventilation with the patient 30° head up or in reverse Trendelenberg position), ventilation resistance may exceed the ability of the EGD to seal and deliver the necessary pressures.

D—*Disrupted or distorted airway:* The key question here is, "If I insert this EGD into the pharynx of this patient, will the device be able to seat itself and seal properly within relatively normal anatomy?" For example, fixed flexion deformity of the spine, penetrating neck injury with hematoma, epiglottitis, and pharyngeal abscess each may distort the anatomy sufficiently to prevent proper positioning of the device.

S—*Stiff:* The stiffness referred to here is as for the MOANS mnemonic, that is, intrinsic resistance to ventilation. Ventilation with an EGD may be difficult or impossible in the face of substantial increases in airway resistance (e.g., asthma) or decreases in pulmonary compliance (e.g., pulmonary edema).

Difficult Cricothyrotomy: SMART

There are no absolute contraindications to performing an emergency cricothyrotomy (see Chapter 18). However, some conditions may make it difficult or impossible to perform the procedure, making it important to identify those conditions in advance and allowing consideration of alternatives rather than assuming or hoping that cricothyrotomy, if necessary, will be successful as a rescue technique. The mnemonic SMART is a modernization of our former algorithm, SHORT, and is used to quickly assess the patient for features that may indicate that a cricothyrotomy might be difficult. A part of patient assessment using this mnemonic, which occurs during the "A" step, is to perform a physical examination of the neck, identifying the landmarks and any barriers to the procedure. The SMART mnemonic is applied as follows:

S—*Surgery (recent or remote):* The anatomy may be subtly or obviously distorted, making the airway landmarks difficult to identify. Scarring may fuse tissue planes and make the procedure more difficult. Recent surgery may have associated edema or bleeding, complicating performance of the procedure.

M—*Mass:* A hematoma (postoperative or traumatic), abscess, or any other mass in the pathway of the cricothyrotomy may make the procedure technically difficult, and requires the operator to meticulously locate the landmarks, which may be out of the midline, or obscured.

A—*Access/anatomy:* Obesity makes surgical access challenging, as it often is difficult to identify landmarks. Similar challenges are presented by subcutaneous emphysema, soft tissue infection, or edema. A patient with a short neck or overlying mandibular pannus presents challenges both with identification of landmarks and access to perform the procedure. Extraneous devices, such as a cervical immobilization collar, or a halo-thoracic brace also may impede access.

R—*Radiation (and other deformity or scarring):* Past radiation therapy may distort and scar tissues making the procedure difficult, often causing tissues that normally are discrete to bond together, distorting tissue planes and relationships.

T—*Tumor:* Tumor, either inside the airway (beware of the chronically hoarse patient) or encroaching on the airway, may present difficulty, both from access and bleeding perspectives.

SUMMARY

- When intubation is indicated, the most important question is, "Is this airway difficult?" The decision to perform RSI, for example, is based on thorough assessment for difficulty (LEMON, MOANS, RODS, and SMART) and appropriate use of the main or difficult airway algorithms.
- If LEMON and MOANS are performed first, in order, then each component of RODS also has been assessed, with the exception of the D: distorted anatomy. In other words, if LEMON and MOANS have identified no difficulties, then all that remains for RODS is the question: "If I insert this EGD into the pharynx of this patient, will the device be able to seat itself and seal properly within relatively normal anatomy?"
- The ability to oxygenate a patient with a bag and mask or an EGD turns a potential CICO situation requiring urgent cricothyrotomy into a *"can't* intubate, *can* oxygenate" situation, in which many rescue options can be considered. The ability to prospectively identify situations in which oxygenation using an EGD or a bag and mask will be difficult or impossible is critical to the decision whether to use neuromuscular blocking agents.
- No single indicator, combination of indicators, or even weighted scoring system of indicators can be relied on to guarantee success or predict inevitable failure for oral intubation. Application of a systematic method to identify the difficult airway and then analysis of the situation to identify the best approach, given the anticipated degree of difficulty and the skill, experience, and judgment of the individual performing the intubation, will lead to the best decisions regarding how to manage the particular clinical situation. In general, it is better to err by identifying an airway as potentially difficult, only to subsequently find this not to be the case, than the other way around.

EVIDENCE

- **What is the incidence of difficult and failed airway?** A poor glottic view is associated with low intubation success. In studies of intubation by direct laryngoscopy in elective anesthesia practice, various definitions of difficult intubation are used. C–L class III and IV glottic visualization occurs in up to 12.5% of elective anesthesia patients.[1] A meta-analysis of elective anesthesia studies found an incidence of difficult laryngoscopy ranging from 6% to 27% among nine studies totaling >14,000 patients.[2] For obese patients, the incidence of difficult intubation certainly is higher, but how much of this is caused by obesity alone, and how much is a product of the presence of various difficult airway markers, such as a poor Mallampati score, is not clear. The Intubation Difficulty Score (IDS) considers the numbers of operators, devices, attempts, the C–L score, vocal cord position (abducted or not), and whether excessive lifting force or external manipulation is required.[3] In one study of 129 lean and 134 obese patients, using an IDS of 5 or greater as the definition of difficult intubation (a relatively high bar), investigators identified difficult intubation in 2.2% of lean patients and 15.5% of obese patients.[4] Only 1% of 663 patients in one British study had grade III glottic views, but 6.5% had grade IIb views (only arytenoids visible) and 2/3 of these were difficult to intubate.[5] In Reed's validation study of the LEMON mnemonic, 11/156 (7%) of patients had C–L grade III glottic views and only 2/156 had grade IV views.[6] The largest emergency department series is from the National Emergency Airway Registry (NEAR) project. In phase 2 of NEAR, reporting on 8,937 intubations from 1997 to 2002, the first chosen method ultimately was not successful in approximately 5% of intubations. Overall airway management success was >99%, and surgical airways were performed on 1.7% of trauma patients and approximately 1% of all cases.[7] Analysis of a subset of almost 8,000 of the NEAR 2 patients showed that about 50% of rescues from failed attempts involved use of RSI after failure of intubation attempts without neuromuscular blockade.[8]

- **What is the evidence basis of LEMON?** Only one external validation of the LEMON mnemonic has been published.[6] The American College of Surgeons adopted the LEMON mnemonic for ATLS in 2008, but mistakenly attributed it to Reed. The gestalt of difficulty provided by the patient obviously is an intuitive notion and will vary greatly with the skills and experience of the intubator. Certainly, it is not a sufficient assessment for intubation difficulty, for many markers, such as limited neck mobility or limited mouth opening, may not be apparent on this first look. There are no studies, of which we are aware, that assess the sensitivity or specificity of this first, quick look. Of interest, in Langeron's study of difficult BMV, clinicians identified in advance only 13/75 difficult BMV patients, a sensitivity of only 17%.[9] We are not aware of the true origin of the 3-3-2 rule. It probably originated from a group of Canadian difficult airway experts, led by Edward Crosby, MD, but, to our knowledge, it was not published before we included it in the first edition of our book in 2000. The 3-3-2 rule has three components. The first is mouth opening, a long-identified and intuitively obvious marker of difficult direct laryngoscopy. The second and third have to do mandibular size and the distance from the floor of the mandible to the thyroid notch. Many studies suggest identifying decreased (and, to a lesser extent, increased) thyromental distance as a predictor of difficult direct laryngoscopy. One study identified that it is relative, but not absolute thyromental distance that matters; in other words, the relevant thyromental distance that predicts difficulty depends on the size of the patient.[1] This reinforces the notion of using the patient's own fingers as a size guide for thyromental distance, but also for the other two dimensions of the 3-3-2 rule. Hyomental distance also has been used, but seems less reliable, causing researchers to explore the value of repeated measurements and ratios involving different head and neck positions.[10] The eponymous Mallampati evaluation has been validated multiple times. The modified Mallampati score, the four-category method that is most familiar, was found highly reliable in a comprehensive meta-analysis of 42 studies, but the authors emphasize, as do we, that the test is important, but not sufficient in evaluating the difficult airway.[2] One study suggested that the Mallampati evaluation gains specificity (from 70% to 80%) without loss of sensitivity if it is performed with the head in extension, but this study involved only 60 patients and performing the Mallampati, even in the neutral position, is challenging enough before emergency intubation, so we do not recommend head extension.[11] Interference with direct laryngoscopy by upper airway obstruction is self-evident. Obesity is uniformly identified as a difficult airway marker but, remarkably, controversy persists regarding obesity, per se, indicates difficult laryngoscopy, or whether obese patients simply have a greater incidence of having other difficult airway markers, such as higher Mallampati scores.[12] An opposing view suggests that, although a higher Mallampati score is associated with difficult intubation in obese patients, other traditional predictors of difficult intubation do not account for the high incidence and degree of difficulty in obese patients.[4] The only two studies to compare obese and lean patients head to head found a similar 5-fold increase in intubation difficulty for obese patients (about 15% vs. about 3% of lean patients), but one study concluded that body mass index (BMI) was important, the other concluded the opposite.[13]

- **What is the evidence basis of MOANS?** Much of the clinical information about difficult bag-mask ventilation came from case reports and limited case series, so were subject to bias and misinterpretation. The first well-designed study of difficult BMV was that of Langeron et al.,[9] where a 5% incidence of difficult BMV occurred in 1,502 patients. They identified five independent predictors of difficult BMV: presence of a beard, high BMI, age >55 years, edentulousness, and a history of snoring. Subsequent studies by other investigators were much larger. Kheterpal et al. used a graded definition of difficult BMV in their study of >22,000 patients. They divided difficult BMV into four classes, ranging from routine and easy (class I) to impossible (class IV). Class III difficulty was defined as inadequate, "unstable," or requiring two providers. They identified class III (difficult) BMV in 313/22,600 (1.4%) and class IV (impossible) in 37 (0.16%) patients. Multivariate analysis was used to identify independent predictors of difficult BMV: presence of a beard, high BMI, age >57 years, Mallampati class III or IV, limited jaw protrusion, and snoring. Snoring and thyromental distance <6 cm were independent predictors of impossible BMV.[14] Subsequently, the same researchers studied 53,041 patients over a 4-year period. Independent predictors of impossible BMV included the following: presence of a beard, male sex, neck radiation changes, Mallampati class III or IV, and sleep apnea.[15] These studies, combined with others, and with our collective experience, are the foundation for the MOANS mnemonic, which we have updated for this edition, reflecting the addition of male sex and Mallampati from the 2009 Kheterpal study. Interestingly, Mallampati class did not fare well as a predictor of difficult BMV in Lee's meta-analysis of 42 studies with >34,000 patients, although it did quite well for difficult intubation.[2] Nevertheless, we feel that Mallampati is a worthy consideration with respect to difficult BMV, as it helps the operator to understand the extent to which the tongue might impede ventilation. Conditions that require increased ventilation pressures, such as reactive airways disease and COPD, and those associated with a decrease in pulmonary compliance, such as ARDS or pulmonary edema, understandably make ventilation with a bag and mask more difficult. Why were these attributes not identified in the elegant studies of predictors of difficult BMV? Likely, patients with these conditions were too ill to be included in any such studies. Nonetheless, we are confident in including this concept in the "S" of MOANS.

- **What is the evidence basis of RODS?** EGDs have not been systematically studied for predictors of difficulty. Original information came from case reports, and now more information is available, principally with respect to seal pressures for the various devices (the airway pressures beyond which leakage occurs, reducing the tidal volume). As such, this mnemonic really represents our expert consensus, rather than an assessment of high-quality evidence. The requirement for minimal mouth opening sufficient to insert the device is self-evident. Obesity and obstruction will interfere with EGD use in similar fashion to their interference with BMV. Devices vary in their utility in various patients, however, and some may be better suited for obese patients than others. One study compared 50 morbidly obese patients to 50 lean patients and identified no increase in difficulty for either ventilation or intubation with the intubating LMA.[16] Distorted anatomy is our own concept, based on the fact that each of these devices is designed to "seat" into normal human anatomy, given that the right size of device is selected. The "S" for stiffness is exactly analogous to that for BMV, perhaps even more compelling here, because greater seal pressures often can be obtained using a bag and mask (with two operators) than with an EGD.

- **How reliable are the factors we evaluate in predicting difficult intubation?** Performing a preintubation assessment confers substantial protection against unexpectedly encountering a difficult intubation. Using a definition of difficult intubation as two failed attempts despite optimal laryngeal manipulation, one study found only 0.9% unexpected difficult intubations among >11,000 patients.[17] Investigators did not report C–L scores, though. In elective anesthesia practice, difficult airway patients often are "selected out" and managed by modified anesthetic technique, such as awake flexible endoscopic intubation. The safety of performing preintubation assessment is reinforced by this practice, however, as difficult and failed bag-mask ventilation and intubation in this population generally are unexpected because of the prescreening, and so probably reasonably predict unexpected (i.e., not detected by preintubation assessment of difficulty) similar events during emergency intubation. In one study of almost 23,000 patients, only about 1.6% had difficult bag-mask ventilation and only 0.37% or 1/300 had a combination of difficult BMV and difficult intubation.[14]

- **Does LEMON apply to video laryngoscopy also?** The short answer is no, or, at least, we do not know. Much of LEMON has to do with the need to see past the tongue, to the glottis, using a straight line of sight. Video laryngoscopy does not involve a straight line of sight, so, for example, we do not have any reason to believe that the 3-3-2 rule applies. Mallampati is not nearly as important, as the video viewer on most video laryngoscopes is positioned beyond the tongue, thus eliminating the tongue from consideration. Mallampati assesses mouth opening, also, though, as does the first "3" of the 3-3-2 rule, and mouth opening remains important for video laryngoscopy, although much less so. Only one study has attempted to identify attributes associated with difficult video laryngoscopy, in this case the GlideScope, and it is difficult to put much weight on any conclusions because 400/400 patients had C–L class I or II views.[18] The evidence for superiority of video laryngoscopy over conventional laryngoscopy is presented in Chapter 13.

REFERENCES

1. Krobbuaban B, Diregpoke S, Kumkeaw S, et al. The predictive value of the height ratio and thyromental distance: four predictive tests for difficult laryngoscopy. *Anesth Analg*. 2005;101(5):1542–1545.

2. Lee A, Fan LT, Gin T, et al. A systematic review (meta-analysis) of the accuracy of the Mallampati tests to predict the difficult airway. *Anesth Analg*. 2006;102(6):1867–1878.

3. Adnet F, Borron SW, Racine SX, et al. The intubation difficulty scale (IDS): proposal and evaluation of a new score characterizing the complexity of endotracheal intubation. *Anesthesiology*. 1997;87:1290–1297.

4. Juvin P, Lavaut E, Dupont H, et al. Difficult tracheal intubation is more common in obese than in lean patients. *Anesth Analg*. 2003;97(2):595–600.

5. Yentis SM, Lee DJ. Evaluation of an improved scoring system for the grading of direct laryngoscopy. *Anaesthesia*. 1998;53(11):1041–1044.

6. Reed MJ, Dunn MJ, McKeown DW. Can an airway assessment score predict difficulty at intubation in the emergency department? *Emerg Med J*. 2005;22(2):99–102.

7. Walls RM, Brown CA III, Bair AE, et al. Emergency airway management: a multi-center report of 8937 emergency department intubations. *J Emerg Med* 2011;41(4):347-54.

8. Bair AE, Filbin MR, Kulkarni RG, et al. The failed intubation attempt in the emergency department: analysis of prevalence, rescue techniques, and personnel. *J Emerg Med.* 2002;23(2):131–140.

9. Langeron O, Masso E, Huraux C, et al. Prediction of difficult mask ventilation. *Anesthesiology.* 2000;92(5):1229–1236.

10. Huh J, Shin HY, Kim SH, et al. Diagnostic predictor of difficult laryngoscopy: the hyomental distance ratio. *Anesth Analg.* 2009;108:544–548.

11. Mashour GA, Sandberg WS. Craniocervical extension improves the specificity and predictive value of the Mallampati airway evaluation. *Anesth Analg.* 2006;103:1256–1259.

12. Brodsky JB, Lemmens HJ, Brock-Utne JG, et al. Morbid obesity and tracheal intubation. *Anesth Analg.* 2002;94(3):732–736.

13. Gonzalez H, Minville V, Delanoue K, et al. The importance of increased neck circumference to intubation difficulties in obese patients. *Anesth Analg.* 2008;106:1132–1136.

14. Kheterpal S, Han R, Tremper KK, et al. Incidence and predictors of difficult and impossible mask ventilation. *Anesthesiology.* 2006;105(5):885–891.

15. Kheterpal S, Martin L, Shanks AM, et al. Prediction and outcomes of impossible mask ventilation: a review of 50,000 anesthetics. *Anesthesiology.* 2009;110(4):891–897.

16. Combes X, Sauvat S, Leroux B, et al. Intubating laryngeal mask airway in morbidly obese and lean patients: a comparative study. *Anesthesiology.* 2005;102(6):1106–1109.

17. Combes X, Le Roux B, Suen P, et al. Unanticipated difficult airway in anesthetized patients: prospective validation of a management algorithm. *Anesthesiology.* 2004;100(5):1146–1150.

18. Tremblay MH, Williams S, Robitaille A, et al. Poor visualization during direct laryngoscopy and high upper lip bite test score are predictors of difficult intubation with the GlideScope videolaryngoscope. *Anesth Analg.* 2008;106(5):1495–1500.

3

The Emergency Airway Algorithms

Ron M. Walls

APPROACH TO THE AIRWAY

This chapter presents and discusses the emergency airway algorithms, which we have used, taught, and refined for >15 years. These algorithms are intended to reduce error and improve the pace and quality of decision making for an event that is uncommonly encountered by most practitioners, and often disrupts attempts at sound and orderly clinical management.

When we first set out to try to codify the cognitive aspects of emergency airway management, we were both liberated and impaired by the complete lack of any such algorithms to guide us. In developing The Difficult Airway Course: Emergency™, The Difficult Airway Course: Anesthesia™, and The Difficult Airway Course: EMS™, and in applying successively each iteration of the emergency airway algorithms to tens of thousands of real and simulated cases involving thousands of providers, we felt guided by both our continuous learning about optimal airway management and the empirical application of these principles on a large scale. They are based on the best evidence available and the opinions of the most reputable experts in the field of emergency airway management. These algorithms, or adaptations of them, now appear in many of the major emergency medicine textbooks and online references. They are used in airway courses, for residency training, and in didactic teaching sessions, both for in-hospital and out-of-hospital providers. They have stood the test of time and have benefited from constant update.

The revolution in video laryngoscopy has caused us to rethink concepts related to the definition and management of the "difficult airway" (see Chapter 2). This current iteration reflects the broader application of flexible endoscopic methods, which formerly were all flexible fiberoptic scopes, now improved by adoption of complementary metal-oxide semiconductor video, which largely will supplant fiberoptic devices. There are new options with extraglottic devices (EGDs), both with and without intubating capability. Surgical airway management, while still an essential skill, moves from uncommon to rare as the sophistication of rescue devices and techniques increases.

Together, as before, these algorithms comprise a fundamental, *reproducible* approach to the emergency airway. The purpose is not to provide a "cookbook," which one could universally and mindlessly apply, but rather to describe a reproducible set of decisions and actions to enhance performance and maximize the opportunities for success, even in difficult or challenging cases.

The specialized algorithms all build from concepts found in the universal emergency airway algorithm, which describes the priority of the key decisions; the determination whether the patient represents a crash airway, a difficult airway, or a failed airway. The algorithms do not attempt to deal with the decision to intubate. This is discussed in Chapter 1. Therefore, the entry point for the emergency airway algorithm is immediately after the decision to intubate has been made.

This iteration of the algorithms introduces a new concept, the "forced to act" situation. There are clinical circumstances in which it is essential to use neuromuscular blocking agents (NMBA) even in the face of an identified difficult airway, simply because there is not sufficient time to attempt any other approach. The operator, *forced to act*, uses an induction agent and an NMBA to create the best possible circumstances for intubation. In other words, to take the one best chance to secure the airway, and for successful rescue should the primary method fail. An example of this might be the morbidly obese difficult airway patient who prematurely self-extubates in the ICU and is agitated, hypoxic, and deteriorating. Although the patient's habitus and airway characteristics normally would argue against the use of rapid sequence intubation (RSI), the need to secure the airway within just a few minutes and the patient's critical deterioration mandate immediate action. By giving an NMBA and induction agent, the operator can optimize conditions for video or direct laryngoscopy, with a plan to either insert a laryngeal mask airway (LMA) or perform a surgical airway if unsuccessful. In some cases, the primary method may be a surgical airway.

The algorithms are intended as guidelines for management of the emergency airway, regardless of the locus of care (emergency department [ED], inpatient unit, operating room, ICU, and out-of-hospital). The goal is to simplify some of the complexities of emergency airway management by defining distinct classes of airway problems. For example, we single out those patients who are essentially dead or near death (i.e., unresponsive, agonal) and manage them using a distinct pathway, the crash airway algorithm. Similarly, a patient with a difficult airway must be

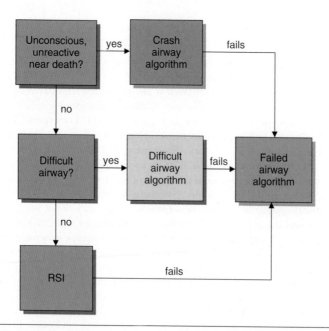

Figure 3-1 ● Universal Emergency Airway Algorithm. This algorithm demonstrates how the emergency airway algorithms work together. For all algorithms, green represents the main algorithm, yellow is the difficult airway algorithm, blue is the crash airway algorithm, red is the failed airway algorithm, and orange represents an end point. (© 2012 The Difficult Airway Course: Emergency™.)

identified and managed according to sound principles. Serious problems can ensue if a NMBA is given to a patient with a difficult airway, unless the difficulty was identified and planned for and the NMBA is part of that planned approach.

In human factors analysis, failure to recognize a pattern is often a precursor to medical error. The algorithms aid in pattern recognition by guiding the provider to ask specific questions, such as "Is this a crash airway?" and "Is this a difficult airway?" The answers to these questions group patients with certain characteristics together and each group has a defined series of actions. For example, in the case of a difficult airway, the difficult airway algorithm facilitates formulation of a distinct, but reproducible plan, which is individualized for that particular patient, yet lies within the overall approach that is predefined for all patients in this class, that is, those with difficult airways.

Algorithms are best thought of as a series of *key questions* and *critical actions*, with the answer to each question guiding the next critical action. The answers are always binary: "yes" or "no" to simplify and speed cognitive factor analysis. Figures 3-1 and 3-2 provide an overview of the algorithms, and how they work together.

When a patient requires intubation, the first question is "Is this a crash airway?" (i.e., is the patient unconscious, near death, with agonal or no respirations, expected to be unresponsive to the stimulation of laryngoscopy?). If the answer is "yes," the patient is managed as a crash airway using the crash airway algorithm (Fig. 3-3). If the answer is "no," the next question is "Is this a difficult airway?" (see Chapter 2). If the answer is "yes," the patient is managed as a difficult airway (Fig. 3-4). If the answer is "no," then neither a crash airway nor a difficult airway is present, and RSI is recommended, as described on the main algorithm (Fig. 3-2). Regardless of the algorithm used initially (main, crash, or difficult), if airway failure occurs, the failed airway algorithm (Fig. 3-5) is immediately invoked. The working definition of the failed airway is crucial and is explained in much more detail in the following sections. It has been our experience that airway management errors occur both because the provider does not recognize the situation (e.g., failed airway), and because, although recognizing the situation, he or she does not know what actions to take.

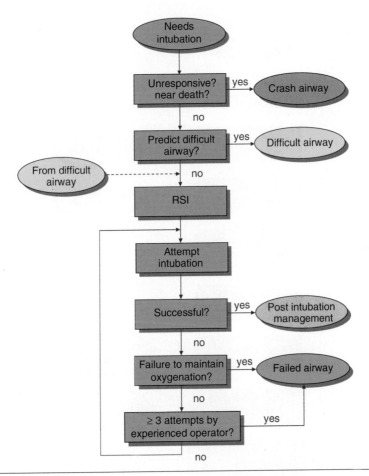

Figure 3-2 ● Main Emergency Airway Management Algorithm. See text for details. (© 2012 The Difficult Airway Course: Emergency™.)

THE MAIN AIRWAY ALGORITHM

The main emergency airway algorithm is shown in Figure 3-2. It begins after the decision to intubate and ends when the airway is secured, whether intubation is achieved directly or through one of the other algorithms. The algorithm is navigated by following defined steps with decisions driven by the answers to a series of key questions:

- **Key question 1: Is this a crash airway?** If the patient presents in an essentially unresponsive state and is deemed to be unlikely to respond to laryngoscopy, then the patient is defined as a crash airway. Here, we are either identifying patients who are in full cardiac or respiratory arrest or those with agonal cardiorespiratory activity (e.g., agonal, ineffective respirations, pulseless idioventricular rhythm). These patients are managed in a manner appropriate for their extremis condition. If a crash airway is identified, exit this main algorithm and begin the crash airway algorithm (Fig. 3-3). Otherwise, continue on the main algorithm.
- **Key question 2: Is this a difficult airway?** If the airway is not identified as a crash airway, the next task is to determine whether it is a difficult airway, which encompasses difficult laryngoscopy and intubation, difficult bag-mask ventilation (BMV), difficult cricothyrotomy, and difficult EGD use. Chapter 2 outlines the assessment of the patient for a potentially difficult airway using the various mnemonics (LEMON, MOANS, RODS, and SMART)

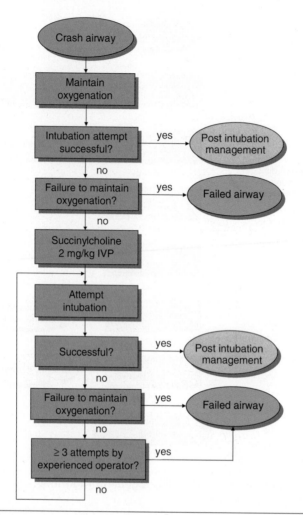

Figure 3-3 ● Crash Airway Algorithm.   See text for details. The portion at the bottom is essentially identical to the corresponding portion of the main emergency airway algorithm. IVP, intravenous push. (© 2012 The Difficult Airway Course: Emergency™.)

corresponding to these dimensions of difficulty. Difficult video laryngoscopy is sufficiently new and rare that useful predictive parameters have yet to be defined. This is discussed further in Chapter 2. It is understood that virtually all emergency intubations are difficult to some extent. However, the evaluation of the patient for attributes that predict difficult airway management is extremely important. If the patient represents a particularly difficult airway situation, then he or she is managed as a difficult airway, using the difficult airway algorithm (Fig. 3-4), and one would exit the main algorithm. Although it is the LEMON assessment for difficult laryngoscopy and intubation that may be the main driver, evaluation for the other difficulties (BMV, cricothyrotomy, and EGD) also is critical at this point. If the airway is not identified as particularly difficult, continue on the main algorithm to the next step, which is to perform RSI.

- **Critical action: Perform RSI.** In the absence of an identified crash or difficult airway, RSI is the method of choice for managing the emergency airway. RSI is described in detail in Chapter 19 and affords the best opportunity for success with the least likelihood of adverse outcome of any possible airway management method, when *applied to appropriately selected*

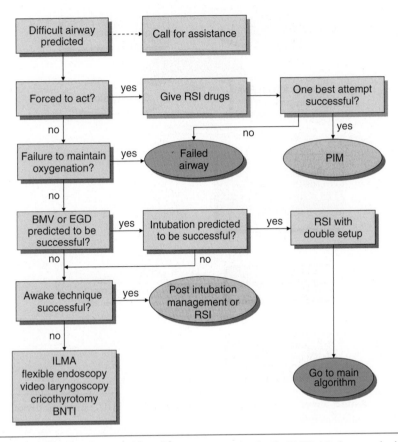

Figure 3-4 • Difficult Airway Algorithm. See text for details. BNTI, blind nasotracheal intubation. (© 2012 The Difficult Airway Course: Emergency™.)

patients. This step assumes that the appropriate sequence of RSI (the seven Ps) will be followed. If the patient is in extreme respiratory distress, or if haste is indicated for any reason, an accelerated or immediate RSI protocol can be used (see Chapter 19). During RSI, intubation is attempted. According to the standard nomenclature of the National Emergency Airway Registry, a multicenter study of emergency intubation, *an attempt is defined as activities occurring during a single continuous laryngoscopy maneuver, beginning when the laryngoscope is inserted into the patient's mouth, and ending when the laryngoscope is removed, regardless of whether an endotracheal tube is actually inserted into the patient.* In other words, if several attempts are made to pass an endotracheal tube (ETT) through the glottis during the course of a single laryngoscopy, these aggregate efforts count as one attempt. If the glottis is not visualized and no attempt is made to insert a tube, the laryngoscopy is still counted as one attempt. These distinctions are important because of the definition of the failed airway that follows.

- **Key question 3: Was intubation successful?** If the first oral intubation attempt is successful, the patient is intubated, postintubation management (PIM) is initiated, and the algorithm terminates. If the intubation attempt is not successful, continue on the main pathway.
- **Key question 4: Can the patient's oxygenation be maintained?** When the first attempt at intubation is unsuccessful, it often is possible and appropriate to attempt a second laryngoscopy without interposed BMV because oxygen saturations often remain acceptable for an extended period of time because of proper preoxygenation. Desaturation may be delayed even further by continuous supplemental oxygen by nasal cannula. In general, supplemental oxygenation with a bag and mask is not necessary until the oxygen saturation falls to

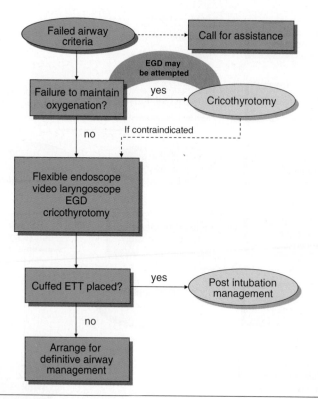

Figure 3-5 ● Failed Airway Algorithm. See text for details. EGD, extraglottic device. (© 2012 The Difficult Airway Course: Emergency™.)

approximately 90%. When the oxygen saturation reaches this level, the appropriate first maneuver is BMV of the patient. This approach underscores the importance of assessing the likelihood of successful BMV (MOANS, see Chapter 2) before beginning the intubation sequence. In the vast majority of cases, especially when neuromuscular blockade has been used, BMV will provide adequate ventilation and oxygenation for the patient, defined as maintenance of the oxygen saturation at 90% or higher. If BMV is not capable of maintaining the oxygen saturation above 90%, better technique, including oral and nasal airways, two-person two-handed technique, and optimal positioning of the patient usually will result in effective ventilation (see Chapter 9). If BMV fails despite optimal technique, the airway is considered a failed airway, and one must exit the main algorithm immediately and initiate the failed airway algorithm (Fig. 3-5). Recognition of the failed airway is crucial because delays caused by persistent, futile attempts at intubation will waste critical seconds or minutes and may sharply reduce the time remaining for a rescue technique to be successful before brain injury ensues.

- **Key question 5: Have three attempts at orotracheal intubation been made by an experienced operator?** There are two essential definitions of the failed airway: (1) "can't intubate, can't oxygenate" (CICO) (described previously); and (2) "three failed attempts by an experienced operator." If three separate attempts at orotracheal intubation by an experienced operator have been unsuccessful, then the airway is again defined as a failed airway, despite the ability to adequately oxygenate the patient using a bag and mask. If an experienced operator has used a particular method of laryngoscopy, such as video laryngoscopy or direct laryngoscopy, for three attempts without success, success with a subsequent attempt is unlikely. The operator must recognize the failed airway and manage it as such using the failed airway algorithm. If there have been fewer than three unsuccessful attempts at intubation, but BMV is successful, then it is appropriate to attempt orotracheal intubation again, provided the oxygen saturation is maintained and the operator can identify an element of the laryngoscopy that can be improved (e.g., patient positioning or different instrument). Similarly, if the initial attempts were made by an inexperienced operator, such as a trainee, and the patient is adequately oxygenated, then it is appropriate to reattempt oral intubation until three attempts by an *experienced* operator have been unsuccessful. Rarely, even a fourth attempt at laryngoscopy may be appropriate before declaring a failed airway. This most often occurs when the operator identifies a particular strategy for success (e.g., better control of the epiglottis by using a larger laryngoscope blade) during the third unsuccessful attempt. Similarly, it is possible that an *experienced* operator will recognize on the *very first attempt* that further attempts at orotracheal intubation will not be successful. In such cases, provided that the patient has been optimally positioned for intubation, good relaxation has been achieved, and it is the operator's judgment that further attempts at laryngoscopy would be futile, the airway should be immediately regarded as a failed airway and the failed airway algorithm initiated. Thus, it is not essential to make three laryngoscopic attempts before labeling an airway as failed, but three failed attempts by an experienced operator should always be considered a failed airway, unless the laryngoscopist identifies a particular problem and potential solution, justifying one more attempt.

THE CRASH AIRWAY ALGORITHM

Entering the crash airway algorithm (Fig. 3-3) indicates that one has identified an unconscious, unresponsive patient with immediate need for airway management. It is assumed that BMV or some other method of oxygenation is occurring throughout.

- **Critical action: Intubate immediately:** The first step in the crash algorithm is to attempt oral intubation immediately by direct or video laryngoscopy, or, less commonly, by flexible endoscopy, without pharmacological assist. In these patient circumstances, direct oral intubation has success rates comparable to RSI, presumably because the patients have flaccid musculature and are unresponsive in a manner similar to that achieved by RSI.
- **Key question 1: Was intubation successful?** If yes, carry on with PIM and general resuscitation. If intubation was not successful, resume BMV or oxygenation using an EGD and proceed to the next step.
- **Key question 2: Is oxygenation adequate?** If oxygenation is adequate using a bag and mask or an EGD, then further attempts at oral intubation are possible. Adequacy of oxygenation with a crash airway usually is not determined by pulse oximetry, but by assessment of patient color, chest rise, and the feel of the bag (reflecting patency of the airway, delivered tidal volume, airway resistance, and pulmonary compliance). *If oxygenation is unsuccessful in the context of a single failed oral intubation attempt with a crash airway, then a failed airway is present.* One further attempt at intubation may be rapidly tried, but no more than one, because intubation has failed, and the failure of oxygenation places the patient in serious and immediate jeopardy. This is a CICO-failed airway, analogous to that described previously. Exit here and proceed directly to the failed airway algorithm (Fig. 3-5).
- **Critical action: Administer succinylcholine 2 mg per kg intravenous push:** If intubation is not successful, it is reasonable to assume that the patient has residual muscle tone and is not optimally relaxed. The dose of succinylcholine is increased here because these patients often have severe circulatory compromise, impairing the distribution and rapidity of the onset of succinylcholine. Bag ventilation is continued for 60 to 90 seconds to allow the succinylcholine to distribute. Remember, it is oxygen the patient requires most, not the ETT. From this point onward, the crash airway algorithm is virtually identical to the corresponding portion of the main airway algorithm, with the exception that the patient has not been adequately preoxygenated, and pulse oximetry is generally incapable of accurately reflecting the state of

oxygenation in the crash airway patient. The sequence and rationale, however, are identical from this point on.

- **Critical action: Attempt intubation:** After allowing time for the succinylcholine to circulate, another attempt is made at oral intubation.
- **Key question 3: Was the intubation successful?** If intubation is achieved, then proceed to PIM. If not, another attempt is indicated if oxygenation is maintained.
- **Key question 4: Is oxygenation adequate?** If oxygenation cannot be maintained at any time, the airway becomes a CICO-failed airway, requiring implementation of the failed airway algorithm.
- **Key question 5: Have there been three or more attempts at intubation by an experienced operator?** This situation is exactly analogous to that described above in the RSI portion of the main airway algorithm (Fig. 3-2). If succinylcholine is administered to a crash patient, count the subsequent intubation attempt as attempt number one.

THE DIFFICULT AIRWAY ALGORITHM

Identification of the difficult airway is discussed in detail in Chapter 2. This algorithm (Fig. 3-4) represents the clinical approach that should be used in the event of an identified potential difficult airway.

- **Critical action: Call for assistance.** The "call for assistance" box is linked as a dotted line because this is an optional step, dependent on the particular clinical circumstances, skill of the airway manager, available equipment and resources, and availability of additional personnel. Assistance might include personnel, special airway equipment, or both.
- **Key question 1: Is the operator forced to act?** In some circumstances, although the airway is identified to be difficult, patient conditions force the operator to act immediately, before there is rapid deterioration of the patient into respiratory arrest. An example of this situation is given earlier in this chapter. Another example is a morbidly obese patient with severe status asthmaticus who is hypoxemic, diaphoretic, agitated, and uncooperative. In such cases, there is not time to consider the use of an "awake" technique (see below and Chapter 2), and all rescue techniques, including a surgical airway, are not possible, given the patient's agitated state. In such circumstances, a prompt decision to give RSI drugs and create circumstances for a *best attempt* at tracheal intubation, whether by laryngoscopy or surgical airway, often is preferable to considering other (likely impossible) approaches as the patient progresses to respiratory arrest and death. Administration of RSI drugs might permit the operator to intubate, perform a surgical airway, place an EGD, or use a bag and mask to oxygenate the patient. The key is for the operator to make the one best attempt that, in the operator's judgment, is most likely to succeed. If the attempt, for example, intubation using video laryngoscopy, is successful, then the operator proceeds to PIM. If the attempt is not successful, a failed airway is present, and the operator proceeds to the failed airway algorithm.
- **Key question 2: Is there adequate time?** In the context of the difficult airway, *oxygen is time*. If ventilation and oxygenation are adequate and oxygen saturation can be maintained over 90%, then a careful assessment and a methodical, planned approach can be undertaken, even if significant preparation time is required. However, if oxygenation is inadequate, then additional oxygenation or BMV is initiated. If oxygenation still is not adequate, move immediately to the failed airway algorithm. This situation is equivalent to a "can't intubate (the identified difficult airway is a surrogate for can't intubate), can't oxygenate (adequate oxygenation saturation cannot be achieved)" failed airway. Certain difficult airway patients will have chronic pulmonary disease, for example, and may not be able to reach an oxygen saturation of 90%, but can be kept stable and viable at, say, 86%. Whether to call this case a failed airway is a matter of judgment, based on the adequacy of oxygenation. If a decision

is made to proceed down the difficult airway algorithm rather than switching to the failed airway algorithm, it is essential to be aware that in cases such as this desaturation will occur rapidly during intubation attempts (see Chapter 19) and to increase vigilance with respect to hypoxemia.

- **Key question 3: Despite the presence of the difficult airway, is RSI indicated?** If the patient is adequately oxygenated, the next step is to consider RSI. This decision hinges on two key factors.

  The first, and most important factor is whether one predicts with confidence that gas exchange can be maintained by BMV or the use of an EGD if RSI drugs are administered rendering the patient paralyzed and apneic. This answer may already be known if BMV has been required to maintain the patient's oxygenation or if the difficult airway evaluation (see Chapter 2) did not identify difficulty for oxygenation using BMV or an EGD. Anticipating successful oxygenation using BMV or an EGD is a virtually essential prerequisite for RSI, except in the "forced to act" situation described above. In some cases, it may be desirable to attempt a trial of BMV, but this approach does not reliably predict the ability to bag-mask ventilate the patient after paralysis.

  Second, if BMV or EGD is anticipated to be successful, then the next consideration is whether intubation is likely to be successful, despite the difficult airway attributes. In reality, many patients with identified difficult airways undergo successful emergency intubation employing RSI, particularly when a video laryngoscope is used. So if there is a reasonable likelihood of success with oral intubation, *despite predicting a difficult airway*, RSI may be undertaken. Remember, this is predicated on the fact that one has already judged that gas exchange (BMV or EGD) will be successful following neuromuscular blockade. In these cases, RSI is performed using a "double setup," in which the rescue plan (often cricothyrotomy) is clearly established, and the operator is prepared to move promptly to the rescue technique if intubation using RSI is not successful (failed airway). In most cases, however, when RSI is undertaken despite identification of difficult airway attributes, appropriate care during the technique and planning related to the particular difficulties present will result in success.

  To reiterate these two fundamental principles, if gas exchange employing BMV or EGD is not confidently assured of success in the context of difficult intubation, *or* if the chance of successful oral intubation is felt to be poor, then RSI is not recommended, except in the "forced to act" scenario.

- **Critical action: Perform "awake" laryngoscopy:** Just as RSI is an essential technique of emergency airway management, "awake" laryngoscopy is the cornerstone of difficult airway management. The goal of this maneuver is to gain a high degree of confidence that the airway will be secured if RSI is performed. Alternatively, the airway can be secured during the "awake look." This technique usually requires moderate sedation of the patient, similar to that used for painful procedures, and the liberal use of local anesthesia (usually topical) to permit laryngoscopy without inducing and paralyzing the patient (see Chapter 23). The principle here is that the patient is awake enough to maintain the airway and effective spontaneous ventilation, but is sufficiently obtunded to tolerate the awake look procedure. Thus, strictly speaking, "awake" is somewhat of a misnomer. The laryngoscopy can be done with a standard laryngoscope, flexible endoscope, video laryngoscope or a semirigid fiberoptic or video intubating stylet, such as the Shikani Optical Stylet. These devices are discussed in detail in Chapters 12 to 16. Two possible outcomes are possible from this awake examination. First, the glottis may be adequately visualized, informing the operator that oral intubation using that device is highly likely to succeed. If the difficult airway is static (i.e., chronic, such as with ankylosing spondylitis), then the best approach might be to proceed with RSI, now that it is known that the glottis can be visualized, using that same device. If, however, the difficult airway is dynamic (i.e., acute, as in smoke inhalation or angioedema), then it likely is better to proceed directly with intubation during this awake laryngoscopy, rather than to back out and perform RSI. This decision is predicated on the possibility that the airway might deteriorate further in the intervening time, arguing in favor of immediate intubation during the awake examination, rather than assuming that the glottis will be visualized with equal ease a few minutes later during an RSI. Intervening deterioration, possibly contributed to by the laryngoscopy itself, might make a subsequent laryngoscopy more difficult or even impossible (see Chapter 34). The second possible outcome during the awake laryngoscopic examination is that the glottis is not adequately visualized to permit intubation. In this case, the examination has confirmed the suspected difficult intubation and reinforced the decision to avoid neuromuscular paralysis. A failed airway has been avoided and several options remain. Oxygenation should be maintained as necessary at this point.

Although the awake look is the crucial step in management of the difficult airway, it is not infallible. In rare cases, an awake look may provide a better view of the glottic structures than is visible after the administration of a neuromuscular blocking drug. Thus, although the likelihood that the glottis will be less well seen after paralysis than during the awake look is remote, it is not zero, and the airway manager must always be prepared for this rare eventuality.

- **Critical action: Select an alternative airway approach:** At this point, we have clarified that we have a patient with difficult airway attributes, who has proven to be a poor candidate for laryngoscopy, and thus is inappropriate for RSI. There are a number of options available here. If the awake laryngoscopy was done using a direct laryngoscope, a video laryngoscope or flexible endoscope likely will provide a superior view of the glottis. The main fallback method for the difficult airway is cricothyrotomy (open or Seldinger technique), though the airway may be amenable to an EGD that facilitates intubation, that is, one of the intubating LMAs (ILMAs). In highly select cases, blind nasotracheal intubation may be possible, but requires an anatomically intact and normal upper airway. In general, blind nasotracheal intubation is used only when flexible endoscopy is not available or is rendered impossible by excessive bleeding in the airway. The choice of technique will depend on the operator's experience, available equipment, the particular difficult airway attributes the patient possesses, and the urgency of the intubation. Whichever technique is used, the goal is to place a cuffed ETT in the trachea.

THE FAILED AIRWAY ALGORITHM

At several points in the preceding algorithms, it may be determined that airway management has failed. The definition of the failed airway (see previous discussion in this chapter and in Chapter 2) is based on one of three criteria being satisfied: (1) a failure of an intubation attempt in a patient for whom oxygenation cannot be adequately maintained with a bag and mask, (2) three unsuccessful intubation attempts by an experienced operator but with adequate oxygenation, and (3) failed intubation using the one *best attempt* in the "forced to act" situation (this is analogous to the "CICO" situation, but oxygenation by bag and mask, or by EGD, may be possible). Unlike the difficult airway, where the standard of care dictates the placement of a cuffed ETT in the trachea providing a definitive, protected airway, the failed airway calls for action to provide emergency oxygenation sufficient to prevent patient morbidity (especially hypoxic brain injury) by whatever means possible, until a definitive airway can be secured (Fig. 3-5). Thus, the devices considered for the failed airway are somewhat different from, but inclusive of, the devices used for the difficult airway (see Chapter 2). When a failed airway has been determined to occur, the response is guided by whether oxygenation is possible.

- **Critical action: Call for assistance.** As is the case with the difficult airway, it is best to call for any available and necessary assistance as soon as a failed airway is identified. Again, this action may be a stat consult to emergency medicine, anesthesia, or surgery, or it may be a call for special equipment. In the prehospital setting, a second paramedic or a medical control physician might provide assistance.

- **Key question 1: Is oxygenation adequate?** As is the case for the difficult airway, this question addresses the time available for a rescue airway. If the patient is a failed airway because of three failed attempts by an experienced operator, in most cases, oxygen saturation will be adequate, and there is time to consider various approaches. If, however, the failed airway is because of a CICO situation, then there is little time left before cerebral hypoxia will result in permanent deficit, and immediate action is indicated. Many, or most, CICO patients will require surgical airway management, and preparation for a surgical airway should be undertaken. It is reasonable, as the first rescue step, to make a single attempt to insert a rapidly placed extraglottic airway device, *simultaneously with the preparation for a cricothyrotomy*. Successful oxygenation using the EGD converts the CICO situation into a *can't* intubate, *can* oxygenate situation, allowing time for consideration of a number of different approaches to securing the airway.
- **Critical action:** Achieve an airway using flexible endoscopy, video laryngoscopy, an EGD, a semirigid intubating stylet, or cricothyrotomy. In the can't intubate, but can oxygenate situation, various devices are available to provide an airway, and most also provide some degree of airway protection. Intubation by flexible endoscopy or video laryngoscopy will establish a cuffed endotracheal in the trachea. Of the EGDs, the ILMAs are preferable because they have a high likelihood of providing effective ventilation and usually permit intubation through the device (see Chapter 10). Cricothyrotomy always remains the final common pathway if other measures are not successful, or if the patient's oxygenation becomes compromised.
- **Key question 2: Does the device used result in a definitive airway?** If the device used results in a definitive airway (i.e., a cuffed ETT in the trachea), then one can move on to PIM. If an EGD has been used, or intubation was not successful through the ILMA, arrangements must be made to provide a definitive airway. A definitive airway may be provided in the operating room, ICU, or ED, once the necessary personnel and equipment are available. Until then, constant surveillance is required to ensure that the airway, as placed, continues to provide adequate oxygenation, with cricothyrotomy always available as a backup.

CONCLUSIONS

These algorithms represent our best thinking regarding a recommended approach to emergency airway management. The algorithms are intended as guidelines only. Individual decision-making, clinical circumstances, skill of the operator, and available resources will determine the final, best approach to airway management in any individual case. Understanding the fundamental concepts of the difficult and failed airway; identification, in advance, of the difficult airway; recognition of the crash airway; and the use of RSI as the airway management method of choice for most emergency intubations will foster in successful airway management while minimizing preventable morbidity.

EVIDENCE

- **Evidence for the algorithms.** Unfortunately, there are no systematized data supporting the algorithmic approach presented in this chapter. The algorithms are the result of careful review of the American Society of Anesthesiologists difficult airway algorithm, the algorithms of the Difficult Airway Society of the United Kingdom, and composite knowledge and experience of the editors and faculty of The Difficult Airway Courses, who function as an expert panel in this regard.[1,2] There has not been, and likely never will be, a study comparing, for example, the outcomes of cricothyrotomy versus alternate airway devices in the CICO situation. Clearly, randomization of such patients is not ethical. Thus, the algorithms are derived from a rational body of knowledge (described previously) and represent a recommended approach, but cannot be considered to be scientifically proven as the only or even necessarily the best way to approach any one clinical problem or patient. Rather, they are designed to help guide a consistent approach to both common and uncommon airway management situations. The evidence for the superiority of RSI over other methods not involving neuromuscular blockade can be found in Chapter 19.

REFERENCES

1. Caplan RA, Benumof JL, Berry FA, et al. Practice guidelines for management of the difficult airway: an updated report by the American Society of Anesthesiologists Task Force on Management of the Difficult Airway. *Anesthesiology*. 2003;98(5):1269–1277.
2. Henderson JJ, Popat MT, Latto IP, et al. Difficult Airway Society guidelines for management of the unanticipated difficult intubation. *Anaesthesia*. 2004;59:675–694.

4

Applied Functional Anatomy of the Airway

Michael F. Murphy

There are many salient features of the anatomy and physiology of the airway to consider with respect to airway management maneuvers. This chapter discusses the anatomical features most involved in the act of intubation, the important vascular structures, and the innervation of the upper airway. Chapter 23 builds on these anatomical and functional relationships to describe anesthesia techniques for the airway. Chapter 24 addresses developmental and pediatric anatomical features of the airway.

We consider each anatomical structure in the order in which it appears as we enter the airway: the nose, the mouth, the pharynx, the larynx, and the trachea (Fig. 4-1).

THE NOSE

The external nose consists of a bony vault, a cartilaginous vault, and a lobule. The bony vault comprises the nasal bones, the frontal processes of the maxillae, and the nasal spine of the frontal bone. The nasal bones are buttressed in the midline by the perpendicular plate of the ethmoid bone that

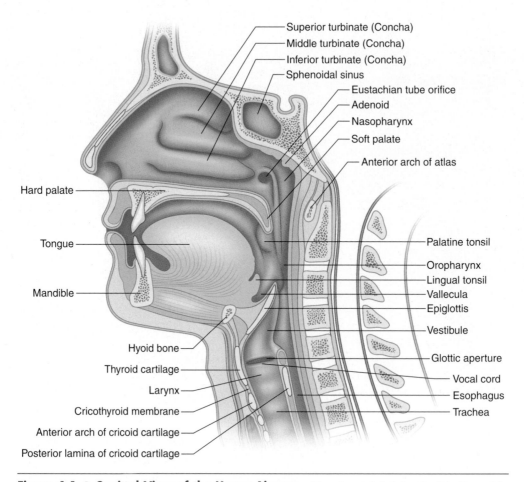

Figure 4-1 ● **Sagittal View of the Upper Airway.** Note the subtle inferior tilt of the floor of the nose from front to back, the location of the adenoid, the location of the vallecula between the base of the tongue and the epiglottis, and the location of the hyoid bone in relation to the posterior limit of the tongue.

forms part of the bony septum. The cartilaginous vault is formed by the upper lateral cartilages that meet the cartilaginous portion of the septum in the midline. The nasal lobule consists of the tip of the nose, the lower lateral cartilages, the fibrofatty alae that form the lateral margins of the nostril, and the columella. The cavities of each nostril are continuous with the nasopharynx posteriorly.

Important Anatomical Considerations

- Kiesselbach's plexus (Little's area) is a very vascular area located on the anterior aspect of the septum in each nostril. Epistaxis most often originates from this area. During the act of inserting a nasal trumpet or a nasotracheal tube (NTT), it is generally recommended that the device be inserted in the nostril such that the leading edge of the bevel (the pointed tip) is away from the septum. The goal is to minimize the chances of trauma and bleeding from this very vascular area. This means that the device is inserted "upside down" in the left nostril and rotated 180° after the tip has proceeded beyond the cartilaginous septum. Although some authors have recommended the opposite (i.e., that the bevel tip approximate the nasal septum to minimize the risk of damage and bleeding from the turbinates), the bevel away from the septum approach makes more sense and is the recommended method.
- The major nasal airway is between the laterally placed inferior turbinate, the septum, and the floor of the nose. The floor of the nose is tilted slightly downward front to back, approximately 10° to 15°. Thus, when a nasal tube, trumpet, or fiberscope is inserted through the nose, it should not be directed upward or even straight back. Instead, it should be directed slightly inferiorly to follow this major channel. Before nasal intubation of an unconscious adult patient, some authorities recommend gently but *fully* inserting one's gloved and lubricated little finger to ensure patency and to maximally dilate this channel before the insertion of the nasal tube. In addition, placing the endotracheal tube (ETT; preferably an Endotrol tube) in a warm bottle of saline or water softens the tube and attenuates its damaging properties.
- The nasal mucosa is exquisitely sensitive to topically applied vasoconstricting medications such as phenylephrine, epinephrine, oxymetazoline, or cocaine. Cocaine has the added advantage of providing profound topical anesthesia and is the only local anesthetic agent that produces vasoconstriction; the others cause vasodilatation. Shrinking the nasal mucosa with a vasoconstricting agent can increase the caliber of the nasal airway by as much as 50% to 75% and may reduce epistaxis incited by nasotracheal intubation, although there is little evidence to support this claim. Cocaine has been implicated in coronary vasoconstriction when applied to the nasal mucosa, so it should be used with caution in patients with coronary artery disease (see "Evidence" section at the end of this chapter).
- The nasal cavities are bounded posteriorly by the nasopharynx. The adenoids are located posteriorly in the nasopharynx just above the nasal surface of the soft palate and partially surround a depression in the mucosal membrane where the eustachian tube enters the nasopharynx. During insertion, the NTT often enters this depression and resistance is encountered. Continued aggressive insertion can cause the NTT to penetrate the mucosa and pass submucosally deep to the naso- and oropharyngeal mucous membrane (Fig. 4-2). Although alarming when one recognizes that this has occurred, no specific treatment is indicated, except that withdrawing the tube and trying the opposite nostril is advised. Despite the theoretical risk of infection, there is no literature to suggest that this occurs. Documentation of the complication and communication to the accepting team on admission is important.
- The soft palate rests on the base of the tongue during quiet nasal respiration, sealing the oral cavity anteriorly.
- The contiguity of the paranasal sinuses with the nasal cavity is believed to be responsible for the infections of the paranasal sinuses that may be associated with prolonged nasotracheal intubation. Although this fact has led some physicians to condemn nasotracheal intubation, fear of infection should not deter the emergency physician from considering nasotracheal intubation when indicated. Securing the airway in an emergency takes precedence over possible later infective complications, and in any case, the intubation can always be changed to an oral tube or tracheostomy, if necessary.

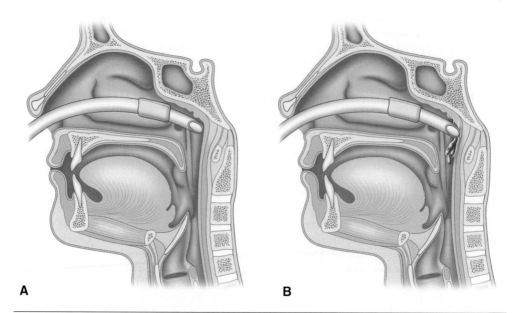

A   **B**

Figure 4-2 ● Mechanism of Nasopharyngeal Perforation and Submucosal Tunneling of the NTT. **A:** The NTT entering the pit of the adenoid where the eustachian tube enters the nasopharynx. **B:** The tube perforating the mucous membrane.

- A nasotracheal intubation is relatively contraindicated in patients with basal skull fractures (i.e., when the maxilla is fractured away from its attachment to the base of the skull) because of the risk of penetration into the cranial vault (usually through the cribriform plate) with the ETT. Careful technique avoids this complication: the cribriform plate is located cephalad of the nares, and tube insertion should be directed slightly caudad (see previous discussion). Maxillary fractures (e.g., LeFort fractures) may disrupt the continuity of the nasal cavities and are a relative contraindication to blind nasal intubation. Again, cautious insertion, especially if guided by a fiberscope, can mitigate the risk.

THE MOUTH

The mouth, or oral cavity, is bounded externally by the lips and is contiguous with the oropharynx posteriorly (Fig. 4-3).

- The tongue is attached to the symphysis of the mandible anteriorly and anterolaterally and the stylohyoid process and hyoid bone posterolaterally and posteriorly, respectively. The posterior limit of the tongue corresponds to the position of the hyoid bone (Fig. 4-1). The clinical relevance of this relationship will become apparent with the 3-3-2 rule described in Chapter 2.
- The potential spaces in the hollow of the mandible are collectively called the mandibular space, which is subdivided into three potential spaces on either side of the midline sublingual raphe: the submental, submandibular, and sublingual spaces. The tongue is a fluid-filled noncompressible structure. During conventional laryngoscopy, the tongue is ordinarily displaced to the left and into the mandibular space, permitting one to expose the larynx for intubation under direct vision. If the mandibular space is small relative to the size of the tongue (e.g., hypoplastic mandible, lingual edema in angioedema, and lingual hematoma), the ability to visualize the larynx may be compromised. Infiltration of the mandibular space by infection (e.g., Ludwig angina), hematoma, or other lesions may limit the ability to displace the tongue into this space and render orotracheal intubation difficult or impossible.

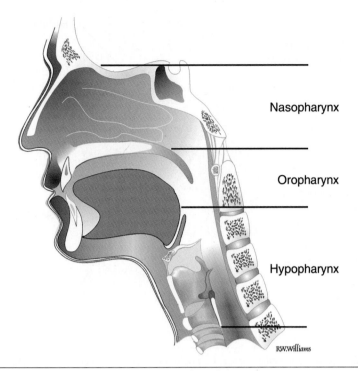

Nasopharynx

Oropharynx

Hypopharynx

R.W.Williams

Figure 4-3 ● **Pharynx Divided into Three Segments: Nasopharynx, Oropharynx, and Hypopharynx.**

- Subtle geometric distortions of the oral cavity that limit one's working and viewing space, such as a high-arched palate with a narrow oral cavity or buckteeth with an elongated oral cavity, may render orotracheal intubation difficult. Chapter 12 elaborates on these issues.
- Salivary glands continuously secrete saliva, which can defeat attempts at achieving sufficient topical anesthesia of the airway to undertake awake laryngoscopy or other active airway intervention maneuvers in the awake or lightly sedated patient—for example, laryngeal mask airway insertion, lighted stylet intubation, and so on.
- The condyles of the mandible articulate within the temporomandibular joint (TMJ) for the first 30° of mouth opening. Beyond 30°, the condyles *translate* out of the TMJ anteriorly onto the zygomatic arches. Once translation has occurred, it is possible to use a jaw thrust maneuver to pull the mandible and tongue forward. This is the most effective method of opening the airway to alleviate obstruction or permit bag-mask ventilation. A jaw thrust to open the airway is not possible unless this translation has occurred (see Chapter 9).

THE PHARYNX

The pharynx is a U-shaped fibromuscular tube extending from the base of the skull to the lower border of the cricoid cartilage where, at the level of the sixth cervical vertebra, it is continuous with the esophagus. Posteriorly, it rests against the fascia covering the prevertebral muscles and the cervical spine. Anteriorly, it opens into the nasal cavity (the nasopharynx), the mouth (the oropharynx), and the larynx (the laryngo- or hypopharynx).

- The oropharyngeal musculature has a normal tone, like any other skeletal musculature, and this tone serves to keep the upper airway open during quiet respiration. Respiratory

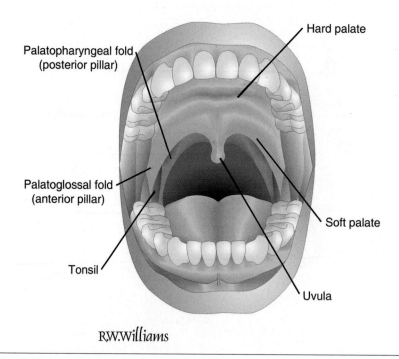

R.W.Williams

Figure 4-4 ● The Oral Cavity.   Note the position of the posterior pillar. The glossopharyngeal nerve runs at the base of this structure.

distress is associated with pharyngeal muscular activity that attempts to open the airway further. Benzodiazepines and other sedative hypnotic agents may attenuate some of this tone. This explains why even small doses of sedative hypnotic medications (e.g., midazolam) may precipitate total airway obstruction in patients presenting with partial airway obstruction.

- An "awake look" is advocated during the difficult airway algorithm (see Chapter 3). Being able to see the epiglottis or posterior glottic structures using topical anesthesia and sedation reassures one that at least this much, and probably more, of the airway will be visualized during an intubation attempt following the administration of a neuromuscular blocking drug. In practice, the glottic view is usually improved following neuromuscular blockade. Rarely, however, the loss of pharyngeal muscle tone caused by the neuromuscular blocking agent leads to the cephalad and anterior migration of the larynx worsening the view at direct laryngoscopy. Although uncommon, this tends to occur more often in morbidly obese or late-term pregnancy patients, in whom there may be submucosal edema.

- The glossopharyngeal nerve supplies sensation to the posterior one-third of the tongue, the valleculae, the superior surface of the epiglottis, and most of the posterior pharynx. This nerve is accessible to blockade (topically or by injection) because it runs just deep to the inferior portion of the palatopharyngeus muscle (the posterior tonsillar pillar) (Fig. 4-4).

THE LARYNX

The larynx extends from its oblique entrance formed by the aryepiglottic folds, the tip of the epiglottis, and the posterior commissure between the arytenoid cartilages (interarytenoid folds) through the vocal cords to the cricoid ring (Fig. 4-5).

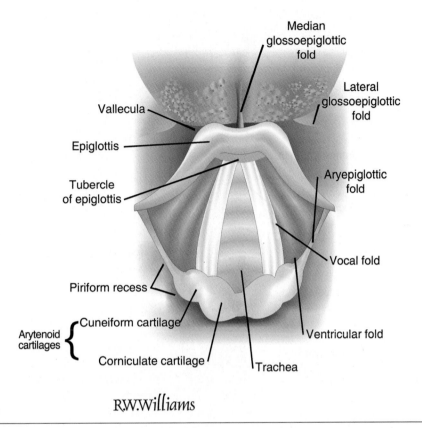

R.W.Williams

Figure 4-5 ● Larynx Visualized from the Oropharynx.   Note the median glossoepiglottic fold. It is pressure on this structure by the tip of a curved blade that flips the epiglottis forward, exposing the glottis during laryngoscopy. Note that the valleculae and the piriform recesses are different structures, a fact often confused in the anesthesia literature. The cuneiform and corniculate cartilages are called the arytenoid cartilages. The ridge between them posteriorly is called the posterior commissure.

- The superior laryngeal branch of the vagus nerve supplies sensation to the undersurface of the epiglottis, all of the larynx to the level of the false vocal cords, and the piriform recesses posterolateral to either side of the larynx (Fig. 4-5). The nerve enters the region by passing through the thyrohyoid membrane just below the inferior cornu of the hyoid bone (Fig. 4-6). It then divides into a superior and an inferior branch; the superior branch passes submucosally through the vallecula, where it is visible to the naked eye, on its way to the larynx; and the inferior branch runs along the medial aspects of the piriform recesses.
- The larynx is the most heavily innervated sensory structure in the body, followed closely by the carina. Stimulation of the unanesthetized larynx during intubation causes tremendous reflex sympathetic activation. BP and heart rate may as much as double. This may lead to the elevation of intracranial pressure, particularly in patients with imperfect autoregulation; aggravate or incite myocardial ischemia in patients with underlying coronary artery disease; or incite or aggravate large vessel dissection or rupture (e.g., penetrating injury to a carotid, thoracic aortic dissection, or abdominal aortic rupture).
- The pyramidal arytenoid cartilages sit on the posterior aspect of the larynx (Fig. 4-5). The intrinsic laryngeal muscles cause them to swivel, opening and closing the vocal cords. An ETT that is too large may, over time, compress these structures, causing

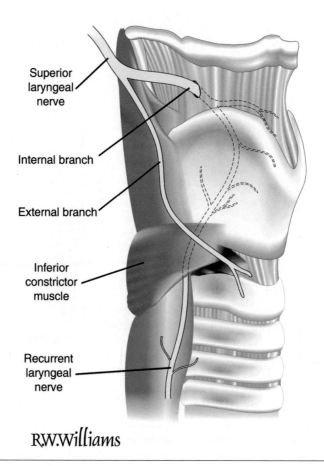

Superior
laryngeal
nerve

Internal branch

External branch

Inferior
constrictor
muscle

Recurrent
laryngeal
nerve

R.W.Williams

Figure 4-6 ● Oblique View of the Larynx.   Note how the internal branch of the superior laryngeal nerve pierces the thyrohyoid membrane midway between the hyoid bone and the superior border of the thyroid cartilage.

mucosal and cartilaginous ischemia and resultant permanent laryngeal damage. A traumatic intubation may dislocate these cartilages posteriorly (more often a traumatic curved blade–related complication) or anteriorly (more often a straight blade traumatic complication), which, unless diagnosed early and relocated, may lead to permanent hoarseness.

- The larynx bulges posteriorly into the hypopharynx, leaving deep recesses on either side called the piriform recesses or sinuses. Foreign bodies (e.g., fish bones) occasionally become lodged there. During active swallowing, the larynx is elevated and moves anteriorly, the epiglottis folds down over the glottis to prevent aspiration, and the bolus of food passes midline into the esophagus. When not actively swallowing (e.g., the unconscious patient), the larynx rests against the posterior hypopharynx such that a nasogastric (NG) tube must traverse the piriform recess to gain access to the esophagus and stomach. Ordinarily, an NG tube introduced through the right nostril passes to the left at the level of the hypopharynx and enters the esophagus through the left piriform recess. Similarly, with a left nostril insertion, the NG tube gains access to the esophagus through the right piriform recess.

- The cricothyroid membrane extends between the upper anterior surface of the cricoid cartilage to the inferior anterior border of the thyroid cartilage. Its height tends to be about the size of the tip of the index finger externally in both male and female adults. Locating the cricoid cartilage and the cricothyroid membrane quickly in an airway emergency is crucial.

It is usually easily done in men because of the obvious laryngeal prominence (Adam's apple). Locate the laryngeal prominence, and then note the anterior surface of the thyroid cartilage immediately caudad, usually about one index finger's breadth in height. There is an obvious soft indentation caudad to this anterior surface with a very hard ridge immediately caudad to it. The soft indentation is the cricothyroid membrane, and the ridge is the cricoid cartilage. Because of the lack of a distinct laryngeal prominence in women, locating the membrane can be much more difficult. In women, place your index finger in the sternal notch. Then drag it cephalad in the midline until the first, and ordinarily the biggest, transverse ridge is felt. This is the cricoid ring. Superior to the cricoid cartilage is the cricothyroid membrane, and superior to that, the anterior surface of the thyroid cartilage, and then the thyrohyoid space and thyroid cartilage. The cricothyroid membrane is higher in the neck in a woman than it is in a man because the woman's thyroid cartilage is relatively smaller than that of the man.

- The cricothyroid membrane measures 6 to 8 mm from top to bottom. If one pierces the membrane in its midportion to perform a retrograde intubation, the puncture point is a mere 3 to 5 mm below the vocal cords, which may not be far enough into the airway to retain the ETT when the wire is cut at the skin. The technique of passing the wire from the outside to the inside of the distal end of the ETT through the Murphy eye enables an additional 4 to 5 mm of insertion, reducing this risk. The proximity of the cricothyroid membrane to the vocal cords is also the driving factor in using small tracheal hooks during surgical cricothyroidotomy to minimize any risk to the cords (see Chapter 18).

TRACHEA

The trachea begins at the inferior border of the cricoid ring. The sensory supply to the tracheal mucosa is derived from the recurrent laryngeal branch of the vagus nerve. The trachea is between 9 and 15 mm in diameter in the adult and is 12 to 15 cm long. It may be somewhat larger in the elderly. The adult male trachea will generally easily accept an 8.5-mm inner diameter (ID) ETT; a 7.5-mm ID ETT may be preferable in women. If the patient being intubated requires bronchoscopic pulmonary toilette after admission (e.g., chronic obstructive pulmonary disease and airway burns), consider increasing to a 9.0-mm ID tube for men and an 8.0-mm ID tube for women.

SUMMARY

Functional anatomy is important to expert airway management. Attention to the nuances and subtleties of anatomy in relation to technique will often mean the difference between success and failure in managing airways, particularly difficult airways. A clear understanding of the relevant anatomical structures, their blood supply, and their innervation will guide the choice of intubation and anesthesia techniques and will enhance understanding regarding the best approach to each patient. It also provides a basis for understanding how complications are best avoided, or if they occur, how they may be detected.

EVIDENCE

- **General.** The reviews by Morris[1] and Redden,[2] as well as a number of others, provide excellent descriptions of the functional anatomy of the upper airway. There is no significant new evidence in these areas.

REFERENCES

1. Morris IR. Functional anatomy of the upper airway. *Emerg Med Clin North Am*. 1988;6:639–669.

2. Redden RJ. Anatomic considerations in anesthesia. In: Hagberg CA, ed. *Handbook of Difficult Airway Management*. Philadelphia, PA: Churchill Livingstone; 2000:1–13.

5

Supplemental Oxygen

Calvin A. Brown III • Steven C. Carleton • Robert F. Reardon

Neuronal and myocardial tissue undergo time-dependent, irreparable damage when deprived of oxygen for relatively brief periods of time, and may function abnormally in low oxygen states. In the context of emergency airway management, the principal purpose of supplemental oxygen is to avoid injury to, or dysfunction of, oxygen-sensitive tissues. Supplemental oxygen also is used to create a high-concentration oxygen reservoir in an effort to maximize the safe apnea period during rapid sequence intubation (RSI) (see Chapter 19). Many misconceptions exist about oxygen therapy, such as the effectiveness of the "100% non-rebreather mask," a device which supplies, at best, 60% to 70% inspired oxygen. This chapter will address the principles of supplemental oxygen delivery and clarify common misunderstandings about this vital drug.

Ventilation and perfusion (V/Q) mismatches or impaired oxygen diffusion across the alveolar membrane reduce systemic arterial oxygen tension by a variety of mechanisms. In cases of reduced pulmonary arterial blood flow, as in pulmonary embolus, oxygen-filled alveoli are not perfused and cannot participate in gas exchange. In conditions with significant airspace disease, such as lobar pneumonia, perfused areas of poorly oxygenated lung fail to oxygenate the pulmonary circulation. Pulmonary edema causes accumulation of airspace fluid and also may impede effective oxygen transport across the alveolar membrane. The most effective way to improve oxygen diffusion is to increase alveolar oxygenation by providing higher oxygen concentrations, often augmented by positive pressure, thereby improving the diffusion gradient and allowing more effective pulmonary arterial oxygenation. This chapter focuses on ambient pressure oxygen supplementation. Positive-pressure oxygenation and ventilation is discussed in Chapter 6.

SUPPLEMENTAL OXYGEN

FiO_2 refers to the fractional concentration of inspired oxygen. Room air FiO_2 is 0.21, corresponding to 21% oxygen concentration. Correct terminology expresses FiO_2 as a fractional number (e.g. 0.4), but common (mis)use is to express it as a percentage (e.g. 40%). For simplicity, we will use the percentage format for FiO_2, as this represents the most common clinical usage. A variety of oxygen delivery systems provide a wide range of supplemental oxygen. Delivery systems are broadly categorized as either low-flow or high-flow, depending both on the inspiratory flow rate provided by each setup and whether inspired oxygen is fixed or variable. High-flow systems provide the entire inspiratory volume with a fixed, but adjustable, concentration of inspired oxygen. Low-flow systems require that the patient breathe variable proportions of room air and supplied oxygen with each breath. The most common oxygen delivery systems in the emergency department (ED) are low-flow types and include nasal cannulas, simple face masks, and face masks with oxygen reservoirs. The most common high-flow device is the Venturi mask. Oxygen supplementation is often delivered in an incremental fashion starting with low-flow systems and subsequently adjusted based on patient need. As a general rule, the least invasive mode of oxygen delivery, and the lowest flow rate needed to maintain normal saturation, should be used.

Low-flow Oxygen Delivery Systems

Nasal cannula

Nasal cannula is a low-flow oxygen delivery system in which oxygen can be administered through small-caliber tubing and narrow nasal prongs. Nasal cannula is often the first line of supplementation and is appropriate in patients with mild oxygen debt. Nasal cannula oxygen creates a high-concentration oxygen reservoir in the nose and posterior nasopharynx, which mixes with room air during inspiration, resulting in a marginal rise in FiO_2. Common initial flow rates are 2 to 4 L per minute. At 6 L per minute, the nasal and nasopharyngeal O_2 reservoirs are full and higher flow rates result in minimal, if any, increases in inspired oxygen. Maximal FiO_2 from nasal cannula is approximately 40%. Other common low-flow systems and their expected maximum achievable FiO_2 can be found in Table 5-1. The effect of nasal cannula oxygen may be tempered by nasal congestion or obstruction, or when used by obligate mouth breathers.

TABLE 5-1
Estimates of Maximum FiO_2 with Various Low-flow Oxygen Delivery Systems

System	100% O_2 flow (L/min)	FiO_2 (approximate) (%)
Nasal cannula	2–4	30–35
	6	40
Simple face mask	6	45
	10	55
Face mask and bag reservoir	10–15	70

Simple face mask

If nasal cannula oxygen does not provide sufficient oxygen saturations, increasing the size of the upper airway reservoir by including the mouth and oropharynx can be achieved by simple face mask oxygen. Additionally, reservoir volume is contained within the mask (approximately 100 to 150 ml). A simple face mask is a non-form-fitting plastic mask that covers the entirety of the nose and mouth. It does not have an external bag reservoir and is attached to small-caliber oxygen tubing similar to that of nasal cannula. Typical flow rates range between 4 and 10 L per minute. The FiO_2 is highly variable and dictated by the patient's respiratory pattern, the amount of room air drawn in around the mask, and the oxygen flow. Peak FiO_2 with a simple face mask is approximately 50%.

Face masks with oxygen reservoir and "non-rebreather" masks

The next step up in oxygen delivery is a face mask attached to an external oxygen bag reservoir (Fig. 5-1). In addition to the anatomic oxygen reservoir and that contained within the mask itself, this arrangement also includes a reservoir bag with approximately 500 to 1,000 ml of volume from which the patient can draw during inspiration. Many masks are assembled with a series of small holes on the side-wall, often arranged in a circle, and covered by a soft plastic disc. The disc sits on a small stalk that allows it to open with exhalation and become opposed to the mask during inspiration, thereby creating a one-way, hence "non-rebreather," valve for exhaled gas. This theoretically limits entrainment of room air into the inspired admixture. Although this does offer higher FiO_2 than a simple face mask, poor mask seal and inconsistent valve function can limit its efficacy. The highest FiO_2 reasonably obtained with traditional non-rebreather masks is approximately 70% at 10 to 15 L per minute of oxygen flow. Newer, more robust, non-rebreather masks (Fig. 5-2) that provide a better mask seal and valve closure may deliver higher FiO_2 than older style versions.

Bag-valve-mask apparatus

If the patient remains hypoxic despite oxygen supplementation with face mask oxygen and a bag reservoir, a higher FiO_2 can be supplied using a bag-valve-mask. Appropriately configured bag-valve-mask's consist of a form-fitting mask designed to provide an airtight seal with the patient's face, an inspiratory valve, a large volume (approximately 1,500 ml) bag reservoir, and a one-way exhalation port (Fig. 5-3). With active patient breathing through the mask with a good facial seal and high-flow rates (10 to 15 L per minute), an FiO_2 of nearly 100% can be achieved. It is critical that the bag-valve-mask apparatus has a one-way exhalation port (Fig. 5-3), allowing efflux of

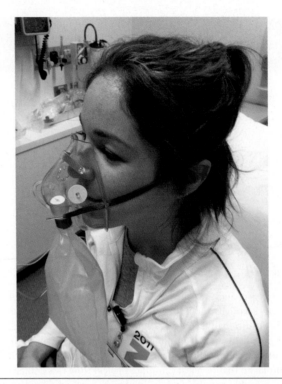

Figure 5-1 ● Non-rebreather face mask with a one-way exhalation valve and bag reservoir.

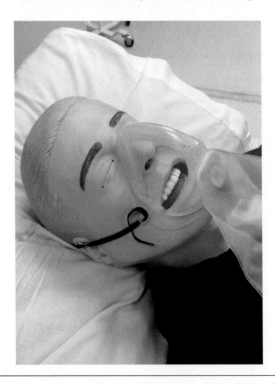

Figure 5-2 ● New version non-rebreather face mask with a more robust mask seal rim and more functional one-way exhalation valve.

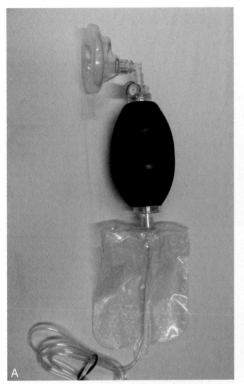
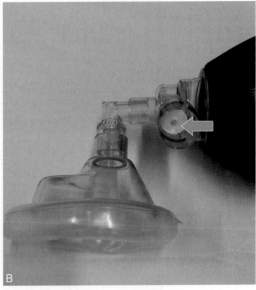

Figure 5-3 ● **A.** Bag-valve-mask apparatus can be applied to a patient for active breathing (no assisted ventilations). **B.** Close up of the one-way exhalation port (arrow) on an appropriately configured bag-valve-mask unit.

exhaled gases, but prohibiting entry of room air, thus ensuring that the entire inspiratory volume is drawn from the oxygen reservoir. Not all resuscitation bags are so equipped, so it is important to inspect the bag to ensure presence of the valve. Without a one-way exhalation valve, large volumes of room air are inspired and mixed with 100% oxygen from the reservoir, reducing the FiO_2, to <40% (Fig. 5-4).

High-flow Oxygen Delivery Systems

Venturi device

High-flow supplemental oxygen systems are less commonly used than low-flow systems in the ED, but frequently are used on inpatient units and in the ICU. The most common of these is the Venturi device. This device is used to entrain a fixed ratio of room air to inspired 100% oxygen in order to ensure a constant rate of oxygen delivery. It is so named because of the underlying physics principle that guides its function (Venturi effect). This device may be helpful when known, titratable amounts of oxygen supplementation are important for patient care or when there is concern about excessive oxygen administration, as in a patient with chronic obstructive pulmonary disease. Venturi devices come in a variety of colors representing the FiO_2 delivered and specify oxygen flow rates, usually 12 to 15 L per minute. Venturi devices supplying an FiO_2 from 24% to 50% are available in the United States. As the FiO_2 increases using a Venturi mask, overall gas flow is reduced because the quantity of entrained room air decreases significantly.

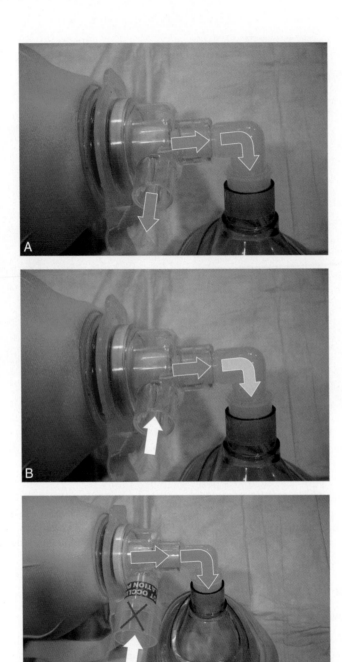

Figure 5-4 ● **A:** Resuscitation bag used with positive pressure (bag is being squeezed) and no active breathing by patient. Whether or not a one-way exhalation valve is present, the patient receives 100% oxygen from the bag reservoir, as long as the mask seal is effective. **B:** Resuscitation bag during active breathing (bag is not being squeezed). Note that there is not a one-way exhalation valve. The exhalation port is open to the ambient air. When the patient inhales, a large amount of room air (FiO_2 21%) is admixed with the 100% oxygen from the bag reservoir, resulting in massive dilution and an FiO_2 as low as 30%. **C:** Resuscitation bag during active breathing with one-way exhalation valve (bag is not being squeezed). Room air cannot enter exhalation port, so FiO_2 approaches 100%.

SUMMARY

Ambient pressure supplemental oxygen can be delivered in a variety of ways, depending on the perceived oxygen requirement. If the patient is critically hypoxemic, oxygen supplementation should begin at the highest level and be reduced as oxygenation targets are reached. For less ill patients, supplementation can follow a step-wise progression from nasal cannula to reservoir face mask to bag-valve-mask apparatus. When it is important to know (or titrate precisely) the delivered oxygen concentration, a Venturi system is preferable. The majority of oxygen delivery systems are low-flow systems, utilizing oxygen flow rates from 4 to 15 L per minute, with variable FiO_2 because of room air admixture. Of the high-flow systems, only the Venturi masks are used in most clinical settings.

EVIDENCE

- **How much oxygen is typically delivered using low-flow oxygen systems?** There is surprisingly little research on the inspired concentrations of oxygen delivered by various standard devices. Consensus, as reflected in standard textbooks in critical care[1] and anesthesia[2] ascribes ranges of FiO_2 with each of a variety of low-flow systems at various flow rates. A brief summary can be found in Table 5-1.
- **What is the appropriate bag-valve-mask configuration to supply the highest FiO_2?** All bag-valve-mask devices deliver close to 100% oxygen when used as a standard resuscitation bag (i.e., positive-pressure ventilation using the bag and without patient inspiratory effort). Depending on the bag configuration, however, there is dramatic variation in the concentration of oxygen delivered when a patient is actively breathing through the mask with no applied positive pressure. All bags have some kind of inspiratory valve, usually a "duckbill" type to prevent exhaled patient gases from mixing with the oxygen in the reservoir bag, and a separate exhalation port allows efflux of exhaled gases into the ambient air. Bag-valve-mask devices can provide >90% FiO_2 during active breathing when the exhalation port is equipped with a working one-way exhalation valve.[3,4] The one-way exhalation valve ensures that room air is not pulled in during active inspiration which would greatly reduce the FiO_2. If the bag is not configured with an exhalation valve or if the valve has been removed, FiO_2 may be lower than that delivered by nasal cannula (approximately 30% to 40%).[4]
- **Can supplemental oxygen applied during intubation help prolong desaturation time?** There are several groups of patients known to desaturate rapidly during the apneic phase of RSI. Obese adults, infants and toddlers, and adult patients who are critically ill will desaturate much more rapidly than the average adult patient.[5] In one study of obese (body mass index 30 to 35 kg per m^2) patients undergoing general anesthesia, those who received continuous oxygenation using nasal cannula at a 5 L per minute flow rate during apnea maintained SpO_2 ≥95% for significantly longer than controls (5.29 vs. 3.49 minutes) and had a significantly higher minimum SpO_2 (94.3% vs. 87.7%).[6] Based on this study, we recommend oxygen supplementation by nasal cannula at 5 L per minute for obese patients during the apneic phase of RSI, and it is reasonable to assume, but not yet proven, that similar benefits will accrue to nonobese patients who are prone to rapid desaturation.

REFERENCES

1. Marino PL, Sutin KM. Oxygen inhalation therapy. *The ICU Book*. Philadelphia, PA: Lippincott Williams & Wilkins; 2007:chap 21:403–418.

2. Miller RD, et al. Respiratory care. *Miller's Anesthesia*. Philadelphia, PA: Lippincott Williams & Wilkins; 2009:chap 93:2879–2898.

3. Cullen P. Self-inflating ventilation bags. *Anaesth Intensive Care*. 2001;29:203.

4. Nimmagadda U, Salem MR, Joseph NJ, et al. Efficacy or preoxygenation with tidal volume breathing: comparison of breathing systems. *Anesthesiology*. 2000;93:693–698.

5. Benumof JL, Dagg R, Benumof R. Critical hemoglobin desaturation will occur before return to an unparalyzed state following 1 mg/kg intravenous succinylcholine. *Anesthesiology*. 1997;87:979–982.

6. Ramachandran SK, Cosnowski A, Shanks A, et al. Apneic oxygenation during prolonged laryngoscopy in obese patients: a randomized, controlled trial of nasal oxygen administration. *J Clin Anesth*. 2010;22:164.

6

Noninvasive Mechanical Ventilation

Kerry B. Broderick • Peter M.C. DeBlieux

Patients with severe respiratory complaints frequently present to the emergency department (ED) and comprise >10% of all presentations. Over the past decade, ED presentations of asthma, pneumonia, and chest pain have increased. A thorough knowledge of mechanical ventilatory support, both invasive and noninvasive, is essential for practicing emergency medicine clinicians. This chapter discusses noninvasive positive-pressure ventilation (NPPV) while Chapter 7 focuses on mechanical ventilation after tracheal intubation. Recently, the use of NPPV has grown steadily as a result of evidence-based research, cost effectiveness, and consideration of patient comfort and complications.

The advantages of NPPV over mechanical ventilation include preservation of speech, swallowing, and physiologic airway defense mechanisms; reduced risk of airway injury; reduced risk of nosocomial infection; and a decreased length of stay in the ICU.

TECHNOLOGY OF NONINVASIVE MECHANICAL VENTILATION

Noninvasive mechanical ventilators have several characteristics that are distinct from standard critical care ventilators. NPPV offers a more portable technology because of the reduced size of the air compressor. Because of this reduction in size, these noninvasive ventilators do not develop pressures as high as their critical care ventilator counterparts do. Noninvasive ventilators have a single-limb tubing circuit that delivers oxygen to the patient and allows for exhalation. To prevent an accumulation of carbon dioxide, this tubing is continuously flushed with supplemental oxygen delivered during the expiratory phase. Exhaled gases are released through a small exhalation port near the patient's mask. During the respiratory cycle, the machine continuously monitors the degree of air leak and compensates for this loss of volume. NPPV is designed to tolerate air leak and compensates by maintaining airway pressures. This is in sharp contrast to the closed system found in invasive, critical care ventilators consisting of a dual, inspiratory and expiratory tubing system that does not tolerate air leak or compensate for lost volume. The device that makes physical contact between the patient and the ventilator is termed the interface. Interfaces for NPPV come in a variety of shapes and sizes designed to cover the individual nares, the nose only, the nose and mouth, the entire face, or the helmet. Ideally, interfaces should be comfortable, offer a good seal, minimize leak, and limit dead space.

MODES OF NONINVASIVE MECHANICAL VENTILATION

In a manner analogous to invasive mechanical ventilation, understanding the modes of NPPV is based on knowledge of three essential variables: the *trigger*, the *limit*, and the *cycle*. The *trigger* is the event that initiates inspiration: either patient effort or machine-initiated positive pressure. The *limit* refers to the airflow parameter that is regulated during inspiration: either airflow rate or airway pressure. The *cycle* terminates inspiration: either a pressure is delivered over a set time period or the patient ceases inspiratory efforts.

Continuous Positive Airway Pressure

Continuous positive airway pressure (CPAP) is a mode for invasive and noninvasive mechanical ventilation. CPAP is not a stand-alone mode of assisted mechanical ventilation. It is equivalent to positive end-expiratory pressure (PEEP) and facilitates inhalation by reducing pressure thresholds to initiate airflow (see Chapter 7). It provides positive airway pressure throughout the respiratory cycle. This static, positive pressure is maintained constantly during inhalation and exhalation. This mode should never be used in patients who may have apneic episodes because of the lack of a backup rate.

Spontaneous and Spontaneous/Timed Modes

In spontaneous mode, the airway pressure cycles between an inspiratory positive airway pressure (IPAP) and an expiratory positive airway pressure (EPAP). This is commonly referred to as bilevel or biphasic positive airway pressure (BL-PAP or BiPAP). The patient's inspiratory effort triggers the switch from EPAP to IPAP. The limit during inspiration is the set level of IPAP. The inspiratory phase cycles off, and the machine switches back to EPAP when it detects a cessation of patient effort, indicated by a decrease in inspiratory flow rate, or a maximum inspiratory time is reached, typically 3 seconds. Tidal volume varies breath to breath and is determined by degree of IPAP, patient effort, and lung compliance. Work of breathing (WOB) is primarily dictated by initiation and maintenance of inspiratory airflow, with additional WOB linked to active contraction of the expiratory muscles.

Spontaneous mode relies on patient effort to trigger inhalation. In this mode, a patient breathing at a low rate can develop a respiratory acidosis. The spontaneous/timed (ST) mode prevents this clinical consequence. The trigger in the ST mode can be the patient's effort, or an elapsed time interval that is predetermined by a set respiratory backup rate. If the patient does not initiate a breath in the prescribed interval, then IPAP is triggered. For machine-generated breaths, the ventilator cycles back to EPAP based on a set inspiratory time. For patient-initiated breaths, the ventilator cycles as it would in the spontaneous mode.

Conceptually, one can consider BiPAP as CPAP with pressure support (PS). The pressure during the inspiratory phase is termed IPAP and is analogous to PS, a pressure boost during inspiratory efforts. The pressure during the expiratory phase is termed EPAP and is analogous to CPAP, or PEEP, positive pressure maintained during the entire respiratory cycle. The IPAP is necessarily set higher than EPAP by a minimum of 5 cm H_2O, and the difference between the two settings is equivalent to the amount of PS provided.

The keys to successfully using NPPV on an emergency basis are patient selection and appropriate aggressiveness of therapy—that is, before resorting to endotracheal intubation and mechanical ventilation.

INDICATIONS AND CONTRAINDICATIONS

The indications for NPPV in the emergency setting are straightforward. The eligible patient must have a patent, nonthreatened airway; be conscious and cooperative; and have an existing, ventilatory drive. Patients who may benefit from NPPV could be hypercarbic, hypoxemic, or both. Patients with an acute exacerbation of chronic obstructive pulmonary disease (COPD), congestive heart failure exacerbation, severe pneumonia, status asthmaticus, or mild postextubation stridor might all be considered for NPPV. NPPV is *contraindicated* if the patient has a threat to the airway, is unable to cooperate, or is apneic. If the patient is in extremis, with very poor oxygen saturations and severe or worsening ventilatory inadequacy, immediate intubation is usually indicated. In such cases, it is not appropriate to delay intubation for a trial of NPPV. This is a relative contraindication, though, and clinical judgment is required. In some cases, the situation permitting, NPPV can be used to enhance preoxygenation of a patient for whom intubation is planned.

The objectives of NPPV are the same as those for invasive mechanical ventilation: to improve pulmonary gas exchange, to alleviate respiratory distress, to alter adverse pressure/volume relationships in the lungs, to permit lung healing, and to avoid complications. Patients on NPPV must be monitored closely, using familiar parameters such as vital signs, oximetry, capnography, chest radiograph, bedside spirometry, and arterial blood gases (ABGs).

INITIATING NONINVASIVE MECHANICAL VENTILATION

Either a face mask or a nasal mask can be used, but a nasal mask is generally better tolerated. There are varying mask sizes and styles, and a respiratory therapist must measure the patient to ensure a good fit and seal. First, explain the process to the patient before applying the mask. Initially supply 3 to 5 cm H_2O of CPAP with supplemental oxygen. Acceptance on the patient's part may improve if the patient is allowed to hold the mask against his or her face. The mask is secured with straps once the patient demonstrates acceptance. Next, explain to the patient that the pressure will change and either sequentially increase the CPAP pressure by 2 to 3 cm H_2O increments every 5 to 10 minutes, or initiate BiPAP to support the patient's respiratory efforts. Recommended initial settings for BiPAP machines in the noninvasive support of patients in respiratory distress or failure are IPAP of 8 cm H_2O and EPAP of 3 cm H_2O, for a PS (IPAP minus EPAP) of 5 cm H_2O. The level of supplemental oxygen flowing into the circuit should be governed by goal pulse oximetry and corroborated by ABG results as necessary. It is appropriate to initiate oxygen therapy with 2 to 5 L per minute, but this amount should be adjusted with each titration of IPAP or EPAP.

As the patient's response to ventilator and other therapy is monitored (using cardiac, respiratory, and BP monitors; oximetry; capnography; ABGs as indicated; and the patient's voiced assessment of tolerance and progress), support pressures are titrated. One approach that has been used successfully in hypoxemic patients in impending respiratory failure is to titrate by raising EPAP and IPAP in tandem in 2 cm H_2O steps, allowing a reasonable trial period (e.g., 5 minutes) at each level before increasing further. If the patient is hypercapnic, it may be better to raise the IPAP in 2 cm H_2O steps, with the EPAP being kept stationary or increased in a ratio to IPAP of approximately 1:2.5 (EPAP:IPAP). The intrinsic PEEP ($PEEP_i$), or auto-PEEP, cannot be measured by a noninvasive ventilator; therefore, EPAP should generally be maintained below 8 to 10 cm H_2O to be certain that it does not exceed $PEEP_i$ in patients with obstructive lung disease. The IPAP must always be set higher than EPAP by at least 5 cm H_2O. The goals are to reduce the patient's WOB, improve comfort, meet oxygen saturation goals, improve gas exchange, foster patient cooperativity, and maintain a respiratory rate of <30 breaths per minute. If the patient is not approaching these goals after the first hour of NPPV, then strong consideration should be made for rapid sequence intubation and institution of invasive mechanical ventilation.

TIPS AND PEARLS

- Patients who need airway protection must be differentiated from those who need intensive ventilatory support. None of the modes of NPPV provide airway protection.
- Patients with both a patent airway and some preserved respiratory drive—even if that drive is clearly insufficient—may be candidates for NPPV.
- Patients most likely to respond to NPPV in the ED (and therefore avoid intubation) are those with more readily reversible etiologies of distress, such as COPD exacerbation with fatigue, pneumonia with hypoxemia-induced fatigue, or cardiogenic pulmonary edema (PE).
- The ventilatory management of patients in frank or impending respiratory failure with NPPV is a *minute-to-minute*, ongoing strategic decision. Virtually every modern ventilator is capable of delivering noninvasive ventilation (NIV) (BiPAP, CPAP) and should be readily accessible to the ED or other critical care areas in the hospital. Physicians, nurses, and respiratory care personnel must be comfortable with NPPV use and knowledgeable of its limitations.
- Patient selection must be made considering the overall condition of the patient, the patient's tolerance of mask support versus intubation, and the anticipated degree of reversal of the underlying insult with ventilatory and pharmacologic support.
- One must be prepared for prompt intubation (i.e., difficult airway assessment completed and drugs and equipment readily at hand) if therapeutic failure occurs.
- NPPV should be accompanied by aggressive medical therapy of the underlying condition (e.g., angiotensin-converting enzyme inhibitors, diuretics, and nitrates for PE, β-adrenergic agonist and anticholinergic aerosols and corticosteroids for reactive airways disease).
- Finally, the patient should be carefully monitored for progress of therapy, tolerance of the mode of support, and any signs of clinical deterioration that indicate a need for intubation with mechanical ventilation.

- Patients treated in the ED with NPPV may require judicious sedation for anxiety in order to tolerate the mask, but doses used, if any, are small because preservation of respiratory drive is essential to the use of these modes.

EVIDENCE

In some published series, patients successfully supported in the ED with NPPV were frequently able to be admitted to telemetry units instead of ICUs, thereby incurring a significant cost savings. Uncontrolled studies without definitive inclusion criteria have found NPPV successful in avoiding intubation and mechanical ventilation in a large variety of patients on whom it has been clinically tested. Most of the studies done with NPPV compare NPPV to standard medical care (SMC) with outcome measures of intubation, length of stay in the ICU, and mortality. Unfortunately, most of the studies are quite small and have either enrollment criteria or end points that are somewhat subjective. Nonetheless, there is a considerable body of literature analyzing the use of NPPV.

- **NPPV and COPD.** Two meta-analysis studies have been performed analyzing the use of NPPV in COPD. The most recent meta-analysis was by Peter et al.[1] in 2002 of 15 randomized control trials of NPPV versus SMC. Eight trials enrolled patients with COPD, and seven trials enrolled patients characterized as a mixed-disease group. NPPV was associated with an overall 8% reduction in mortality ($p = .03$), 19% reduced need for intubation ($p = .001$), and 2.74 days shorter hospital stay ($p = .004$). The COPD group had more significant reductions with 13% decrease in mortality ($p = .001$), 18% decreased need for MV ($p = .02$), and decrease in hospital stay by 5.66 days ($p = .01$). In 1997, Keenan et al.[2] published a meta-analysis of such trials and identified only 7 out of 212 that met rigorous inclusion criteria for analysis. The analysis showed NPPV to have a decreased mortality (odds ratio, 0.29; 95% confidence interval [CI], 0.15 to 0.59), and a decreased need for intubation (odds ratio, 0.20; 95% CI, 0.11 to 0.36).[2] Early fiberoptic bronchoscopy in NIV patients with COPD and community acquired pneumonia has demonstrated promising decreases in rates of complications, and lower rates of tracheostomy.[9]
- **NPPV and asthma.** Shivaram et al.[3,4] demonstrated both a decreased WOB and an increased patient comfort level during CPAP support of acute asthma exacerbations. A recent RCT showed that patients in the NIV arm ($n = 28$) versus standard medical treatment arm ($n = 25$) had lower rates of ICU and hospital stays as well as lower doses of bronchodilators.[8] These small studies should not be considered to constitute evidence that NPPV is of benefit in acute asthma, and NIVS should be used in asthma only with extreme caution.
- **NPPV and PE.** There have been three recent meta-analyses that have reviewed the application of NPPV in cases of acute PE. Peter et al.[10] reviewed 23 trials comparing standard care for acute PE versus NPPV, both CPAP and BiPAP. CPAP was associated with a significantly lower mortality rate than standard therapy (relative risk, 0.59; 95% CI, 0.38 to 0.90; $p = .015$). A nonsignificant trend toward reduced mortality was seen in the comparison between bilevel ventilation and standard therapy (relative risk, 0.63; 95% CI, 0.37 to 1.10; $p = .11$). There was no substantial difference in mortality risk between bilevel ventilation and CPAP ($p = .38$). The need for mechanical ventilation was reduced with CPAP (relative risk, 0.44; 95% CI, 0.29 to 0.66; $p = .0003$) and with bilevel ventilation (relative risk, 0.50; 95% CI, 0.27 to 0.90; $p = .02$), when compared with standard therapy; but no significant difference was seen between CPAP and bilevel ventilation ($p = .86$). Weak evidence of an increase in the incidence of new myocardial infarction with bilevel ventilation versus CPAP was recorded (relative risk, 1.49; 95% CI, 0.92 to 2.42; $p = .11$). Ho and Wong compared CPAP and BiPAP using a meta-analysis and found no difference with regard to rate of myocardial infarction. In 2008, Masip[12] published a meta-analysis of NPPV in acute PE and documented a reduced need for intubations and an improvement in respiratory distress.

- **NIV and obesity.** As rates of obesity climb so will rates of difficult intubation.NIV is a potential alternative in this special population. A recent study showed that obese patients required higher end-expiratory pressure levels and more time to reduce their $PaCO_2$ levels below 50 mm Hg.[13] Another study showed that NIV was more successful in obese patients with lower age, weight, and body mass index.[14]

REFERENCES

1. Peter JV, Moran JL, Phillips-Hughes J, et al. Noninvasive ventilation in acute respiratory failure—a meta-analysis update. *Crit Care Med.* 2002;30:555–562.

2. Keenan SP, Kernerman PD, Cook DJ, et al. Effect of noninvasive positive pressure ventilation on mortality in patients admitted with acute respiratory failure: a meta-analysis. *Crit Care Med.* 1997;25:1685.

3. Shivaram U, Donath J, Khan FA, et al. Effects of continuous positive airway pressure in acute asthma. *Respiration.* 1987;52:157.

4. Shivaram U, Miro AM, Cash ME, et al. Cardiopulmonary responses to continuous positive airway pressure in acute asthma. *J Crit Care.* 1993;8:87.

5. Meduri GU. Noninvasive positive-pressure ventilation in patients with acute respiratory failure. *Clin Chest Med.* 1996;17:513.

6. Bersten AD, Holt AW, Vedig AE, et al. Treatment of severe cardiogenic pulmonary edema with continuous positive airway pressure delivered by face mask. *N Engl J Med.* 1991;325:1825–1830.

7. Hoffman B, Welte T. The use of noninvasive pressure support ventilation for severe respiratory insufficiency due to pulmonary oedema. *Intensive Care Med.* 1999;25:15–20.

8. Gupta D, Nath A, Agarwal R, et al. A prospective randomized controlled trial on the efficacy of noninvasive ventilation in severe acute asthma. *Respir Care.* 2010;55(5):536–543.

9. Scala R, Naldi M, Maccari U. Early fiberoptic bronchoscopy during non-invasive ventilation in pateints with decompensated chronic obstructive pulmonary disease due to community-acquired-pneumonia. *Crit Care.* 2010;14:R80.

10. Peter JV, Moran JL, Phillips-Hughes J, et al. Effect of non-invasive positive pressure ventilation (NIPPV) on mortality in patients with acute cardiogenic pulmonary oedema: a meta-analysis. *Lancet.* 2006;367:1155–1163.

11. Ho KM, Wong K. A comparison of continuous and bi-level positive airway pressure non-invasive ventilation in patients with acute cardiogenic pulmonary oedema: a meta-analysis. *Crit Care.* 2006;10:R49.

12. Masip J. Noninvasive ventilation in acute cardiogenic pulmonary edema. *Curr Opin Crit Care.* 2008;14(5):531.

13. Gursel G, Aydogdu M, Gulbas G, et al. The influence of severe obesity on non-invasive ventilation (NIV) strategies and responses in patients with acute hypercapnic respiratory failure attacks in the ICU. *Minerva Anestesiol.* 2011;77:17–25.

14. Duarte AG, Justino E, Bigler T, et al. Outcomes of morbidly obese patients requiring mechanical ventilation for acute respiratory failure. *Crit Care Med.* 2007;35:732–737.

7

Mechanical Ventilation

Peter M.C. DeBlieux • Alan C. Heffner

Initiating mechanical ventilation is a common task and a required skill for all emergency physicians. The etiologies for respiratory failure are expansive, and the choice between invasive and noninvasive mechanical ventilation can be a challenging clinical decision. This chapter focuses on patients requiring invasive mechanical ventilation following endotracheal intubation, and introduces the concepts essential for the initiation of invasive mechanical ventilation. Chapter 6 focuses on respiratory distress and the institution of noninvasive mechanical ventilation.

Spontaneous ventilation draws air into the lungs under negative pressure, whereas mechanical ventilation uses positive pressure to provide airflow. In either case, the amount of negative or positive pressure required to deliver the breath (tidal volume [V_t or TV]) must overcome resistance to airflow. Positive-pressure ventilation alters normal pulmonary physiology by decreasing venous return to the thorax, changing ventilation-perfusion matching in the lung, and increasing airway pressures.

TERMINOLOGY OF MECHANICAL VENTILATION

The following terms are used in mechanical ventilation:

- V_t or TV is the volume of a single breath. Conventional goal TV is approximately 7 ml per kg ideal body weight (IBW). Note that IBW is more a function of patient height than weight or overall size. TVs may be reduced (to 4 to 6 ml per kg IBW) in certain circumstances to minimize ventilator-induced lung injury (VILI) associated with excessive airway pressure and overdistention of functional lung units.

  The airway conduits do not exchange gas and therefore represent anatomical dead space that accounts for a fixed volume of each tidal breath. The remaining volume in each breath participates in gas exchange and constitutes alveolar ventilation. As TV is reduced, anatomical dead space makes up a proportionally larger portion of each breath. It is important to increase minute ventilation through enhanced respiratory rate (RR) to balance the decrease of effective alveolar ventilation with TV reduction.

- RR or frequency (f) is simply the number of breaths per minute. Usual starting RR is 12 to 20 breaths per minute in adults. Higher rates are typical in neonates, infants, and small children.

  Given our attention to low-TV ventilation, even in patients without lung injury, minute ventilation is typically modified by increasing RR rather than TV. In addition to compensating for the relative proportion of dead space mentioned above, enhanced RR may be used to provide compensation for metabolic acidosis or enhanced carbon dioxide (CO_2) production (e.g., fever/hyperthermia, sepsis, and hypermetabolic conditions).

  In reactive airways diseases, the concept of permissive hypercapnia refers to the use of a low RR (8 to 10 breaths per minute), which allows for a prolonged expiratory time, combined with low TVs (6 to 7 ml per kg IBW) to diminish the risk of hyperinflation.

- Fractional concentration of inspired oxygen (FiO_2) ranges from the concentration of oxygen in room air (0.21 or 21%) to that of pure oxygen (1.0 or 100%). When initiating mechanical ventilation, start with an FiO_2 of 100% and reduce the oxygen based on pulse oximetry.

- Inspiratory flow rate (IFR) is the rate at which a TV is delivered during inspiration. In an adult, this is typically set at 60 L per minute. Cases of reactive airways disease may require peak IFR to be increased to 90 to 120 L per minute to shorten the inspiratory time (Ti) and thus increase expiratory time and diminish dynamic hyperinflation.

- Positive end-expiratory pressure (PEEP) provides a static pressure to the airways during inspiration and expiration, and is typically set at a minimum of 5 cm H_2O. PEEP increases functional residual capacity, total lung volumes, and total lung pressures. When a patient is unable to meet oxygenation goals using an FiO_2 >50%, PEEP can be progressively increased to augment mean airway pressure and oxygenation. Excessive PEEP can cause overdistention and contribute to VILI and compromised venous return with consequent hemodynamic deterioration.

- Peak inspiratory pressure (PIP) and plateau pressure (P_{plat}): The PIP, the greatest pressure reached at any point during the inspiratory phase, is a function of the ventilator circuitry, endotracheal tube (ETT), peak flow, and the patient's lung and thoracic compliance. It is useful for rapidly assessing the patient when acute change has occurred, but does not accurately reflect the risk of VILI. The risk for VILI is best represented by the P_{plat}, measured at the end of inspiration during an inspiratory pause. The pause enables equilibration of pressures between the ventilator and lung units to measure the P_{plat} of the system. P_{plat} correlates best with the risk of VILI and the current recommendation is to maintain the P_{plat} <30 cm H_2O. P_{plat} >30 cm H_2O are best managed by reducing either TVs or PEEP.

VENTILATION MODES

There are a variety of modes in invasive mechanical ventilation, and the key to understanding the differences between these modes centers on three variables: the trigger, the limit, and the cycle.

- The trigger is the event that initiates inspiration: either patient effort or machine-initiated positive pressure.
- The limit refers to the airflow parameter that is used to regulate inspiration: either airflow rate or airway pressure.
- The cycle terminates inspiration: either a delivered set volume (volume cycled ventilation), a delivered pressure over a set time period (pressure cycled ventilation [PCV]), or termination of inspiratory effort by the patient (pressure support [PS] ventilation).
- The best mode in a given circumstance depends on the needs of the patient.

Commonly used ventilation modes are as follows:

- Control mode ventilation (CMV) is almost exclusively relegated to the operating room in sedated and paralyzed patients, but an understanding of this mode provides appreciation of the support provided through other modes. In CMV, all breaths are triggered, limited, and cycled by the ventilator. The clinician sets the TV, RR, IFR, PEEP, and FiO_2. The ventilator then delivers the prescribed V_t (the cycle) at the set IFR (the limit). Even if the patient wanted to initiate an additional breath, the machine would not respond. In addition, if the patient has not completely exhaled before initiation of the next breath, the machine would generate the required pressure to deliver the full V_t breath. For these reasons, CMV is only used in those patients who are sedated and paralyzed.
- Assist control (AC) is the preferred mode for patients in respiratory distress. The clinician sets the V_t, RR, IFR, PEEP, and FiO_2. In contrast to all other modes, the trigger that initiates inspiration can be either patient effort or an elapsed time interval. When either occurs, the ventilator delivers the prescribed TV. The ventilator synchronizes set RRs with patient efforts, and if the patient is breathing at or above the set RR, then all breaths are patient initiated. The work of breathing is primarily limited to the patient's effort to trigger the ventilator and can be altered by adjusting the sensitivity threshold.
- Synchronized intermittent mandatory ventilation (SIMV with or without PS) is commonly misunderstood and can lead to excessive patient work of breathing. The physician sets the V_t, RR, IFR, PEEP, and FiO_2. Importantly, the trigger that initiates inspiration depends on the patient's RR relative to the set RR. When the patient is breathing at or below the set RR, the trigger can be patient effort or elapsed time. In these cases, the ventilator operates similar to an AC mode. If the patient is breathing above the set RR, the ventilator does not automatically assist the patient efforts and the TV is determined by effort and resistance to airflow through the ETT and ventilator circuit. In these instances, work of breathing can be excessive.

Addition of PS to the SIMV mode provides a set inspiratory pressure that is applied during patient-initiated breaths, which exceed the set RR. Appropriate PS balances the inherent resistance of the artificial airways and supports the patient's physiologic situation to limit undue work of breathing. Insufficient PS is associated with high RR and low V_t, also known as rapid, shallow breathing. Typically, RR is the best marker for the appropriate level of PS. RR should be maintained at <30 breaths per minute and ideally below 24 breaths per minute. SIMV provides no clear benefit over AC mode ventilation. Although previously used as a weaning mode wherein the set rate is progressively decreased to allow the patient to assume increased work of breathing, the absence of additional pressure support (PSV) substantially increases work of breathing and is frequently overtaxing. Spontaneous breathing trials using minimal pressure support ventilation (PSV), without SIMV, is the current standard approach to assess readiness for liberation from mechanical ventilation.

- Continuous positive airway pressure (CPAP) is not a true mode of invasive mechanical ventilation. It is equivalent to PEEP in that it provides a static positive airway pressure throughout the entire respiratory cycle.

In a fashion similar to SIMV, PS can be added to CPAP to function as an assisted form of ventilation. In the CPAP-PS mode, the patient determines the RR, initiating and terminating each breath. The TV is dependent on patient effort and the degree of PS relative to the resistance of the airway circuit. This mode should never be used in patients at risk for hypoventilation or apnea because there is no mandatory backup rate to support the patient in case of failure.

VENTILATOR TV DELIVERY

Volume Cycled Ventilation

In this method of delivering a breath, the operator sets the TV of each breath. The pressure required to deliver this volume varies by the flow rate selected and the resistance of the airway circuit and lungs and compliance of lungs and thorax. In adults, the initial peak flow is usually set to 60 L per minute.

Volume cycled ventilation (VCV) also allows selection of the flow characteristics of a delivered breath. The waveform may be square or decelerating (Fig. 7-1). A square wave

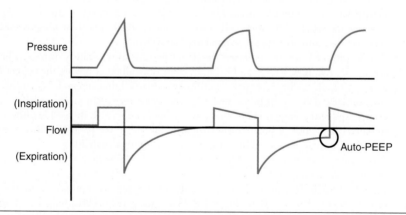

Figure 7-1 ● **Volume-Control Ventilation (VCV).** The lower trace demonstrates a square flow waveform first. The next waveform is a decelerating waveform. Note that the peak pressure generated by the square waveform exceeds that of the decelerating waveform. The third waveform demonstrates inspiration being initiated before expiratory flow has reached zero. This is how breath stacking and auto-PEEP occur.

delivers the V_t at a constant peak flow throughout inspiration. This waveform usually generates a higher peak pressure than the decelerating waveform, but has the advantage of a shorter Ti, providing more time for expiration. A decelerating flow wave delivers the initial V_t at a selected peak flow and then decelerates flow linearly as the breath is delivered. Because resistance to flow normally increases during inspiration, the decelerating waveform generally results in lower PIP. This approach increases the Ti, at the expense of expiratory time, potentially trapping gas in the lung, causing dynamic hyperinflation and auto-PEEP. For this reason, the peak flow set for decelerating flow wave is usually higher than that used in a square wave flow pattern. When setting up the ventilator, one can switch back and forth from one waveform to another in attempting to determine which offers best patient synchrony.

Pressure Cycled Ventilation

PCV should not be confused with PS ventilation, described previously. The limit during PCV is a set airway pressure. Instead of V_t, the cycle during PCV is a set Ti. Some PCV ventilator models require a set RR and inspiratory to expiratory (I:E) ratio. Ti is then calculated by the ventilator based on these settings. The clinician specifies an inspiratory pressure and an inspiratory–expiratory (I/E) ratio predicted to provide a reasonable V_t and RR, based on the patient's expected resistance and compliance. TV may vary breath to breath based on airway resistance, lung compliance and patient effort, but it should generally meet the same 7 ml per kg IBW goal previously discussed.

In this mode, the peak flow of the administered tidal breath and the flow waveform vary according to airway and lung characteristics. Early in inspiration, the ventilator generates a flow rate that is sufficiently rapid to reach the preset pressure, and then automatically alters the flow rate to stay at that pressure, and cycles off at the end of the predetermined Ti. The flow waveform created by this method is a decelerating pattern (Fig. 7-2). A normal I/E ratio is 1:2. If the RR is 10 breaths per minute evenly distributed over a minute, each cycle of inspiration and expiration is 6 seconds. With an I/E ratio of 1:2, inspiration is 2 seconds, and expiration is 4 seconds.

The I/E ratio is usually determined by simply observing the pressure and flow waveforms on the ventilator monitor. After the inspiratory pressure is adjusted to meet the goal V_t, the Ti is

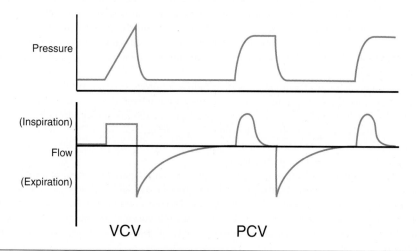

Figure 7-2 ● Pressure-Control Ventilation. These waveforms demonstrate the differing waveform characteristics between volume-control ventilation (VCV) and PCV. Note that PCV generates lower peak pressures than VCV.

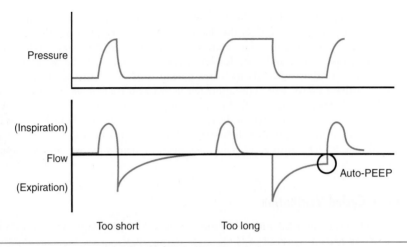

Figure 7-3 ● **Pressure-Control Ventilation and Inspiratory–Expiratory Ratio.** The first waveform set demonstrates an inspiratory time that is so short that the tidal volume is likely insufficient. The second and third waveform sets demonstrate how an inspiratory time that is too long may lead to breath stacking and auto-PEEP, as illustrated in Figure 7-1.

adjusted while monitoring end-expiratory flow. Terminal end-expiratory flow should approach zero to confirm expiration is complete, and there is no retained V_t in the thorax. Even small volumes of retained V_t are quickly compounded by the ventilator and lead to dynamic hyperinflation with eventual increased intrathoracic pressure known as auto-PEEP (Fig. 7-3). In contrast, overly brief Ti can lead to low-TVs and hypoventilation.

INITIATING MECHANICAL VENTILATION

The patient who is spontaneously breathing possesses a complex series of physiologic feedback loops that control the volume of gas moved into and out of the lungs each minute (minute ventilation). They automatically determine the RR and the volume of each breath necessary to effect gas exchange and maintain homeostasis. The patients who are entirely dependent on ventilators have no such "servocontrol" mechanism and must rely on the individuals setting the ventilatory parameters to meet their physiologic needs. In the past, this required frequent blood gas determinations. Now we rely on noninvasive techniques such as pulse oximetry and end-tidal CO_2 monitoring.

A certain amount of ventilation is required each minute (minute ventilation or minute volume) to remove the CO_2 produced by metabolism and delivered to the lungs by the circulatory system each minute. This minute volume approximates 100 ml per kg, provided the metabolic rate is normal. Hypermetabolic and febrile patients can produce up to 25% more CO_2 compared with a patient in a normal steady state. Minute ventilation would need to increase proportionally to accommodate this increased production.

Our recommended initial ventilator settings for adult patients are shown in Box 7-1. For the vast majority of patients, this formula produces reasonable gas exchange to provide adequate oxygenation and ventilation. Obviously, the components of minute ventilation (V_t and RR) can be manipulated to provide adequate minute volume. Smaller TVs may be desired, but this typically requires a compensatory increase in respiratory frequency (see earlier discussion).

Supranormal TV and high airway pressure risk VILI during mechanical ventilation. This underlies the recommended starting V_t. For some patients, the most difficult task in optimizing

---

Box 7-1 Recommended initial ventilator settings for adult patients. See text for abbreviations.

- Mode   AC
- V_t 7 ml per kg IBW
- f 12 to 20 breaths per minute
- FiO_2 1.0
- PEEP   5.0 cm
- IFR   60 L per minute

---

mechanical ventilation is balancing TV and distending lung pressure. Patients with unilateral pulmonary disease such as pneumonia or traumatic contusion or diffuse bilateral disease such as pulmonary edema or acute lung injury/acute respiratory distress syndrome (ALI/ARDS) warrant modifications to minimize VILI induced by excessive airway pressure and overdistention of functional lung units. Measured airway pressure correlates with the risk of VILI and current recommendations aim to maintain P_{plat} <30 cm H_2O. Because many of these patients require PEEP augmentation for oxygenation, this is best managed by reducing TV in a range of 4 to 6 ml per kg IBW.

Positive-pressure breathing increases intrathoracic pressure that is transmitted to the great vessels and can compromise venous return. In some situations, this can seriously compromise cardiovascular performance and precipitate shock or cardiac arrest (i.e., pulseless electrical activity).

In other situations, ventilator modifications aim to balance minute ventilation with airflow dynamics. The intubated patient with obstructive lung disease such as asthma is a good example. Minute volume aims to provide reasonable minute ventilation relative to CO_2 production, but must be balanced to support complete TV expiration to avoid inadequate gas emptying and dynamic hyperinflation. Frequency has the greatest impact on expiratory time and should start as low as 8 breaths per minute. The inspiratory cycle can also be shortened by increasing the IFR to maximize expiratory time. Following these manipulations, the flow-time graphic should be interrogated to confirm complete expiration (i.e., return to zero flow). Initiation of the next breath occurs before complete expiration is known as "breath stacking," and leads to dynamic hyperinflation. In extreme cases, deliberate hypoventilation is performed to avoid dynamic hyperinflation and associated high-intrathoracic pressure (i.e., barotraumas and cardiovascular compromise). In return, permissive hypercapnia (respiratory acidosis with pH > 7.15) is tolerated. Equipment considerations are important when there is outflow obstruction, as in asthma or COPD. This is one case where attention to detail can make a material difference. Recommendations are shown in Box 7-2.

For details regarding ventilation of patients with specific disorders and initiating mechanical ventilation for those conditions, refer to Section 8 of this book.

Box 7-2 Recommendations for mechanical ventilation for adult patients with outflow obstruction. See text for abbreviations.

- Use as large an ETT as possible.
- Cut the ETT to minimize the length.
- Set RR of 8 to 10 breaths per minute.
- Set V_t of 6 to 7 cc per kg IBW.
- Increase the IFR to 90 to 120 L per minute.

TIPS AND PEARLS

- Have a respiratory therapist (RT) review the features and graphics of ventilators available at your particular institution. Make sure that your RTs are familiar with the ARDSnet protocol, P_{plat} measurements and the concept of permissive hypercapnia.
- When a ventilator alarms, you should know how to take a patient off the ventilator and resume bag ventilation until an RT can assist. To do this, you must be able to turn the ventilator on and off and know how to silence the alarms. These minimal steps will preserve calm until the RT can respond. Bag ventilation can be used to deal with temporary problems and provides the additional feedback of "feel."
- Understand the typical resistance and compliance characteristics of various respiratory disorders. This information may help predict specific TV and rate settings for your patients.
- Use AC as your primary mode following initial intubation. This provides support for apneic patients and relieves the patient of the work of breathing. SIMV-PS may be used for patients without evidence of respiratory distress.
- Consider disconnecting the patient from the breathing circuit and provide bag ventilation support during transport, unless a small transport ventilator is used. The circuit is heavy and may drag the ETT out, especially in infants and children.

EVIDENCE

- **What is permissive hypercapnia, and is there evidence that it is safe?** All patients are capable of trapping inspired air if the expiratory period is inadequate. Patients with obstructive lung disease are particularly vulnerable. Maximizing expiratory periods through ventilator modifications (i.e., low RR and V_t and rapid IFR) to maintain physiologic minute ventilation may not be the safest approach in all patients. Permissive hypercapnia is the technique of providing intentional hypoventilation to avoid dynamic hyperinflation that leads to intrinsic- or auto-PEEP. Significant respiratory acidosis (pH > 7.15) is well tolerated.[1–3] Patients require significant sedation and often paralysis to maintain sufficient bradypnea during this technique.
- **What is the current ventilator management strategy to limit lung injury in ARDS?** Contemporary mechanical ventilation aims to minimize VILI induced by lung overdistention. The ARDSnet study group showed that use of low-TV (6 vs. 12 cc per kg) reduced mortality and ventilator days.[4–8] Recognizing that TV is distributed predominantly to healthy, patent lung, lower TV prevents overdistention and injury of these functional lung units. P_{plat} (goal <30 cm H_2O) is used as the surrogate measure of lung compliance to individualize the appropriate reduction of V_t. The low-TV method is now routinely applied to mechanical ventilation of patients with ALI/ARDS.[9]

REFERENCES

1. Moore BB, Wagner R, Weiss KB. A community-based study of near fatal asthma. *Ann Allergy Asthma Immunol.* 2001;86(2):190–195.

2. Williams TJ, Tuxen DV, Scheinkestel CD, et al. Risk factors for morbidity in mechanically ventilated patients with acute severe asthma. *Am Rev Respir Dis.* 1992;146:607–615.

3. Leatherman JW, McArthur C, Shapiro RS. Effect of prolongation of expiratory time on dynamic hyperinflation in mechanically ventilated patients with severe asthma. *Crit Care Med.* 2004;32:1542–1545.

4. Brower RG, Shanholtz CB, Fessler HE, et al. Prospective, randomized, controlled clinical trial comparing traditional versus reduced tidal volume ventilation in acute respiratory distress syndrome patients. *Crit Care Med.* 1999;27:1492–1498.

5. Stewart TE, Meade MO, Cook DJ, et al. Evaluation of a ventilation strategy to prevent barotrauma in patients at high risk for acute respiratory distress syndrome. *N Engl J Med.* 1998;338:355–361.

6. Donahoe M. Basic ventilator management: lung protective strategies. *Surg Clin North Am.* 2006;86:1389–1408.

7. The Acute Respiratory Distress Syndrome Network Authors. Ventilation with lower tidal volumes as compared with traditional tidal volumes for acute lung injury and the acute respiratory distress syndrome. *N Engl J Med.* 2000;342:1301–1308.

8. Girard TD, Bernard GR. Mechanical ventilation in ARDS: a state-of-the-art review. *Chest.* 2007;131(3):921–929.

9. Determann RM, Royakkers A, Wolthuis EK, et al. Ventilation with lower tidal volumes as compared with conventional tidal volumes for patients without acute lung injury: a preventive randomized controlled trial. *Crit Care.* 2010;14(1):R1.

8

Oxygen and Carbon Dioxide Monitoring

Alan C. Heffner • Robert F. Reardon

PULSE OXIMETRY

The amount of oxygen reversibly bound to hemoglobin in arterial blood is described as hemoglobin saturation (SaO_2), which is a critical element of systemic oxygen delivery. Unfortunately, clinical detection of hypoxemia is unreliable. Pulse oximeters enable in vivo, noninvasive, and continuous measurement of arterial oxygen saturation at the bedside. Reliable interpretation of the information provided by these devices requires appreciation of their technology and limitations.

Principles of Measurement

Pulse oximetry relies on the principle of spectral analysis, which is the method of analyzing physiochemical properties of matter based on their unique light-absorption characteristics. For blood, absorbance of transmitted light is dependent on the concentration of hemoglobin species.

Oximeters are made up of a light source, photodetector, and microprocessor. Light-emitting diodes (LED) emit high-frequency signals at 660 nm (red) and 940 nm (infrared) wavelengths. When positioned to traverse (transmittance) or reflect from (reflectance) a cutaneous vascular bed, the opposed photodetector measures light intensity of each transmitted signal. Signal processing exploits the pulsatile nature of arterial blood to isolate arterial saturation. The microprocessor averages these data over several pulse cycles and compares the measured absorption to a reference standard curve to determine hemoglobin saturation, which is displayed as percentage of oxyhemoglobin (SpO_2). SpO_2 and SaO_2 correlation vary with manufacturer but exhibit high accuracy ($\pm2\%$) within normal physiologic range and circumstances.

Two oximetry techniques are used in clinical practice. Transmission oximetry deploys the LED and photodetector on opposite sides of a tissue bed (e.g., digit, nares, and ear lobe) such that the signal must traverse tissue. Reflectance oximeters position the LED and photodetector side by side on a single surface and can be placed in anatomic locations without an interposed vascular bed (e.g., forehead). This facilitates more proximal sensor placement with improved response time relative to core body SaO_2.

Indications

Pulse oximetry provides important real-time physiologic data and is the standard noninvasive measure of arterial saturation. Widespread adoption has contributed to its label and integration as the fifth vital sign. Continuous monitoring is indicated for any patient at risk or in the midst of acute cardiopulmonary decompensation. Reliable continuous oximetry is mandatory for patients requiring airway management and should be a component of each preintubation checklist. The probe is preferably placed on an extremity without a BP cuff.

Limitations and Precautions

Pulse oximeters have a number of important physiologic and technical limitations that influence bedside use and interpretation (Table 8-1).

Signal Reliability

Proper pulse oximetry requires pulse detection to distinguish light absorption from arterial blood relative to the background of other tissues. Abnormal peripheral circulation as a consequence of shock, vasoconstriction, and hypothermia may prevent pulsatile flow detection. Heart rate and plethysmographic waveform display verify arterial sensing, and SpO_2 should be considered inaccurate unless corroborated by these markers. Varying pulse amplitude is easily recognized on the monitor and represents the measure of arterial pulsality at the sampled vascular bed. Quantification in the form of perfusion index is being incorporated into some software to verify signal reliability and gauge microvascular flow.

TABLE 8-1
Etiology and Examples of Unreliable Pulse Oximetry

Etiology	Examples
Sensor location	Critical illness (forehead probe is best)
	Extraneous light exposure
Motion artifact	Exercise
	CPR
	Seizure
	Shivering
	Tremor
	Prehospital transport
Signal degradation	Poor peripheral perfusion
	Hypotension
	Hypoperfusion
	Vasoconstriction
	Nail polish (position probe transversely)
Physiologic range	Increasingly inaccurate when systolic BP <80 mm Hg
	Increasingly inaccurate when SaO_2 <75%
Dyshemoglobinemia	CO-Hgb (overestimates SpO_2)
	Met-Hgb (variable response)
Intravenous dye	Methylene blue
	Indocyanine green

Even with verified signal detection, measurement bias limits SpO_2 reliability during physiologic extremes. Reliability deteriorates with progressive hypotension below systolic BP of 80 mm Hg. Readings generally underestimate true SaO_2. Severe hypoxemia with SaO_2 <75% is also associated with increased measurement error. However, patients with this severity of hypoxemia are typically receiving maximized intervention, and closer discrimination in this range rarely imparts new information that alters management.

A number of physical factors affect pulse oximetry accuracy. Signal reliability is influenced by sensor exposure to extraneous light, excessive movement, synthetic fingernails, nail polish, intravenous dyes, severe anemia, and abnormal hemoglobin species. Diligent probe placement and shielding the probe from extraneous light should be routine. Surface extremity warming may improve local perfusion to enable arterial pulse sensing, but SpO_2 accuracy using this technique is not confirmed. Transverse digital sensor orientation overcomes limitations resulting from nail abnormalities.

Carboxyhemoglobin (CO-Hgb) and methemoglobin (Met-Hgb) absorb light at different wavelengths. Co-oximeters (and some new generation pulse oximeters) use four wavelengths of light stimulus to selectively discriminate these species. However, CO-Hgb absorbance is close to oxyhemoglobin such that most conventional pulse oximeters sum their measurement and give artifactually high SpO_2 reading. Met-Hgb produces variable error, depending on the true oxy- and Met-Hgb levels. SpO_2 classically approximates 85% in severe toxicity.

Response Time

Pulse oximetry readings lag the patient's physiologic state. Signal averaging of 4 to 20 seconds is typical of most monitors. Delay because of sensor anatomic location and abnormal cardiac performance compound the lag relative to central SaO_2. Forehead and ear probes are closer to the heart and respond more quickly than distal extremity probes. Response difference compared to central SaO_2

is also compounded by hypoxemia (i.e., starting on the steep portion of the oxyhemoglobin dissociation curve) and slower peripheral circulation such as low cardiac output states. As such, forehead reflectance probes are often preferred in critically ill patients. All of these response delays become more clinically important during rapid desaturation such as may occur during airway management.

Physiologic Insight and Limitations

Hemoglobin saturation is just one part of the assessment of systemic oxygenation. Although monitoring is continuous, SpO_2 provides momentary information on arterial saturation without detailing insight into systemic oxygenation and respiratory reserve. The physiologic context of oximetry is critical for appropriate interpretation and assists estimation of a patient's cardiopulmonary reserve for planning and execution of an airway management plan.

Oximetry measures arterial hemoglobin saturation but not the arterial oxygen tension or oxygen content of blood. The oxyhemoglobin dissociation curve describes the relationship of oxygen partial pressure (PaO_2) and saturation (SaO_2). Its sigmoidal shape hinges on varying hemoglobin affinity with successive oxygen binding. It is important to note that SpO_2 provides poor correlation with PaO_2 in the normal range. Normal SaO_2 is associated with a wide range of PaO_2 (80 to 400 mm Hg), which includes two extremes of oxygen reserve. Similarly, oximetry is insensitive at detecting progressive hypoxemia in patients with high-baseline PaO_2 (Table 8-1). Correlation is established in the hypoxemic range at and below the upper inflection point of the oxyhemoglobin curve (PaO_2 <60 mm Hg approximating SaO_2 90% at normal pH) where desaturation is rapid with declining PaO_2.

Hemoglobin saturation must also be interpreted in the context of inspired oxygen fraction (FiO_2) to provide insight into gas exchange and physiologic reserve. Simple observation at the bedside provides qualitative assessment. More formal calculation of the SpO_2/FiO_2 (SF) ratio is advocated. For the same reasons previously discussed, SF ratio correlates with PaO_2/FiO_2 (PF) ratio in the hypoxemic range (SpO_2 <90%) but not in the normal range. As such, observation of the patient's condition before supplemental oxygen escalation or preoxygenation provides more insight into the physiologic state. Correct interpretation of SpO_2 relative to FiO_2 is also important in assessing for failure of noninvasive ventilation. Hypoxemia and/or requirement of oxygen escalation above FiO_2 >70% leaves a thin margin of physiologic reserve for preoxygenation and execution of safe, uncomplicated endotracheal intubation.

Although PaO_2 (with or without conscious calculation of PF ratio) is a traditional and reliable gauge of pulmonary gas exchange and reserve, measurement of PaO_2 through arterial blood gas sampling before airway management is not generally helpful. The aim to maximize preoxygenation in all patients supersedes this strategy. However, knowledge of these principles and relationships provides insight into physiologic events and the fallibility of current technology during the management of critical illness.

The context of cardiac performance is also vital to interpretation of oximetry data. Although saturated hemoglobin accounts for the majority of blood oxygen content, systemic oxygen delivery is largely regulated (and limited) by cardiac performance. Pertinent to airway management, rapid desaturation and delayed response to pulmonary oxygenation should be anticipated in the setting of low cardiac output.

Finally, oxygen saturation is an unreliable gauge of ventilation, $PaCO_2$ level or acid–base status. Normal arterial saturation does not ensure appropriate ventilation. Oxygenation often is adequate with minimal volume of gas exchange, whereas carbon dioxide (CO_2) removal relies on pulmonary ventilation. Arterial blood gas analysis is the traditional means to measure $PaCO_2$, but alternative noninvasive CO_2 monitoring provides additional insight.

END-TIDAL CO$_2$ MONITORING

CO_2 is a normal byproduct of systemic metabolism. The quantity of expired CO_2 is dependent on three factors: metabolic production, venous return and pulmonary circulation to deliver CO_2 to the lungs, and alveolar ventilation. Capnography therefore provides insight into each of these factors. The corollary is that interpretation of exhaled CO_2 is not always straightforward as a consequence of its dependence on these three functions.

Basics of CO_2 Monitoring

CO_2 monitors measure the partial pressure of CO_2 (in millimeters of mercury) in expired gas. A variety of methods and devices are available. Qualitative (or semiquantitative) colorimetric monitors simply detect expired CO_2 above a threshold concentration. Quantitative devices include nonwaveform capnometers and waveform capnographers, which display the partial pressure of CO_2 in each breath. When measured at the end of expiration, this is referred to as end-tidal CO_2 (ETCO$_2$), which approximates alveolar CO_2. Waveform capnographers display a continuous waveform, representing exhaled CO_2 concentration over time and therein provide the most comprehensive data on metabolism, perfusion, and ventilation.

Colorimetric CO_2 Detectors

Colorimetric CO_2 detectors use pH-sensitive filter paper impregnated with metacresol purple, which changes color from purple (<4 mm Hg CO_2) to tan (4 to 15 mm Hg CO_2) to yellow (>20 mm Hg CO_2), depending on the concentration of exhaled CO_2. The indicator, housed in a plastic casing, is typically interposed between the endotracheal tube (ETT) and ventilator bag. Qualitative colorimetric detectors are inexpensive and easy to use, making them an excellent choice for ETT confirmation. One important limitation of qualitative colorimetric detectors is that they have a 25% false-negative rate (no color change with correct intubation) in the setting of (usually prolonged) cardiac arrest resulting from the absence of circulatory distribution of CO_2 to the lungs.

Quantitative CO_2 Monitors

Quantitative monitors include nonwaveform capnometers, which display ETCO$_2$ of each breath, and waveform capnographers which display ETCO$_2$ and a continuous waveform representing exhaled CO_2 over time (Fig. 8-1). Most of these devices use an infrared sensor, which measures the amount of infrared light absorbed by CO_2 in the exhaled gases.

There are two types of capnographers: sidestream monitors withdraw gas samples from the airway with a thin tube and mainstream monitors sample gas with an in-line sensor. Both types can be used for intubated patients. Nonintubated patients undergoing sedation are usually monitored with a sidestream capnographer through a nasal cannula. Capnography face masks that use both sidestream and mainstream technology are also available for monitoring nonintubated patients.

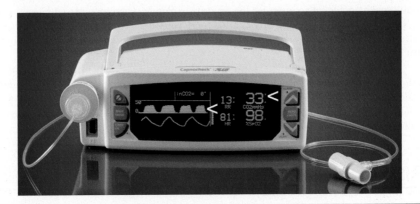

Figure 8-1 • Waveform capnographer, displaying the ET CO$_2$ value (<) with each breath and a waveform (<) representing exhaled CO_2 concentration over time.

Capnography Interpretation

In healthy patients, a close correlation exists between $ETCO_2$ and arterial CO_2 ($PaCO_2$) such that $ETCO_2$ is approximately 2 to 5 mm Hg less than $PaCO_2$ (normal $ETCO_2$ is 35 to 45 mm Hg). Unfortunately, changes in ventilation and perfusion alter the alveolar to arterial gradient such that absolute $PaCO_2$ can be difficult to predict based on capnography. This does not detract from the utility of capnographic waveform and trend analysis (Table 8-2).

Monitors can display capnograph waveforms at a high-recording rate, which improves waveform assessment, or a low-recording rate for assessing $ETCO_2$ trends (Figs. 8-2 and 8-3). A normal capnogram waveform has a characteristic rectangular shape and should start from 0 mm Hg and return to 0 mm Hg. Elevation of the baseline above zero implies CO_2 rebreathing or hypoventilation. The upstroke should be rapid and almost vertical. A slurred upstroke occurs with expiratory obstruction caused by bronchospasm, chronic lung disease, or

---

TABLE 8-2
Abnormal $ETCO_2$ Values

$ETCO_2$	Physiology	Clinical Condition
Increased	Decreased CO_2 clearance	Classic hypoventilation
	Increased circulation	ROSC in cardiac arrest
	Increased CO_2 production	Increased metabolism (fever and seizure)
Decreased	Increased CO_2 clearance	Hyperventilation
	Lack of CO_2 in gas	Hypopneic hypoventilation
	Sample decreased circulation	Low cardiac output
	Decreased CO_2 production	Pulmonary embolism
		Decreased metabolism (hypothermia)
Zero	No ventilation	Esophageal intubation
		Accidental extubation
		Apnea
	No circulation	Cardiac arrest

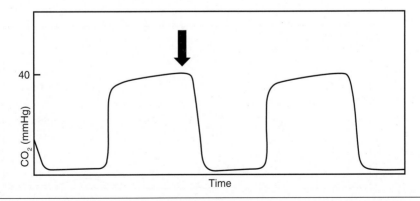

Figure 8-2 ● Normal capnography waveform at a high-recording rate (12.5 mm per second) with a characteristic rectangular shape. The upstroke and downstroke are nearly vertical, the plateau rises slightly throughout expiration and the ET CO_2 value (about 40 mm Hg) is measured at the end of expiration (*arrow*).

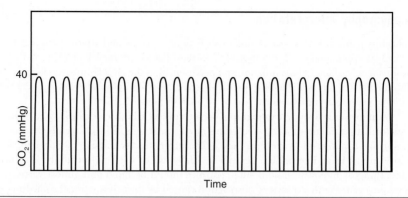

Figure 8-3 ● Normal capnography waveform at a low-recording rate (25 mm per minute). The low-recording rate is useful for monitoring ET CO_2 trends, not waveform shape.

a kinked ETT. The plateau tends to slope gently upward to the end of expiration where the $ETCO_2$ value is measured. Beginning with inspiration, there is a rapid vertical drop back to the baseline.

Clinical Utility of Quantitative Capnometry and Capnography

Confirmation of ETT placement and detection of accidental extubation

Continuous waveform capnography and nonwaveform capnometry are the most accurate methods for confirming ETT placement (See chapter 12.). Esophageal intubation results in an absent or abnormal $ETCO_2$ value or waveform after the first few breaths (Fig. 8-4). Correct ETT placement results in a reasonable $ETCO_2$ value and a characteristic rectangular waveform. The $ETCO_2$ value and waveform can be continuously monitored during prehospital and intrahospital transport. Sudden waveform loss is the earliest sign of accidental extubation and may precede oxygen desaturation by minutes.

Capnography during cardiopulmonary resuscitation

Capnography is a sensitive indicator of cardiovascular status. Exhaled CO_2 is dependent on pulmonary circulation, which is absent during untreated cardiac arrest. The 2010 American Heart Association (AHA) guidelines encourage the use of continuous waveform capnography to optimize

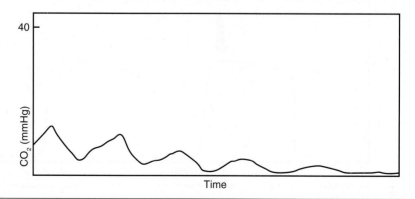

Figure 8-4 ● Esophageal intubation. Note that there is a minimal abnormal waveform that disappears within five to six breaths.

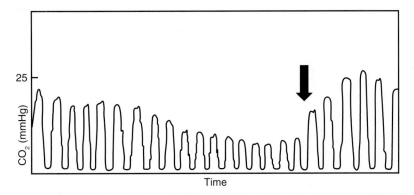

Figure 8-5 ● Capnography waveform during CPR displayed at a low-recording speed for trend analysis. $ETCO_2$ values during CPR are closely correlated with circulation. This trend waveform shows an increase in $ETCO_2$ with improved chest compressions (arrow). ROSC also will result in an abrupt rise in $ETCO_2$.

chest compressions during CPR. Effective chest compressions lead to an immediate rise in $ETCO_2$ as a result of effective pulmonary circulation (Fig. 8-5). $ETCO_2$ <10 mm Hg signals ineffective circulation despite CPR or a prolonged arrest with poor prognosis. Return of spontaneous circulation (ROSC) is unlikely if $ETCO_2$ persists <10 mm Hg after correct ETT placement and optimal CPR. An abrupt increase in $ETCO_2$ to normal values (>30 mm Hg) during CPR is an early indicator of ROSC and often precedes other clinical signs. Be aware that intravenous bicarbonate administration liberates CO_2 and causes a transient rise in $ETCO_2$ that should not be misinterpreted as optimized CPR or ROSC.

Monitoring ventilation during procedural sedation

In the setting of procedural sedation, capnography is the most sensitive indicator of hypoventilation and apnea. Several studies show that patients undergoing procedural sedation have a high rate of acute respiratory events including hypoventilation and apnea, and clinical assessment of chest rise is not sensitive for detecting these events. Oxygen desaturation is a late finding in hypoventilation, especially in patients receiving supplemental oxygen. Addition of capnography to standard monitoring provides advanced warning and reduces hypoxic events.

When using capnography to assess for respiratory depression, it is important to understand that hypoventilation can result in an increase or decrease in $ETCO_2$. Capnographic evidence of respiratory depression includes $ETCO_2$ >50 mm Hg, a change of $ETCO_2$ of 10% from baseline (or absolute change of 10 mm Hg), or loss of waveform. Bradypneic (classic) hypoventilation results in a waveform of increased amplitude and width (Fig. 8-6). Hypopneic hypoventilation (shallow ineffective breathing) results in a low-amplitude waveform, despite rising alveolar CO_2 (Fig. 8-7). In this case, the measured $ETCO_2$ value will decline because of the relative decrease in the volume of exhaled gas relative to the fixed volume of dead-space gas, thus diluting the CO_2 in the sample. as indicated.

Analogous to its use in procedural sedation, capnography can be used to gauge adequacy of spontaneous ventilation whenever there is a concern for respiratory depression, as in patients with depressed mental status caused by disease, trauma, or pharmacologic agents.

Surveillance and monitoring of mechanically ventilated patients

Capnography is useful for determining adequacy of ventilation in mechanically ventilated patients. Although $ETCO_2$ is an unreliable gauge of $PaCO_2$ because of variation in alveolar-arterial gradient, $ETCO_2$ can be incorporated as a surrogate for $PaCO_2$ to minimize routine blood gas analysis. An initial

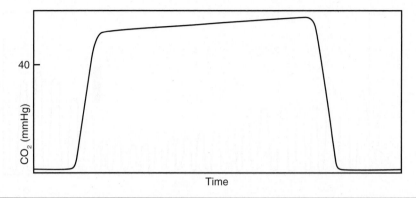

Figure 8-6 ● Bradypneic (classic) hypoventilation. Note that the waveform is wide and has increased amplitude, with an ET CO_2 >50 mm Hg.

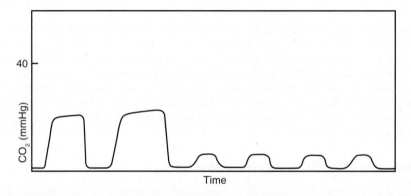

Figure 8-7 ● Hypopneic hypoventilation. Very shallow breathing results in a low-amplitude waveform and a low ET CO_2, despite a rising alveolar CO_2.

arterial blood gas sample allows comparison of $PaCO_2$ and $ETCO_2$ and establishes calibration so that $ETCO_2$ monitoring provides a continuous gauge of $PaCO_2$, assuming no major clinical change in patient condition. This is especially helpful for maintaining normocapnia in intubated patients who may be harmed by hypercapnea or hyperventilation, such as those with intracranial hypertension or brain injury.

Assessment and monitoring of patients in respiratory distress

Capnography can be useful for monitoring patients presenting with respiratory distress. A large pulmonary embolism can cause a decrease in $ETCO_2$ because of a lack of pulmonary perfusion, but most patients with severe respiratory distress are hypercapnic. Chronic obstructive lung disease and bronchospasm display a characteristic waveform with a slurred upstroke. The waveform shape may normalize with treatment of the underlying disease. Increasing $ETCO_2$ usually indicates worsening of respiratory distress, and decreasing $ETCO_2$ usually indicates improvement of respiratory distress. $ETCO_2$ values and waveform trends may help guide management decisions, such as endotracheal intubation or intensive care observation, in patients with respiratory distress from any etiology.

EVIDENCE

- **What key points of pulse oximetry monitoring are particularly pertinent during emergency airway management?** Rapid change in arterial saturation is common during airway management. Although pulse oximetry is continuous, there is a delay in peripheral cutaneous oximetry relative to central SaO_2. Monitor averaging, measurement location, circulatory status, oxygenation status, and rate of desaturation all contribute to the degree of correlation. Sensor anatomic location is an easily modifiable factor. Forehead probes are closer to the heart and respond more quickly than distal extremity probes. Although most sensors lose reliability during hypotension, hypoperfusion, and hypothermia, forehead reflectance probes maintain reliability during these conditions.[1–3] As such, they are often preferred in the management of critically ill patients.[4]

- **What are published guidelines for $ETCO_2$ monitoring in emergency settings?** The 2010 AHA guidelines recommend the use of $ETCO_2$ monitoring for confirmation of correct ETT placement, monitoring CPR quality, and indicating ROSC.[5] Continuous waveform capnography is recommended as the most reliable method of confirming and monitoring correct ETT placement (Class I, Level of Evidence A). Colorimetric exhaled CO_2 detectors and nonwaveform $ETCO_2$ capnometers are recommended as alternatives for initial confirmation of ETT placement, when waveform capnography is not available (Class II, LOE B).[5] Colorimetric detectors are less accurate for confirming correct ETT placement during cardiac arrest. However, colorimetric and nonwaveform capnometers are nearly 100% accurate for confirming correct ETT placement in patients with circulation.[6] AHA guidelines also recommend quantitative waveform capnography to optimize CPR performance (Class IIb, LOE C).[7] ROSC is unlikely when $ETCO_2$ values are persistently low (<10 mm Hg) in intubated patients receiving good quality CPR.[8] A sudden increase in $ETCO_2$ to normal values (>30 mm Hg) during CPR is an early indication of ROSC (Class IIa, LOE B).[7]

  Capnography during procedural sedation is common in anesthesiology and recommended by the American Society of Anesthesiologists and the American Academy of Pediatrics.[9] It is not routinely used by emergency physicians during procedural sedation, but should be used if deep sedation is planned. Waveform capnography is an early indicator of hypoventilation and apnea, and its use decreases the incidence of hypoxia during procedural sedation.[10,11]

ACKNOWLEDGMENTS

The authors wish to thank Robb Poutre for his assistance with this chapter.

REFERENCES

1. Hinkelbein J, Genzwuerker HV, Fiedler F. Detection of a systolic pressure threshold for reliable readings in pulse oximetry. *Resuscitation*. 2005;64:315–319.

2. MacLeod DB, Cortinez LI, Keifer JC, et al. The desaturation response time of finger pulse oximeters during mild hypothermia. *Anaesthesia*. 2005;60:65–71.

3. Schallom L, Sona C, McSweeney M, et al. Comparison of forehead and digit oximetry in surgical/trauma patients at risk for decreased peripheral perfusion. *Heart Lung*. 2007;36:188–194.

4. Branson RD, Mannheimer PD. Forehead oximetry in critically ill patients: the case for a new monitoring site. *Respir Care Clin N Am*. 2004;10:359–367, vi–vii.

5. Neumar RW, Otto CW, Link MS, et al. Part 8: adult advanced cardiovascular life support: 2010 American Heart Association Guidelines for Cardiopulmonary Resuscitation and Emergency Cardiovascular Care. *Circulation*. 2010;122:S729–S767.

6. Ornato JP, Shipley JB, Racht EM, et al. Multicenter study of a portable, hand-size, colorimetric end-tidal carbon dioxide detection device. *Ann Emerg Med*. 1992;21:518–523.

7. Falk JL, Rackow EC, Weil MH. End-tidal carbon dioxide concentration during cardiopulmonary resuscitation. *N Engl J Med.* 1988;318:607–611.

8. Levine RL, Wayne MA, Miller CC. End-tidal carbon dioxide and outcome of out-of-hospital cardiac arrest. *N Engl J Med.* 1997;337:301–306.

9. American Society of Anesthesiologists. Standards for basic anesthetic monitoring. http://www.asahq.org/. Published 2010 (accessed 11-16-2011).

10. Deitch K, Miner J, Chudnofsky CR, et al. Does end tidal CO_2 monitoring during emergency department procedural sedation and analgesia with propofol decrease the incidence of hypoxic events? A randomized, controlled trial. *Ann Emerg Med.* 2010;55:258–264.

11. Waugh JB, Epps CA, Khodneva YA. Capnography enhances surveillance of respiratory events during procedural sedation: a meta-analysis. *J Clin Anesth.* 2011;23:189–196.

9

Bag-Mask Ventilation

Steven C. Carleton • Robert F. Reardon • Calvin A. Brown III

Bag-mask ventilation (BMV) is a foundational skill in airway management. BMV is a consideration in every airway intervention, and evaluation for potential difficulty in bagging is a fundamental component of every airway assessment. Effective BMV reduces both the urgency to intubate and the anxiety that accompanies challenging laryngoscopy and intubation, buying time as one works through the potential solutions for a difficult or failed airway. The confident application of BMV is particularly critical when muscle relaxants are used to facilitate intubation; competence with BMV should be considered a prerequisite to using paralytic agents for this purpose. The ability to oxygenate and ventilate a patient with a bag and mask effectively eliminates the "can't oxygenate" portion of the can't intubate, can't oxygenate scenario (see Chapter 2), leaving three unsuccessful attempts at intubation, or a failed best attempt after induction and paralysis in the "forced to act" scenario as the only pathways to a failed airway.

In spite of its importance, there is a paucity of literature that adequately describes effective BMV. Most health care providers mistakenly think that they are proficient at it, and it is given less attention in many airway texts and courses than are more glamorous, but less frequently applied, airway techniques. Nonetheless, BMV is among the most difficult airway skills to master, requiring a clear understanding of functional airway obstruction, familiarity with the required equipment, mechanical skill, teamwork, and an organized approach when initial efforts are suboptimal.

Successful BMV depends on three factors: (1) a patent airway, (2) an adequate mask seal, and (3) proper ventilation. A patent airway permits the delivery of appropriate tidal volumes with the least possible positive pressure. Basic methods for opening the airway include head extension, and the chin lift and jaw thrust maneuvers. Creating an adequate mask seal requires an understanding of the design features of the mask, the anatomy of the patient's face, and the interrelationship between the two. Proper ventilation involves delivering an appropriate volume at a rate and force that minimize gastric insufflation and the potential for breath stacking and barotrauma.

The specific type of bag used is critically important. Self-inflating bags are useful in the emergency situation because of their low cost and simplicity. The bags vary in volume depending on their intended use, with adult bags typically having a volume of 1,500 ml, whereas those for children and infants have volumes of 500 and 250 ml, respectively. Bags that minimize dead space, incorporate unidirectional inspiratory and expiratory airflow valves, and have an oxygen reservoir are essential to optimize oxygenation during BVM (see Chapter 5). Bags with a pop-off pressure valve minimize the potential for barotrauma; most with this feature allow the valve to be manually disabled when high pressures are required for ventilation.

Face masks for BMV in the emergency department and prehospital setting are usually disposable, plastic models. Three sizes (small, medium, and large) are sufficient to accommodate most adults and school-aged children. Choice of size is empiric. Smaller masks are available for use in toddlers, infants, and newborns. A selection of face masks is shown in Figure 9-1. Note that it is generally easier to establish an adequate mask seal if the mask is too large than if it is too small because the mask must cover both the mouth and nose. A typical mask consists of three components:

- A round orifice that fits over the standard 22-mm outside diameter connector on the bag assembly.
- A hard shell or body; this is often clear, to allow continuous monitoring of the patient's mouth and nose for regurgitation.
- A circumferential cushion or inflatable cuff, which evenly distributes downward pressure onto the patient's face, filling irregular contours and promoting an effective seal.

Although newer, ergonomically designed face masks may be more effective in reducing mask leaks than standard, disposable face masks, such masks are not widely available and have yet to be evaluated in the emergency clinical setting.

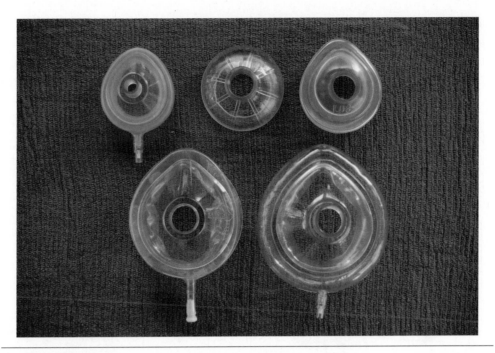

Figure 9-1 ● Face masks of various types in sizes from infant to large adult.

OPENING THE AIRWAY

The airway should be opened *before* placing the mask on the face. Functional occlusion of the airway is common in supine, obtunded patients, particularly when neuromuscular blocking agents have been given. This results from posterior displacement of the tongue into the oropharynx as the supporting mandible and hyoid bone relax, but also may result from occlusion of the hypopharynx by the epiglottis, or circumferential collapse of the pharynx as supporting muscles relax. Airway collapse is exacerbated by flexion of the head on the neck, and by opening the mouth. Maneuvers to open the airway are directed at counteracting these conditions by anterior distraction of the mandible and hyoid. The head tilt/chin lift is an initial maneuver that may be used in any patient in whom cervical spine injury is not a concern. In this technique, the clinician applies downward pressure to the patient's forehead with one hand while the index and middle fingers of the second hand lift the mandible at the chin, pulling the tongue from the posterior pharynx, and slightly extending the head on the neck. Airway caliber may be augmented by coupling atlanto-occipital extension with slight flexion of the lower cervical spine (i.e., the "sniffing position") similar to positioning for direct laryngoscopy (see Chapter 12). Although chin lift may be sufficient in some patients, the jaw thrust maneuver more effectively displaces the tongue anteriorly with the mandible and hyoid, minimizing its obstructing potential. The jaw thrust is achieved by forcibly and fully opening the mouth to translate the condyles of the mandible out of the temporomandibular joints, then pulling the mandible forward (Fig. 9-2A–D). This is most easily accomplished from the head of the bed, by placing the fingers of both hands on the body, angle, and ramus of the mandible with the thumbs on the mental processes. The forward position of the mandible can be maintained, and anterior traction on the hyoid and tongue can be increased, by closing the mandible on the bite-block of an oropharyngeal airway (OPA). It is useful to think of the jaw thrust maneuver as "creating an underbite," with the bottom incisors placed anterior to the upper incisors. The fingers maintain the thrusted position while the mask is applied to the face. The jaw thrust is the safest first approach to opening the airway of a patient with a potential cervical spine injury; properly performed, it can be accomplished without moving the head or neck. Jaw thrust should also be

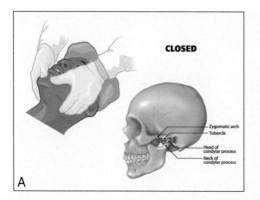

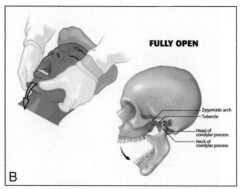

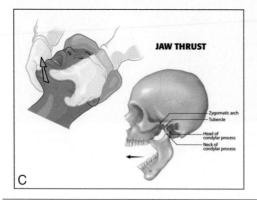

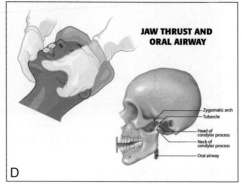

Figure 9-2 ● Relieving upper airway obstruction by "creating an underbite" with the jaw thrust maneuver. This is the most important technique for opening and maintaining the airway. **A:** From the head of the bed, the closed mandible is grasped between the thumbs and fingers of both hands. **B:** The mandible is widely opened. **C:** The open mandible is displaced anteriorly out of the temporomandibular joint. **D:** The mandible is closed on the bite block of an OPA to maintain the jaw thrust with the lower teeth in front of the upper teeth.

applied in any patient where chin lift and head tilt incompletely open the airway. The effectiveness of these airway maneuvers has been substantiated in multiple studies. Reduced emphasis on the jaw thrust technique in advanced cardiac life support is intended to lessen the complexity of CPR for laypersons, rather than representing opposition to its use.

ORAL AND NASAL PHARYNGEAL AIRWAYS

Once an open airway has been established, it must be maintained. OPAs and nasopharyngeal airways (NPAs) are important adjuncts in achieving this goal. Both prevent the tongue from occluding the airway and provide an open conduit for ventilation. OPAs are available in a variety of lengths, measured in centimeters (Fig. 9-3A). They are intended to extend from the central incisors to just short of the epiglottis and posterior pharyngeal wall. The appropriate size can be estimated by choosing an OPA that extends from the lips to just beyond the angle of the mandible when held alongside the face. Sizes from 8 to 10 cm suffice for the majority of adults. Two methods of insertion are in common use. In one, the OPA is inserted into the open mouth in an inverted position with its tip sliding along the palate. As the insertion is completed, the OPA is rotated 180° into its final position with the flange resting against the lips. This method is designed to minimize the likelihood of the OPA impinging the tongue and displacing it posteriorly. In the second method,

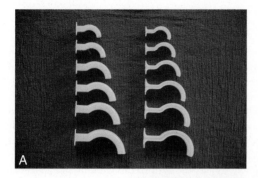

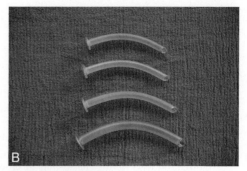

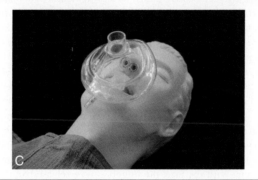

Figure 9-3 ● **A:** Guedel **(left)** and Berman **(right)** OPAs. **B:** NPAs. **C:** OPA and two NPAs in place within the body of the mask to optimize airway maintenance.

the tongue is pulled forward with a tongue blade or laryngoscope blade, and the OPA is inserted in its normal orientation until the flange rests against the lips. The latter technique has less potential for causing trauma to oral structures but requires additional hands and equipment. NPAs are available in various sizes based on internal luminal diameter (Fig. 9-3B). Sizes from 6 to 8 mm accommodate most adult patients. The appropriate size is commonly stated as the diameter of the patient's small finger, or 0.5 to 1.0 mm smaller than the endotracheal tube size for the patient, but neither method of estimation has been validated. For the purpose of augmenting BMV while minimizing the potential for nasal trauma, the smallest effective tube should be used; generally, this is 6 mm in adult females and 7 mm in adult males. When time permits, the larger nostril should be chosen based on inspection, and decongested with oxymetazoline or neosynephrine spray. Topical anesthesia spray, such as 4% lidocaine, also can be applied. A generously lubricated NPA is then inserted through the inferior nasal meatus parallel to the palate until the flange rests at the nostril. A slight rotary motion during insertion may facilitate passage. If resistance is met, the tube should either be downsized, or insertion should be attempted through the contralateral nostril. An NPA should never be forced when resistance is encountered, as bleeding almost inevitably results. Relative contraindications to NPA insertion should be observed, including bleeding diathesis and suspected traumatic disruption of bony cranial floor structures.

OPAs generally facilitate airway maintenance more reliably than NPAs, but OPAs are tolerated poorly in patients with intact gag and cough reflexes. Use of an NPA, particularly when time permits topical anesthesia of the nose, may be tolerated in this circumstance. When airway patency during BMV is difficult to maintain with an OPA, it can be supplemented by one, or even two, NPAs (Fig. 9-3C). The following cannot be stated strongly enough: At a minimum, an OPA should be inserted whenever BMV is used to support oxygenation and ventilation in an unresponsive patient and, absent contraindications, an NPA should be strongly considered when supporting respirations by BMV in a responsive patient, or to augment airway maintenance with an OPA.

POSITIONING AND HOLDING THE MASK

Once the airway is opened, the mask is placed to obtain a seal on the face. This should be accomplished with the mask *detached* from the bag to permit optimal positioning free from the unbalanced weight and bulk of the complete assembly. The cuff on the mask is intended to seat on the bridge of the nose, the malar eminences of the maxillae, the maxillary and mandibular teeth, the anterior body of the mandible, and the groove between the mentum and alveolar ridge of the mandible. This ensures that the mouth and nose will be covered entirely and that the majority of the cuff will be supported by bony structures. In general, the seal between the mask and face is least secure laterally, over the cheeks. This is particularly true in edentulous patients where the unsupported soft tissue of the cheeks may incompletely contact the cuff. In this circumstance, adequate facial support for the cuff can be maintained by leaving dentures in place during BMV, or restored by packing gauze rolls into the cheeks. Medial compression of the soft tissue of the face against the outside margins of the cuff can also mitigate leakage from the cuff, and shifting the mask such that the caudal edge of the cuff rests inside the lower lip may improve the seal between the mask and face in edentulous patients (Fig. 9-4).

Optimal placement of the mask is facilitated by grasping its body between the thumbs of both hands, and then spreading the cuff with the fingers (Fig. 9-5). Initially, the nasal part of the mask is placed on the bridge of the nose, and the mask is adjusted superiorly or inferiorly to optimize coverage. The body of the mask is then lowered onto the patient's face, and the cuff released once in firm contact with the skin. This effectively pulls the soft tissue of the face into the body of the mask, improving the mask seal. In masks with inflatable cuffs, the cuff volume can be adjusted with a syringe to further augment the seal if leakage is encountered. Once the mask is in full contact with the face, the fingers can be released and used to pull the lower face upward into the mask as the grip on the mask is maintained with the thumbs. The bag is then attached, and ventilation initiated. Avoid the tendency to rest the ulnar surfaces of either hand or the cuff on the orbits during BMV. Compression of the eyes may cause ocular injury or a vagal response.

With proper technique, the mask is not pushed down onto the patient's face during BMV. Rather, the patient's face is pulled upward into the mask. This has significant implications on the most effective method of holding the mask after the initial seal is obtained.

Single-Handed Mask Hold

Securing the mask to the face using one hand may be necessary when personnel are limited. Single-handed BMV can be successful in selected, unchallenging patients, particularly when the

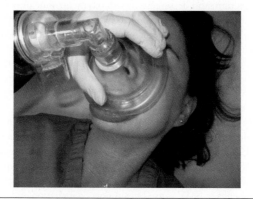

Figure 9-4 ● Lower-lip positioning of the face mask. This position may improve the mask seal in edentulous patients. (Photograph courtesy of Tobias D. Barker, MD.)

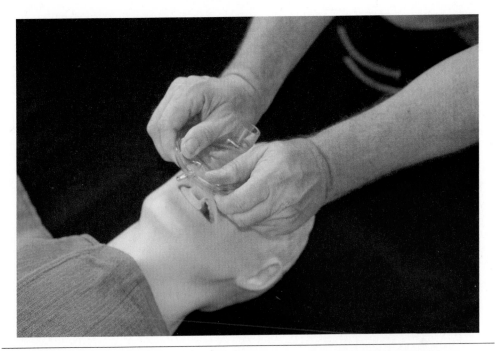

Figure 9-5 ● Spreading the cuff of the mask before seating it on the face to improve the mask seal.

operator's hands are large and strong enough to maintain a robust seal for extended periods of time. However, when it is difficult to achieve or maintain a good mask, seal, a two-person, two-handed technique is used. In the one-handed technique, the operator's dominant hand is used to hold and compress the bag, while the nondominant hand is placed on the mask with the thumb and the index finger partially encircling the mask connector, as if making an "OK" sign. The grasping hand and mask are then rocked gently from side to side to achieve the best seal. The ring and little fingers should lie comfortably on the body of the mask with their respective finger pads contacting the body of the mandible to pull it upward toward the mask (Fig. 9-6A). Ordinarily, the tip of the long finger is placed beneath the point of the chin to maintain the previously applied chin lift or jaw thrust. When the operator's hands are of sufficient size, the pad of the little finger can be placed posterior to the angle of the mandible to augment the jaw thrust. The three fingers grasping the mandible contact only its bony margin to avoid pressure on the submandibular and submental soft-tissues, which may occlude the airway. When holding the mask with one hand, it may be necessary to gather the cheek with the ulnar aspect of the grasping hand and compress it against the mask cuff to establish a more effective seal. One-handed bagging can be extremely fatiguing. A common tendency, especially if there is difficulty effectively bagging the patient, or the operator is fatiguing, is to deform the body of the mask by squeezing it between the thumb and index fingers, creating or worsening a mask leak.

Two-Handed Mask Hold

The two-handed mask hold is the most effective method of opening the airway while achieving and maintaining an adequate mask seal. It is the method of choice in the emergency situation, whenever two operators are available. The two-handed, two-person technique mandates that one operator's sole responsibilities are to ensure proper placement of the mask, an effective mask seal, and a patent airway. Usually, the more experienced member should handle the mask. The other member provides ventilation with the bag.

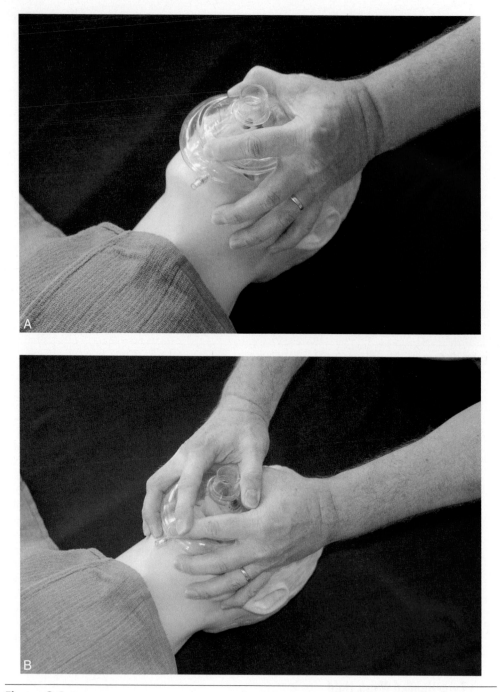

Figure 9-6 ● **A:** Single-handed mask hold with the "OK" grip. **B:** Two-handed mask hold with the conventional, double "OK" grip.

The operator's hands may be placed on the mask in one of two ways. The traditional method involves placing the index fingers and thumbs of each hand on the body of the mask in an identical fashion as for one-hand, "OK" mask grip (Fig. 9-6B). The tips of the remaining three fingers of each hand are used to capture the mandible and perform a simultaneous jaw thrust and chin lift, opening the airway, pulling the face upward into the mask, and creating a mask seal. This method provides a more effective seal than the one-handed technique, but is still subject to hand fatigue if bagging is difficult or prolonged. In the second method, both thenar eminences are positioned on the body of the mask, parallel to one another, with the thumbs pointing caudally. The cuff of the mask is placed on the bridge of the nose, and the remainder of the mask is lowered onto the face (Fig. 9-7A). The index, long, and ring fingers of both hands grasp the body of the mandible, while the fifth fingers grasp the angles, and pull the mandible forward into the mask to produce a seal. The jaw thrust maneuver produced in this manner is much more effective than that produced with the conventional two-handed grip, and the mask seal is more robust than in either alternative described technique. The two-handed, thenar mask hold is also more comfortable and less tiring compared with the other methods. When extremely difficult BMV is encountered, a more aggressive version of the thenar grasp may be useful. Here, the operator stands on a stool, or has the bed lowered until the arms are straight, with the second through fifth fingers pointing straight toward the floor as the thenar grip on the mask is maintained. The angles of the mandible are grasped with the long fingers of both hands to perform the jaw thrust. In this posture, the operator can recruit their truncal and proximal shoulder musculature to provide the lifting force, and utilize their strongest fingers to open the airway.

If clinical circumstances require that the operator perform BMV from a position facing the patient, the thenar mask grip, reversed so that the thumbs point cephalad, is the best method in this setting, and can also be applied successfully in seated patients (Fig. 9-7B). In circumstances where there is a lone rescuer and difficulty is encountered in obtaining a mask seal, the care provider can free both hands for the two-hand, thenar mask grip and still provide ventilation by compressing the bag between their elbow and lateral torso if standing, or between their knees if kneeling on the floor. When the prospective assessment for difficult bagging is highly unfavorable, or a single rescuer anticipates insurmountable difficulty performing one-person technique, consideration should be given to bypassing BMV in favor of placing a laryngeal mask airway or other extraglottic device as the initial means of ventilation (see Chapters 10 and 11).

VENTILATING THE PATIENT

Once the airway is opened and an optimal mask seal obtained, the bag is connected to the mask and ventilation is initiated. The entire volume of the self-inflating resuscitation bag cannot, and should not, be delivered. Overzealous volume delivery may exceed the opening pressures of the upper and lower esophageal sphincters (approximately 20 to 25 cm H_2O pressure), insufflating gas into the stomach and increasing the risks of regurgitation and aspiration. It also may result in barotrauma to the lungs and breath stacking. The goal for effective oxygenation and ventilation without excessive inspiratory pressure is to deliver 10 to 12 reduced tidal volume breaths (5 to 7 ml per kg; approximately 500 ml in an adult) per minute over 1 to 2 seconds each. Factors which increase peak inspiratory pressures include shorter inspiratory times, larger tidal volumes, incomplete airway opening, increased airway resistance, and decreased lung or chest compliance. Several of these factors are controllable, and assiduous attention should be paid by the clinician to maintenance of airway patency, delivery of inspiration over a 1- to 2-second period, and limiting tidal volume to that sufficient to produce visible chest rise.

SELLICK MANEUVER

During BMV, studies demonstrate that application of Sellick maneuver (see Chapter 19) may significantly reduce gastric insufflation. If resources permit, we recommend applying Sellick maneuver during bag ventilation of an unresponsive patient. Sellick maneuver involves pressing the cricoid cartilage posteriorly, attempting to occlude the cervical esophagus against the anterior vertebral bodies. Two errors are commonly committed. The first is to apply pressure to the thyroid cartilage instead of the cricoid cartilage, failing to compress the esophagus and potentially occluding the airway. The second is to over-enthusiastically apply cricoid pressure, resulting in distortion of the airway and more difficult ventilation.

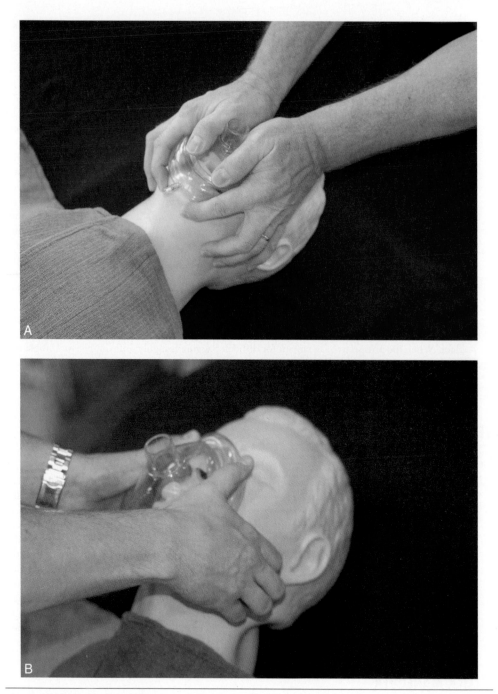

Figure 9-7 ● **A:** Two-handed, thenar mask grip. This grip provides a superior face seal, better airway maintenance, and is less fatiguing than the alternative methods. **B:** The two-handed, thenar mask grip applied from the side in a semi-seated patient.

SUMMARY

BMV is a dynamic process. The patency of the airway, position of the mask, and adequacy of gas exchange must be assessed continually. Listening and feeling for mask leaks, monitoring the compliance of the bag during delivery of breaths, and observing the rise and fall of the chest are crucial to success. The most important role falls to the person holding the mask, but coordination of the efforts of this individual, the person ventilating with the bag, and the person performing Sellick maneuver is essential to optimal BMV. Two-handed technique with the thenar mask grip is our preferred method for maintaining both airway patency and the mask seal. In addition to optimizing the jaw thrust and mask seal, this grip allows a lateral mask leak to be felt by the care provider's hypothenar eminences. Compression of the cheek into the lateral mask cuff may occlude the leak. Note that it may be necessary to periodically rock the mask upward, downward, or from side-to-side to achieve the best seal. It also may be necessary to reapply the jaw thrust maneuver to re-establish airway patency because of the tendency of the mandible to fall back into the temporo-mandibular joint. When delivering tidal volumes with the bag, the operator should simultaneously feel for the resistance of the bag to compression, and observe the patient's chest for rise and fall during ventilation. This feedback can provide clues to the compliance of the patient's chest and lungs, and influence bagging technique in response. Other signs of satisfactory ventilation are adequate oxygen saturation, and the appearance of an appropriate waveform on a capnograph, or color change on a colorimetric end-tidal carbon dioxide detector.

Occasionally after a breath is delivered, passive expiration fails to occur. This generally indicates closure of the airway because of an inadequate jaw thrust. Removal of the mask from the face and re-application of a vigorous jaw thrust will generally relieve the airway occlusion and permit expiration.

Whenever BMV fails to establish or maintain adequate oxygen saturation, the bag and mask technique must be adjusted to compensate. Simply stated, when bagging fails, bag better. Bagging better requires a systematic reappraisal of the adequacy of airway opening, the mask seal, and the mechanics of ventilation with the bag. If a single-handed mask hold is being used by a lone care provider, the mask grip should immediately shift to two-handed thenar technique and the bag should be compressed by one of the alternative methods described earlier. If two care providers are available, two-person, two-handed thenar technique should be used and the providers should focus on the following questions:

1. Does the jaw thrust maneuver need to be redone to more effectively open the airway? Optimal jaw thrust is facilitated by positioning the person holding the mask at the head of the bead, with the bed at a height that allows the provider to comfortably maintain the upward pull required to open the airway. Jaw thrust is easier when performed by an individual with large hands; if an experienced operator with large hands is available, recruit them for this task.
2. Is the mask seal optimal? If not, can this be improved by applying water-soluble jelly or an occlusive plastic membrane to a beard, packing fluffed gauze inside the cheeks to create a better mask seal, reinserting the patient's dentures, gathering and compressing both cheeks inside the body of the mask, ensuring that the entire mouth and nose are within the body of the mask, rocking the mask to re-establish cuff contact with the face, or considering lower-lip mask positioning in the edentulous patient? Note, however, that the application of excessive jelly to a bearded patient can cause the face to become extremely slippery, rendering stabilization of the mask difficult. Positioning a morbidly obese patient in a semi-seated position during BMV may improve pulmonary dynamics and ease difficult bagging. However, this may require the person holding the mask to use a stool or to move to the side of the bed, and adjust their mask grip accordingly.
3. Are airway adjuncts being properly used? The most common error in BMV is the failure to use OPAs and NPAs. A minimum of one of these adjuncts should *always* be used during BMV of an unresponsive patient. An OPA and two NPAs should be used in cases where persistent difficulty is encountered in delivering adequate ventilation and oxygenation.
4. Does a more experienced person need to be recruited to optimize efforts at BMV? The learning curve for proficiency with BMV is long. Novice providers may fail to achieve the most effective

possible ventilation, and should be replaced by the most experienced available operator when difficult bagging fails to respond to simple countermeasures.

EVIDENCE

- **What is the best method for maintaining a mask seal during BMV?** Simulation studies suggest that two-handed mask techniques facilitate delivery of greater tidal volumes and peak airway pressures than the one-handed technique in both child[1] and adult manikin models.[2] The traditional two-handed, and two-handed thenar mask grips yielded similar results in the adult study, but fatigue with prolonged bagging was not evaluated. A recent clinical trial comparing the two-handed grip where the mask was grasped with the thumbs, and standard one-handed technique, clearly documents the superiority of the two-handed grip in delivering greater tidal volumes in apneic patients.[3] Mask seal in edentulous patients may be improved by modifying placement of the caudal margin of the mask cuff to a position inside of the lower lip, bearing on the alveolar ridge.[4] Further more, in edentulous patients with dentures, ventilation and gas flow during BMV are facilitated by leaving the dentures in place during bagging.[5] Newer, ergonomically designed masks improve the mask seal with the face in comparison to standard, disposable masks with inflatable cuffs during simulated BMV.[6]

- **What is the optimal technique to ventilate the patient during BMV?** The primary goal is oxygenation without gastric inflation. This is best accomplished by avoiding high airway pressures during BMV (e.g., longer inspiratory times, smaller tidal volume, and optimal airway opening).[7,8] The recommended adult tidal volume of approximately 500 ml is best achieved by squeezing the bag with the hands, rather than compressing it between the arm and torso.[9]

- **Should Sellick maneuver be performed during BMV?** If the necessary personnel are available, it may be helpful to use this technique during BMV. Proper application of cricoid pressure does appear to reduce the volume of air entering the stomach when BMV is performed with low to moderate inspiratory pressures.[10] Other literature indicates that this technique may not reliably occlude the esophagus,[11] or may impair ventilation by partially obstructing the airway.[12] Further more, there are studies that suggest that Sellick maneuver may either improve[13] or worsen[14,15] laryngoscopic view of the glottis.

- **How easily can competence in BMV be achieved?** An evaluation of the number of repetitions required for novice physicians to achieve a success rate of 80% for BMV found that 25 training runs were necessary.[16] It should be noted that an 80% success rate is an insufficiently rigorous goal for a frequently applied, life-sustaining procedure, highlighting the necessity for frequent, scrupulous training in BMV.

REFERENCES

1. Davidovic L, LaCovey D, Pitetti RD. Comparison of 1- versus 2-person bag-valve-mask techniques for manikin ventilation of infants and children. *Ann Emerg Med*. 2005;46:37–42.

2. Reardon R, Ward C, Hart D, et al. Assessment of face-mask ventilation using an airway simulation model. *Ann Emerg Med*. 2008;52(4):S114.

3. Joffe AM, Hetzel S, Liew EC. A two-handed jaw-thrust technique is superior to the one-handed "EC-clamp" technique for mask ventilation in the apneic, unconscious person. *Anesthesiology*. 2010;113:873–875.

4. Racine SX, Solis A, Hamou NA, et al. Face mask ventilation in edentulous patients. A comparison of mandibular groove and lower lip placement. *Anesthesiology*. 2010;112:1190–1193.

5. Conlon NP, Sullivan RP, Herbison PG, et al. The effect of leaving dentures in place on bag-mask ventilation at induction of general anesthesia. *Anesth Analg.* 2007;105:370–373.

6. Bauman EB, Joffe AM, Lenz L, et al. An evaluation of bag-valve-mask ventilation using an ergonomically designed facemask among novice users: a simulation-based pilot study. *Resuscitation.* 2010;81:1161–1165.

7. American Heart Association. 2005 American Heart Association guidelines for cardiopulmonary resuscitation and emergency cardiovascular care. *Circulation.* 2005;112(suppl I):IV.

8. Uzun L, Ugur MB, Altunkaya H, et al. Effectiveness of the jaw-thrust maneuver in opening the airway: a flexible fiberoptic endoscopic study. *ORL J Otorhinolaryngol Relat Spec.* 2005;67:39.

9. Wolcke B, Schneider T, Mauer D, et al. Ventilation volumes with different self-inflating bags with reference to the ERC guidelines for airway management: comparison of two compression techniques. *Resuscitation.* 2000;47:175–178.

10. Petito SP, Russell WJ. The prevention of gastric inflation—a neglected benefit of cricoid pressure. *Anaesth Intensive Care.* 1988;16:139.

11. Smith KJ, Dobranowski JD, Yip G, et al. Cricoid pressure displaces the esophagus: an observational study using magnetic resonance imaging. *Anesthesiology.* 2003;99:60–64.

12. Hartsilver EL, Vanner RG. Airway obstruction with cricoid pressure. *Anaesthesia.* 2000;55:208.

13. Levitan RM, Kinkle WC, Levin WJ, et al. Laryngeal view during laryngoscopy: a randomized trial comparing cricoid pressure, backward-upward-rightward pressure, and bimanual laryngoscopy. *Ann Emerg Med.* 2006;47:548–555.

14. Snider DD, Clarke D, Finucane BT. The "BURP" maneuver worsens the glottic view when applied in combination with cricoid pressure. *Can J Anaesth.* 2005;52:100–104.

15. Harris J, Ellis DY, Foster L. Cricoid pressure and laryngeal manipulation in 402 pre-hospital emergency anaesthetics: essential safety measure or a hindrance to rapid safe intubation? *Resuscitation.* 2010;81:810–816.

16. Komatsu R, Kayasu Y, Yogo H, et al. Learning curves for bag-and-mask ventilation and orotracheal intubation: an application of the cumulative sum method. *Anesthesiology.* 2010;112:1525–1531.

10

Laryngeal Mask Airways

Michael F. Murphy • Jennifer L. Avegno

INTRODUCTION

The laryngeal mask airway (LMA) is an extraglottic device (EGD) (i.e., a device that provides ventilation without any part of it passing through the vocal cords) that was introduced in 1981 as an alternative to mask anesthesia. Some 30 years later, LMA-type devices enjoy widespread use in a variety of patient and clinical settings and have become accepted adjuncts in emergency management of both routine and difficult airways.

TERMINOLOGY

The terminology of the EGDs is not standardized and has been confusing. Some authors refer to a device either as a *supraglottic* device (SGD) or as a retroglottic device (RGD), the latter also sometimes referred to as an infraglottic device (IGD). The term RGD or IGD has been used to refer to those devices that pass behind and beyond the larynx to enter the upper esophagus (e.g., Combitube, King LT airway, and EasyTube). Only certain designs are truly supraglottic, such as the various LMAs and the CobraPLA (PeriLaryngeal Airway).

We refer to any member of this entire family of devices as an EGD, and consider two subclasses: the SGDs, which sit above and surround the glottis (almost all of which are some type of LMA) and RGDs (or, less precisely, IGDs), which enter the upper esophagus (e.g., Combitube). Most EGDs are single-use, but some are available in reusable variants.

EGDs differ from face mask gas delivery apparatus in that they are inserted through the mouth to a position where they provide a direct conduit for air to flow through the glottis and into the lungs. They vary in size and shape, and most have balloons or cuffs that when inflated provide a reasonably tight seal in the upper airway to permit positive-pressure ventilation with variable limits of peak airway pressure.

Although bag-mask ventilation (BMV) is relatively simple in concept, it is difficult or impossible to perform in selected patients (see Chapter 9), even in the hands of experts. Use of an EGD is a more easily acquired skill than BMV for the nonexpert airway practitioner. Similarly, tracheal intubation is the "gold standard" for effective ventilation and airway protection from aspiration, but the skill is not easily mastered or maintained. EGDs are a viable alternative to tracheal intubation in many emergency settings, particularly in prehospital care.

Finally, airway management difficulty and failure are associated with significant morbidity and mortality. Certain EGDs have a potential role in both the difficult (LMA) and failed (most EGDs) airway (see Chapters 2 and 3).

Thus, the indications for these devices have expanded over the past three decades and include potential for use as

- An airway rescue device when BMV is difficult and intubation has failed.
- A "single attempt" rescue device performed simultaneously with preparation for cricothyrotomy in the "*can't* intubate, *can't* oxygenate" (CICO) failed airway (see Chapter 3).
- An easier and more effective alternative to BMV in the hands of basic life support providers or nonmedical rescue personnel.
- An alternative to endotracheal intubation by advanced life support providers.
- An alternative to endotracheal intubation for elective airway management in the operating room (OR) for appropriately selected patients.
- A conduit to facilitate endotracheal intubation (various types of intubating LMAs [ILMAs]).

SUPRAGLOTTIC DEVICES

The Laryngeal Mask Company developed the original SGD, the LMA Classic (Fig. 10-1), which serves as the prototype for much of the supraglottic class, although other designs exist. The

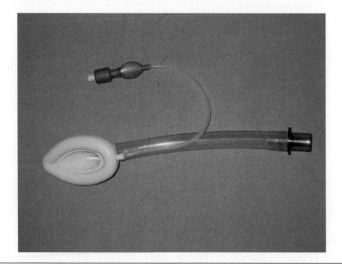

Figure 10-1 ● LMA Classic. Note the aperture bars at the end of the plastic tube intended to limit the ability of the epiglottis to herniate into this opening.

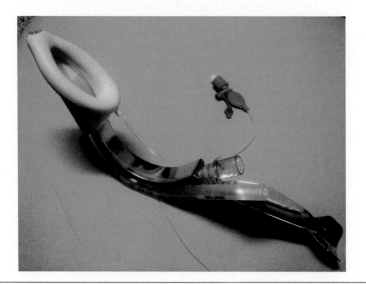

Figure 10-2 ● LMA ProSeal. Note the drain tube and distal orifice to permit gastric tube passage and drainage.

company also makes several other versions of the LMA, including both reusable and nonreusable (disposable) devices:

- LMA Unique (disposable variant of the LMA Classic)
- LMA Flexible (reinforced tube variant of the LMA Classic)
- LMA ProSeal (reusable) (Fig. 10-2)
- LMA Supreme (disposable) (Fig. 10-3)
- Fastrach or ILMA (reusable and disposable) (Fig. 10-4)

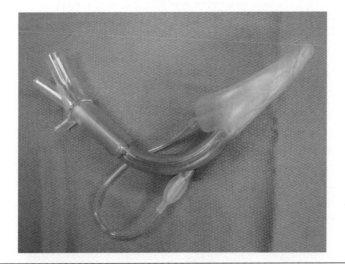

Figure 10-3 ● LMA Supreme.   The rigid construction of the tube and the curvature of the device enhance insertion characteristics and the immediacy of the seal obtained once inflated.

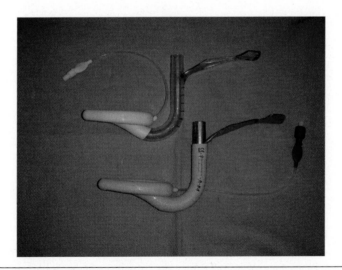

Figure 10-4 ● LMA Fastrach or ILMA.   Both the reusable (bottom) and disposable (top) variants are pictured. The most unique feature of this device that confers a particular advantage is the handle to permit positioning in the hypopharynx to improve airway seal and the capacity for adequate gas exchange. This factor may be crucial in rescuing a failed airway.

Other companies also make SGDs, both LMA type and non-LMA type, including

- A variety of disposable LMA Classic type designs (e.g., Portex and Solus)
- Ambu LMA (ALMA) family of devices (AuraOnce, Aura Straight, Aura-i; disposable and reusable) (Fig. 10-5)
- CobraPLA (disposable) (Fig. 10-6)
- Cookgas ILA (reusable) and Air Q (disposable) (Fig. 10-7A and B)
- I-Gel (Fig. 10-8)

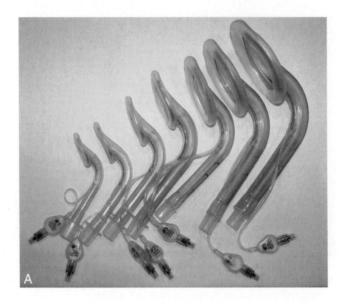

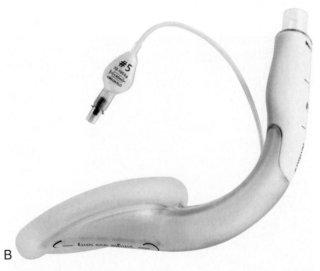

Figure 10-5 ● A: Range of sizes of the Ambu AuraOnce LMA. B: Ambu Aura-i LMA, specifically designed to be used with the Ambu A Scope for endoscopic intubation.

The LMA-type SGDs are easy to use, generally well tolerated, produce little in the way of adverse hemodynamic responses on insertion, and play a significant role in both routine and rescue emergency airway management. Ventilation success rates near 100% have been reported in OR series, although patients with difficult airways were excluded. It is likely that emergency airway ventilation success rates are somewhat lower. Intubation success rates through the ILMA are consistently in the 95% range, comparable to success rates with flexible endoscopic intubation and significantly better than through the standard LMA (about 80%). However, an LMA does not constitute *definitive airway management*, defined as a protected airway (i.e., a cuffed endotracheal tube [ETT] in the trachea). Although they do not reliably prevent the gastric insufflation or the regurgitation and aspiration of gastric contents, LMAs confer some protection of the airway from aspiration of blood and saliva from the mouth and pharynx.

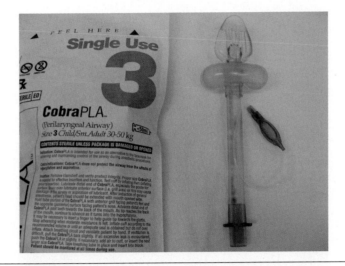

Figure 10-6 ● CobraPLA.

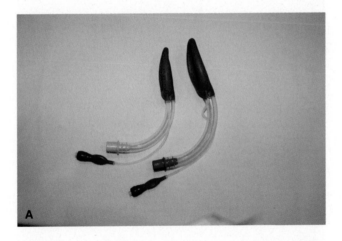

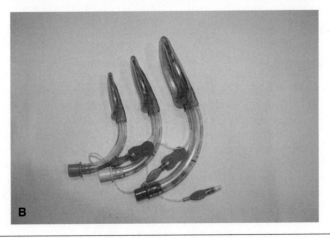

Figure 10-7 ● **A:** The reusable Cookgas ILA. **B:** The disposable Air Q variant.

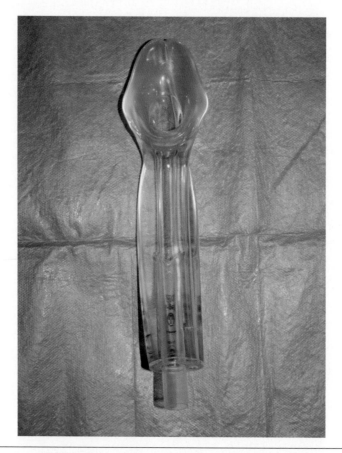

Figure 10-8 ● The I-Gel Device.   Note the esophageal drainage tube.

Maximal success is only achievable when the patient has effective topical airway anesthesia (see Chapter 23) or is significantly obtunded (e.g., by rapid sequence intubation medications) to tolerate insertion of these devices.

LARYNGEAL MASK COMPANY DEVICES

Standard, Non-ILMAs

The original LMA, now called the LMA Classic, was introduced into clinical practice in 1981 and looks like an ETT equipped with an inflatable, elliptical, silicone rubber collar (laryngeal mask) at the distal end (Fig. 10-1). The laryngeal mask component is designed to surround and cover the supraglottic area, providing upper airway continuity. Two rubber bars cross the tube opening at the mask end to prevent herniation of the epiglottis into the tube portion of the LMA.

The LMA Classic is a multiuse (reusable) device. The disposable and much less costly variety of this device is called the LMA Unique. A similar product, the LMA Flexible, incorporates wire reinforcement in the tube portion of the device to prevent kinking as the tube warms. We do not recommend the LMA Flexible for management of the emergency airway.

The reusable LMA ProSeal incorporates an additional lumen through which one can pass a suction catheter into the esophagus or stomach. In addition to the standard perilaryngeal cuff, it also has a "directional sealing cuff" dorsally. This design modification results in higher sealing

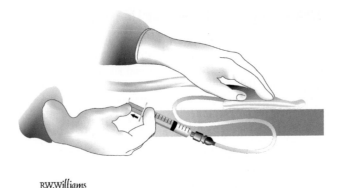

R.W.Williams

Figure 10-9 ● Correct Method of Deflating the LMA Cuff.

pressure capacity than the LMA Classic (28 vs. 24 cm H_2O), theoretically conferring an advantage for ventilating patients requiring higher airway pressures, although the difference may not be clinically significant. Because of its expense, relatively difficulty with insertion characteristics, and marginal benefit in the emergency situation, the LMA ProSeal does not currently have a place in emergency airway management.

A disposable device similar to the LMA Classic called the LMA Supreme has compelling design characteristics that may make it suitable for emergency airway management. It is easy to insert, seals readily, has a built-in bite block, and has a channel through which a gastric tube can be passed. This device can be considered as a replacement for BMV and endotracheal intubation in the hands of nonexpert airway managers and is the preferred device for emergency airway management if a nonintubating style of LMA is desired.

Intubating LMAs

The LMA Fastrach, also called the ILMA, is the most important version of the LMA for emergency airway management because it combines the high insertion and ventilation success rate of the other LMAs with specially designed features to facilitate blind intubation. It has an epiglottic elevating bar and a rigid guide channel that directs an ETT in a superior direction into the larynx, enhancing the success rate when passed blindly. The LMA Fastrach device is a substantial advance in airway management, particularly as a rapidly attempted rescue device in the CICO situation while preparations for cricothyrotomy are underway. It is supplied in both reusable and disposable forms.

Indications and Contraindications

The standard LMA is now widely used in anesthetic practice instead of mask anesthesia, and the LMA Fastrach is an accepted device in emergency and failed airway management.

The LMA and LMA Fastrach have two principal roles in rescue emergency airway management: (1) as a rescue device in a "*can't* intubate, *can* oxygenate" situation, and (2) as a single attempt to effect gas exchange in the CICO failed airway as one concurrently prepares to perform a cricothyrotomy (see Chapter 3). The success rate of LMA-facilitated ventilation in the difficult airway may be eroded if multiple preceding intubation attempts have traumatized the upper airway.

The handle of the LMA Fastrach enhances its insertion characteristics and allows for manipulation to achieve optimum seal once the cuff is inflated. The LMA Fastrach can be used as a rescue device for *a* CICO airway when upper airway anatomy is believed to be normal, thus allowing for a proper "seat." These devices have been used successfully in pediatrics, by novice intubators, during CPR, and in emergency medical services (EMS).

Technique: LMA Classic, LMA Unique, and LMA Supreme

The LMA Classic, Unique, and Supreme can all be rapidly inserted as primary airway management devices, or to rescue a failed airway. First, the appropriate size of LMA should be selected
based on patient characteristics. The LMA Classic and Unique come in sizes 1 to 6 (ranging from
neonates <5 kg to adults >100 kg); the Supreme sizes range from 1 to 5. For adults, the simplest
sizing formula is weight-based, regardless of patient size: size 3, 30 to 50 kg; size 4, 50 to 70 kg; and
size 5, >70 kg. For patients on the borderline between one mask size and another, it is generally
advisable to select the larger mask because it provides a better seal.

1. Place the device so that the collar is on a flat surface and inflate; then deflate the mask by aspirating the pilot balloon (Fig. 10-9). Completely deflate the cuff and ensure that it is not folded.
   Inflating the mask, and then deflating it while pressing the ventral surface of the inflatable
   collar firmly against a flat surface, produces a smoother and "flipped-back" leading edge, enhancing insertion characteristics. The collar is designed to flip backward so the epiglottis is not
   trapped between the collar and the glottic opening and to minimize "tip roll." Lubricate both
   sides of the LMA with water-soluble lubricant to facilitate insertion.
2. Open the airway by using a head tilt as one would in basic airway management, if possible.
   Some, including the device inventor, recommend that a jaw lift be performed to aid insertion.
3. Insert the LMA into the mouth with the laryngeal surface directed caudally and the tip of your
   index or long finger resting against the cuff-tube junction (Fig. 10-10). Press the device onto the
   hard palate (Fig. 10-11) and advance it over the back of the tongue as far as the length of your
   index or long finger will allow (Fig. 10-12). Then use your other hand to push the device to its
   final seated position (Fig. 10-13), allowing the natural curve of the device to follow the natural
   curve of the oro- and hypopharynx to facilitate its falling into position over the larynx. The
   dimensions and design of the device allow it to wedge into the esophagus with gentle caudad
   pressure and to stop in the appropriate position over the larynx.
4. Inflate the collar with air—20 ml, no. 3; 30 ml, no. 4; and 40 ml, no. 5—or until there is no leak
   with bag ventilation (Fig. 10-14). If a leak persists, ensure that the tube of the LMA emerges
   from the mouth in the midline, ensure that the head and neck are in anatomical alignment (i.e.,
   neither flexed nor extended), withdraw the device approximately 6 cm with the cuff inflated,
   readvance it (the "up–down" maneuver, intended to free a folded or trapped epiglottis), reinsert
   the device, or go to the next larger size.

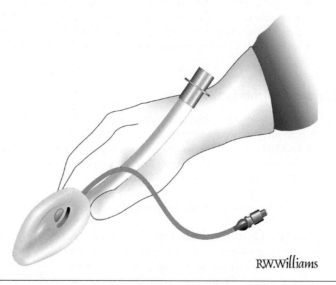

R.W.Williams

Figure 10-10 ● **Correct Position of the Fingers for LMA Insertion.**

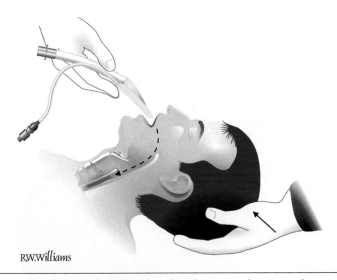

R.W.Williams

Figure 10-11 ● **Starting Insertion Position for the LMA Classic and LMA Unique.**

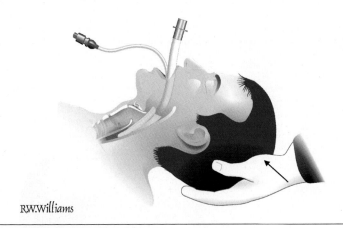

R.W.Williams

Figure 10-12 ● Insert the LMA to the limit of your finger length.

Technique: LMA Fastrach

Although the LMA devices mentioned above enjoy ventilation success rates comparable to that of the LMA Fastrach, they are not as effective as the LMA Fastrach for facilitating intubation. In fact, the LMA Fastrach is often easier to insert because of the handle and metal tube design. The LMA Fastrach comes in three sizes: no. 3, no. 4, and no. 5, with corresponding ETT sizes of 6.0 to 8.0. The no. 3 will fit a normal-size 10- to 12-year-old child and small adults, and sizing is as recommended above.

The intention is to rescue a patent airway initially and recover the oxygen saturations by ventilating through the LMA Fastrach device. Once the saturations are adequate, the operator intubates through the device using the manufacturer-supplied silicone-tipped ETT (although conventional ETTs can be used as well). Intubation can be done blindly or by using a flexible endoscope.

1. Select the appropriate-sized LMA Fastrach. Deflate the cuff of the mask (Fig 10-9), and apply a water-soluble lubricant to the anterior and posterior surfaces and the greater curvature of the

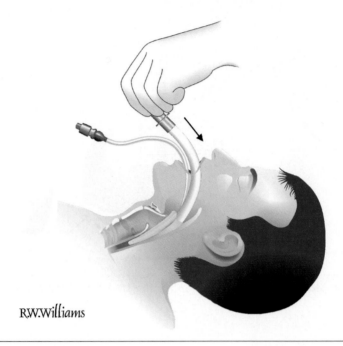

Figure 10-13 ● Complete the insertion by pushing the LMA in the remainder of the way with your other hand.

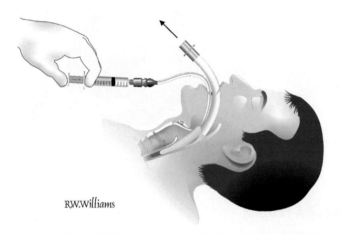

Figure 10-14 ● Inflate the Collar of the LMA.

bend of the rigid "stem." Hold the device in the dominant hand by the metal handle and open the airway. Insert the collar in the mouth, ensuring that the curved tube portion of the device is in contact with the chin and the mask tip is flat against the palate before rotation (Fig. 10-15A).

2. Rotate the mask into place with a circular motion, maintaining firm pressure against the palate and posterior pharynx (Fig. 10-15 B-C). Insert the device until resistance is felt and only the proximal end of the tube protrudes from the airway.

3. Inflate the cuff of the LMA Fastrach and hold the metal handle firmly in the dominant hand, using a "frying pan" grip. Ventilate the patient through the device. While ventilating, manipulate the mask with the dominant hand by a lifting motion in a direction similar to that used for direct laryngoscopy (i.e., toward the ceiling over the patient's feet, Fig. 10-16). This may enhance mask seal and intubation success. Best mask positioning will be identified by essentially noiseless ventilation, almost as if the patient is being ventilated through a cuffed ETT.

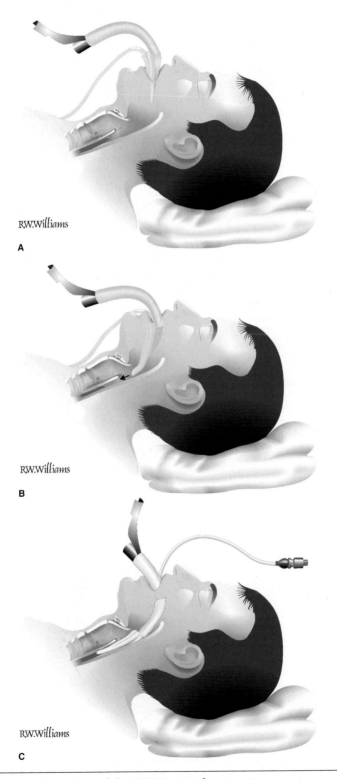

Figure 10-15 ● A–C: Insertion of the LMA Fastrach. Note that only a short segment of the tubular portion of the device extends beyond the lips. This metal tube accepts a bag-mask device fitting to enable BMV.

4. Visually inspect and test the cuff of the silicone-tipped ETT that is supplied with the LMA Fastrach. *Fully deflate* the cuff (important), lubricate the length of the ETT liberally, and pass it through the LMA Fastrach. With the black vertical line on the ETT facing the operator (indicates that the leading edge of the bevel will advance through the cords in an A–P orientation), insert the ETT to the 15-cm-depth marker, which corresponds to the transverse black line on the silicone-tipped ETT. This indicates that the silicone tip of the tube is about to emerge from the LMA Fastrach, pushing the epiglottic elevating bar up to lift the epiglottis. Use the handle to gently lift the LMA Fastrach as the ETT is advanced (Fig. 10-16). Carefully advance the ETT until intubation is complete. Do not use force of the ETT. Inflate the ETT cuff and confirm intubation. Then deflate the cuff on the LMA Fastrach.

5. After intubation, the LMA Fastrach can be removed fairly easily, leaving just the ETT in place. The key to successful removal of the mask is to remember that one is attempting to keep the ETT precisely in place and to remove the mask over it. First remove the 15-mm connector from the ETT. Then immobilize the ETT with one hand and gently ease the deflated LMA Fastrach out over the ETT with a rotating motion until the proximal end of the mask channel reaches the proximal end of the ETT. Use the stabilizer rod provided with the device to hold the ETT in position as the LMA Fastrach is withdrawn over the tube (Fig. 10-17). Remove the stabilizer rod from the LMA Fastrach and grasp the ETT at the level of the incisors (Fig. 10-18). *The stabilizer bar must be removed to allow the pilot balloon of the ETT to pass through the LMA Fastrach* (Fig. 10-19). Failure to do so may result in the pilot balloon being avulsed from the ETT, rendering the balloon incompetent and necessitating reintubation, preferably over an ETT changer.

Complications and Limitations

Unfortunately, the distal collar tip of the Laryngeal Mask Company Limited devices can "roll up" on insertion, creating a partial "insertion block" hindering optimal placement. This feature also likely contributes to pharyngeal abrasion and bleeding that is sometimes seen with these devices. Some authorities recommend partial inflation of the cuff to minimize tip roll, although there is

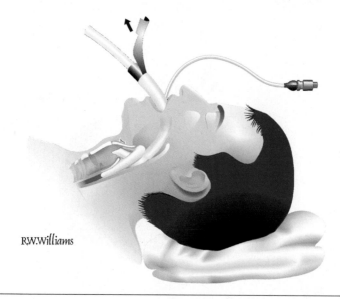

R.W.Williams

Figure 10-16 ● Lift the handle of the LMA Fastrach as the ETT is about to pass into the larynx to improve the success rate of intubation. This is called the Chandy maneuver after Dr. Archie Brain's associate Dr. Chandy Vergese.

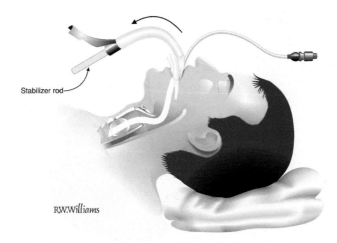

Figure 10-17 ● Use of the stabilizer rod to ensure the ETT is not inadvertently dragged out of the trachea as the LMA Fastrach is removed.

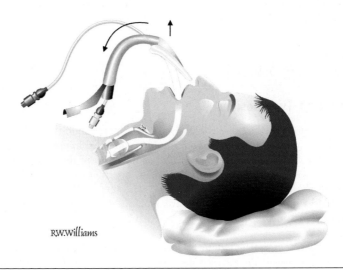

Figure 10-18 ● The stabilizer rod is removed from the LMA Fastrach to permit the pilot balloon of the ETT to go through the LMA Fastrach and prevent it from being avulsed from the ETT.

little evidence that this helps; others suggest the up/down maneuver (see above). Insertion of the LMA Classic and LMA Unique "upside down" and rotating into place once in the hypopharynx has also been described and is preferred by some. Our preferred method is as we described above.

Achieving a seal sufficient to enable positive-pressure ventilation with an LMA may be difficult. Keeping the tube portion of the device in the midline and altering the position of the head and neck from flexion (more usual) to neutral or extension may be of help. Overall, ventilation success rates are very high with all LMA-type devices. Optimal positioning improves ventilatory effectiveness and, in the case of the LMA Fastrach, facilitates intubation.

It is not known to what extent the LMA protects the airway against the aspiration of gastric contents, so the device is considered a temporizing measure only. This limits its usefulness in prehospital and emergency airway care, except when the LMA Fastrach is used to achieve intubation. Cricoid pressure has variously been reported to hinder and help in achieving proper seat and seal of the LMA.

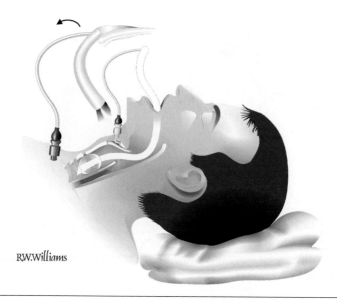

R.W.Williams

Figure 10-19 ● The pilot balloon of the ETT emerges from the end of the LMA Fastrach intact.

OTHER SUPRAGLOTTIC DEVICES

Disposable LMA-Type Designs

Several manufacturers produce disposable devices have appear almost identical to the LMA Classic. Although they do not incorporate the vertical bars intended to prevent epiglottic intrusion as are present in the LMA Classic and LMA Unique, the effect of this absence is not clear. These devices have the same indications, contraindications, insertion techniques, and complications as similar Laryngeal Mask Company Limited devices.

The ALMA (Fig. 10-5A) devices have several unique design features that may confer particular insertion and seal advantages:

- The device is semi-inflated in the package. This feature provides an "immediate seal" once inserted, eliminating the inflation step and speeding the time to ventilation.
- The leading tip of the inflatable collar is reinforced and "spatulated" to minimize tip roll and improve insertion characteristics.
- The AuraOnce LMA incorporates a tube that is flexible at the curved portion and more rigid proximally to improve insertion characteristics. In a recent design modification, the plastic in the curved portion of the tube was softened in response to concerns that this portion of the tube might compress the hypopharyngeal mucous membrane and lead to ischemia. Evidence suggests that this device and the LMA Supreme are the most easily inserted and rapid to seal of the disposable nonintubating LMA-type devices.

Ambu has recently introduced the Ambu Aura-i (Fig. 10-5B). This device is single use, virtually identical in design to the Ambu AuraOnce and is specifically modified to be used with the Ambu A Scope System, a disposable intubating endoscope (see Chapter 15.)

Cookgas ILA and Air Q

Like the LMA Fastrach, the Cookgas ILA device (Fig. 10-7A) is a supraglottic ventilatory device that also permits endotracheal intubation. Conventional ETTs (size 5.0 to 8.5) are used for intubation as opposed to a unique ETT as is supplied with the LMA Fastrach. The Air Q (Fig. 10-7B) is a disposable version of the Cookgas ILA. Like the Fastrach, the Cookgas device may be removed over the ETT (once ETT placement is confirmed) with use of a special stabilizing rod.

CobraPLA

The CobraPLA (Fig. 10-6) is an SGD with a cuffed pharyngeal (rather than perilaryngeal) seal. It consists of a breathing tube with a circumferential inflatable cuff proximal to the ventilation outlet portion, a 15-mm standard adapter, and a distal widened "cobra head," which holds soft tissues apart and allows ventilation of the trachea. Once in place, the cobra head should lie in front of the laryngeal inlet. Inside the cobra head is a ramp that directs breathing gases into the trachea. Over the distal, anteriorly placed breathing hole of the cobra head, there is a soft grill. This feature helps direct the epiglottis off the cobra head anteriorly. The bars of the grill are flexible enough to allow the passage of an ETT. The cuff is shaped to reside in the hypopharynx at the base of the tongue, and when inflated, raises the base of the tongue exposing the laryngeal inlet, as well as effecting an airway seal. The CobraPLA is available in eight sizes according to the weight of the patient. When one is unsure of size, or when learning placement technique, it is advisable to pick the *smaller size*. There is little evidence regarding use of these devices in emergency airway management, routine, or rescue.

I-Gel Airways

The I-Gel family of devices (Fig. 10-8) all contain preshaped, noninflatable seals made of a soft, gel-like substance that theoretically reduces insertion trauma. They include an integral bite block and gastric channel, and are available in a range of sizes from small infant to large adult. Advantages include ease of insertion without a cuff inflation step and decreased minor adverse effects; however, the preformed sizes may make an exact fit more difficult than other SGDs.

EVIDENCE—SGDS

- **Is the LMA effective in emergency, difficult, and failed airway management?** There is ample evidence that LMAs are useful in emergency airway management, both for the management of the difficult airway and rescue of the failed airway,[1-3] provided one is concurrently preparing to undertake a surgical airway. Furthermore, numerous studies have demonstrated that the LMA is at least as effective as other methods of airway management for patients requiring CPR.[4]
- **What success rates have been achieved intubating through the ILMAs (Fastrach and Cookgas)?** Success rates for blind intubation through these devices range from 70% to 99%.[5,6] Some authors report using a lighted stylet to guide intubation through the ILMA, but there is very limited experience with this technique.[7] Some studies have described the technique of coupling the LMA Fastrach or LMA Classic with a fiberscope to ensure intubation success in both infants and adults.[8]
- **Is the LMA effective in the pediatric population?** There is ample evidence that the LMA is appropriate and widely accepted as a rescue device in children.[9] Some authors have described guidelines for selecting the appropriate size in children, and the manufacturer provides a pocket card to guide clinicians. There is also evidence to support the use of ILMAs in both routine and difficult pediatric airway management.[10]
- **How easy is it for nonexperts to successfully use these LMA devices?** A variety of authors have described successful insertion and use of the device by minimally trained rescuer nonmedical personnel, prehospital care providers, nurses, and respiratory therapists, and naive airway managers.[11,12] Some of the EMS literature has questioned the ease of use of the device as a primary method of airway management in EMS,[13] although analysis has shown that training is key to its successful use.
- **Can the LMA fail to provide adequate ventilation, and what complications with short-term use might I expect?** The incidence of major airway adverse events with an LMA is quite low, and thought to be significantly less than standard tracheal intubation or bag-valve

mask.[14] The LMA may fail to provide a seal sufficient to permit adequate ventilation, often attributed to the sensitivity of the seal to head and neck position. The head and neck should be neutral to slightly flexed, the tube of the LMA in the midline, and the natural anterior curve of the device maintained during ventilation.[15] Insufflation of the stomach may occur.[16] Although the LMA may not offer total protection from the aspiration of regurgitated gastric contents,[17] it does offer protection from the aspiration of material produced above the device. This material that accumulates above the cuff of an ETT is suspected to be a major cause of ventilator-associated pneumonia in ventilated ICU patients. Cricoid pressure may or may not interfere with proper functioning of an LMA,[18] although in practice each case is evaluated individually. Negative-pressure pulmonary edema (mentioned previously) is caused by a patient sucking hard to inspire against an obstruction, where fluid is sucked into the alveolar spaces. This complication has been reported with patients biting down on the LMA[19] and can be prevented by placing folded gauze flats between the molar teeth on either side. This also serves to keep the device in the midline, enhancing the seal.

- **How do the preformed cuffless devices compare to more traditional cuffed LMAs?** The I-Gel has compared favorably in most aspects to other LMA products. Compared to the LMA Classic/Unique, physiologic response to insertion is equivalent or improved, there is less gastric insufflation and increased leak pressures.[20] However, evidence is mixed regarding ease of insertion and first-pass success, and the I-Gel seal adequacy has been found to be inferior compared with some of the LMA devices.[21]

- **How do the ILMA devices compare to one another?** Both the Cookgas and LMA Fastrach devices have been shown to have excellent insertion success rates and ventilatory function as an SGD; however, the blind endotracheal intubation rates are consistently >90% for the Fastrach only.[22]

REFERENCES

1. American Society of Anesthesiologists Task Force on Management of the Difficult Airway. Practice guidelines for management of the difficult airway: an updated report by the American Society of Anesthesiologists Task Force on Management of the Difficult Airway. *Anesthesiology*. 2003;98(5):1269–1277.

2. Parmet JL, Colonna-Romano P, Horrow JC, et al. The laryngeal mask airway reliably provides rescue ventilation in cases of unanticipated difficult tracheal intubation along with difficult mask ventilation. *Anesth Analg*. 1998;87:661–665.

3. Brimacombe J, Berry A. LMA for failed intubation. *Can J Anaesth*. 1993;40:802–803.

4. Grayling M, Wilson IH, Thomas B. The use of the laryngeal mask airway and Combitube in cardiopulmonary resuscitation: a national survey. *Resuscitation*. 2002;52:183–186.

5. Fukutome T, Amaha K, Nakazawa K, et al. Tracheal intubation through the intubating laryngeal mask airway (LMA-Fastrach) in patients with difficult airways. *Anaesth Intensive Care*. 1998;26:387–391.

6. Karim YM, Swanson DE. Comparison of blind tracheal intubation through the intubating laryngeal mask airway (LMA Fastrach) and the Air-Q. *Anaesthesia*. 2011;66:185–190.

7. Agro F, Hung OR, Cataldo R, et al. Lightwand intubation using the Trachlight: a brief review of current knowledge. *Can J Anaesth*. 2001;48:592–599.

8. Kannan S, Chestnutt N, McBride G. Intubating LMA guided awake fibreoptic intubation in severe maxillo-facial injury. *Can J Anaesth*. 2000;47:989–991.

9. Greif R, Theiler L. The use of supraglottic airway devices in pediatric laparoscopic surgery. *Minerva Anestesiol*. 2010;76:575–576.

10. Jagannathan N, Roth AG, Sohn LE, et al. The new air-Q intubating laryngeal airway for tracheal intubation in children with anticipated difficult airway: a case series. *Paediatr Anaesth*. 2009;19:618–622.

11. Braun P, Wenzel V, Paal P. Anesthesia in prehospital emergencies and in the emergency department. *Curr Opin Anaesthesiol*. 2010;23:500–506.

12. Howes BW, Wharton NM, Gibbison B, et al. LMA Supreme insertion by novices in manikins and patients. *Anaesthesia*. 2010;65:343–347.

13. Paal P, Gruber E, Beikircher W, et al. Sunset of bag-valve mask and rise of supra-glottic airway ventilation devices during basic life support. *Resuscitation*. 2009;80:1240–1243.

14. Cook TM, Woodall N, Ferk C; on behalf of the Fourth National Audit Project. Major complications of airway management in the UK: results of the fourth national audit project of the Royal College of Anaesthetists and the Difficult Airway Society. Part I: anesthesia. *Br J Anaesth*. 2011;106:617–631.

15. Brimacombe J, Berry A. Leak reduction with the LMA. *Can J Anaesth*. 1996;43:537.

16. Latorre F, Eberle B, Weiler N, et al. Laryngeal mask airway position and the risk of gastric insufflation. *Anesth Analg*. 1998;86:867–871.

17. Brimacombe JR, Berry A. The incidence of aspiration associated with the laryngeal mask airway: a meta-analysis of published literature. *J Clin Anesth*. 1995;7:297–305.

18. Aoyama K, Takenaka I, Sata T, et al. Cricoid pressure impedes positioning and ventilation through the laryngeal mask airway. *Can J Anaesth*. 1996;43:1035–1040.

19. Bhavani-Shankar K, Hart NS, Mushlin PS. Negative pressure induced airway and pulmonary injury. *Can J Anaesth*. 1997;44:78–81.

20. Ismail SA, Bisher NA, Kandil HW, et al. Intraocular pressure and haemodynamic responses to insertion of the i-gel, laryngeal mask airway or endotracheal tube. *Eur J Anaesthesiol*. 2011;28:443–448.

21. Chew EE, Hashim NH, Wang CY. Randomised comparison of the LMA Supreme with the I-Gel in spontaneously breathing anaesthetized adult patients. *Anaesth Intensive Care*. 2010;38:1018–1022.

22. Erlacher W, Tiefenbrunner H, Kästenbauer T, et al. CobraPLUS and Cookgas air-Q versus Fastrach for blind endotracheal intubation: a randomised controlled trial. *Eur J Anaesthesiol*. 2011;38:181–186.

11

Extraglottic Devices

Erik G. Laurin • Michael F. Murphy

INTRODUCTION

The term extraglottic device (EGD), and its subclasses, supraglottic device (SGD), infraglottic device (IGD), and retroglottic device (RGD) are defined and discussed in Chapter 10. This chapter reviews the non-laryngeal mask airway (LMA) EGDs, all of which can be classified as RGDs, our preferred term, or, less precisely, as IGDs. For the balance of this chapter, we refer to these devices collectively as EGDs, recognizing that the LMAs, a distinct class of EGDs, have been discussed in Chapter 10. The uses and contraindications of these retroglottic EGDs, however, are comparable to those for the supraglottic (LMA-type) EGDs, and are discussed in Chapter 10.

These devices share the following contraindications with the SGDs:

- Responsive patients with intact airway-protective reflexes
- Patients with known esophageal disease
- Caustic ingestions
- Upper airway obstruction because of laryngeal foreign bodies or pathology

Modern EGDs represent a dramatic improvement over the esophageal obturator airway and the esophageal gastric tube airway of the 1970s and 1980s, which have no place in modern emergency airway management. Instead, several of these devices have demonstrated their effectiveness and safety in rapidly establishing oxygenation and ventilation in a variety of emergency situations. This chapter will focus on the devices that have sufficient data to support their use in emergency airway management, as opposed to nonemergency operating room cases. Some of the currently available EGDs that lack a track record in emergency airway practice will require more evaluation before their potential role can be understood.

RETROGLOTTIC DEVICES

To many practitioners, the most familiar EGD is the esophageal tracheal Combitube (Esophageal-Tracheal Combitube (ETC) or Combitube [Tyco-Healthcare-Kendall-Sheridan, Mansfield, MA]). It has been in use since 1987, and has substantial evidence supporting its use. It creates a seal above and below the laryngeal inlet, and provides a direct conduit for gas exchange that is easier to use and more effective than a bag and a mask, and less invasive than an endotracheal tube (ETT) in that it is not intended to enter the trachea. The success of the Combitube has spawned the development of devices based on the same principles, attempting to replicate or improve on its safety, ease of use, and ability to facilitate oxygenation and ventilation.

The devices in this class commonly are collectively called EGDs, or, more precisely, RGDs, and include the following:

- ETC or Combitube (Fig. 11-1)
- King LT airway (King Systems Corp, Noblesville, IN; also known as laryngeal tube airway) (Fig. 11-2)
- Rusch EasyTube (Fig. 11-3)
- LaryVent (LV Teleflex Medical Rusch, Research Triangle Park, Raleigh, NC, USA)
- Airway management device (AMD)

These devices are intended to be passed behind the larynx and glottis (hence, retroglottic) and inserted blindly into the esophagus. Each is designed with two high-volume, low-pressure cuff balloons. One balloon seals the oropharynx above and the other the esophagus below, trapping the laryngeal inlet between the two. The Combitube and the EasyTube use two separate inflation ports to enable independent balloon inflation; the King LT has a single inflation port that inflates both the upper and lower portions of the balloon. Two somewhat similar devices, the LV and the AMD, have not achieved a body of evidence at the time of writing to recommend their use in emergency airway management and are therefore not further discussed.

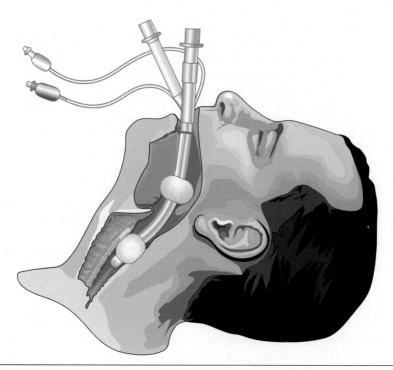

Figure 11-1 ● The Combitube Inserted and Seated. Note how the laryngeal aperture is trapped between the two balloons.

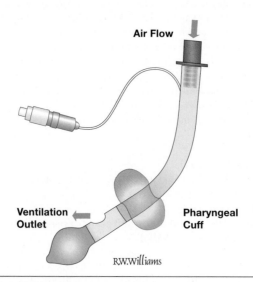

Figure 11-2 ● The King LT Airway. Note that there is only one inflation port to inflate both balloons.

When compared with LMAs, some of these EGDs may offer advantages. For instance, these balloon-type devices typically have higher cuff leak pressures (up to 40 cm H_2O) than LMA-type devices (up to 25 cm H_2O), which may be advantageous in patients requiring high peak airway pressures (asthma and obesity) or if glottic anatomy is distorted from hematoma, infection, or mass,

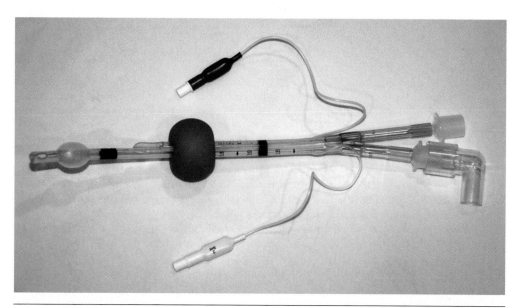

Figure 11-3 ● Rusch EasyTube.

requiring increased inflation pressure. None of these EGDs, however, is specifically designed to be a conduit through which a definitive airway can be established, like the intubating LMA.

Combitube

The Combitube (Fig. 11-1) has been in clinical use for a much longer period of time than any of the other EGDs has, and therefore it has accumulated the largest body of evidence describing its indications, contraindications, benefits, and risks.

The Combitube is a dual-lumen, dual-cuff, disposable airway intended to be inserted into the esophagus, although it can rarely enter the trachea on insertion (<5% of insertions), and is designed to function adequately in either position. The Combitube is supplied in two sizes: 37F SA (small adult) to be used in patients 4 ft (1.22 m) to 5 ft 6 in (1.67 m) tall, and 41F, which is for use in patients more than 5 ft 6 in tall. There is no Combitube suitable for use in children or patients <4 ft tall. In addition to the indications listed earlier, use of the Combitube has been described in upper gastrointestinal or upper airway hemorrhage that threatens airway and tracheal patency and in a case of severe facial burns.

Insertion Technique

Insertion of the Combitube is a blind technique, although a laryngoscope may be used, permitting insertion under direct vision. Although the Combitube can be inserted in almost any conceivable patient position, including sitting, semi-prone, etc., the technique described here assumes the patient is in the supine position.

1. With the patient supine and the head and neck in a neutral position, lift the tongue and jaw upward (jaw lift) with the nondominant hand.
2. Insert the device in the midline, allowing the curve of the device to follow the natural curve of the airway, and advance the device until the upper incisors (or alveolar ridge if the patient is edentulous) lie between the imprinted black circular bands on the device. Moderate force is required to enable the device to pass through the pharyngeal constrictor muscles into the esophagus. Substantial resistance should prompt the operator to withdraw and readvance.

3. Inflate the proximal large oropharyngeal balloon with approximately 100 ml of air (Combitube SA: 85 ml) through the blue pilot balloon port labeled no. 1.

4. Inflate the white distal balloon with 5 to 15 ml of air (Combitube SA: 5 to 12 ml) through the white pilot balloon port labeled no. 2.

5. Begin ventilation using the longer blue connecting tube (labeled no. 1). The presence of air entry into the lung, the detection of end-tidal carbon dioxide, and the absence of gastric insufflation by auscultation indicate that the Combitube is in the esophagus, which occurs with virtually every insertion. With the Combitube in the esophageal position, aspiration of gastric contents and gastric decompression is possible by passing the provided suction catheter through the clear connecting tube (labeled no. 2) into the stomach.

6. If bag ventilation using the longer blue tube no. 1 results in no breath sounds in the chest, absence of end-tidal carbon dioxide detection, and the presence of gastric insufflation sounds, then the Combitube is in the trachea (a distinctly rare event), and ventilation should be performed through the shorter clear connection tube no. 2.

7. The absence of any sounds on auscultation may indicate that the device has been inserted too far and should be repositioned after the proximal balloon is deflated.

After the Combitube is placed in the esophagus, oxygenation and ventilation can occur, but there is no way to establish a definitive airway when the device is in use. To intubate, the operator has to deflate and remove the Combitube entirely, or deflate just the proximal balloon and intubate around the Combitube, which remains in place in the esophagus. If the Combitube is placed in the trachea, an ETT changer or gum-elastic bougie (i.e., intubating introducer) can be placed through the ventilating tube and down the trachea, the Combitube balloons deflated and device removed, and a standard ETT advanced over the tube changer into the trachea. Even with tracheal placement of the Combitube, it is advisable to exchange it with a standard ETT within hours because of concerns of mucosal ischemia from the firm walls of the Combitube against the pharynx, even with the pharyngeal cuff deflated.

Complications

The Combitube has been shown to be an effective device that is easy to position properly. The Combitube appears in one study to be superior to the LMA Classic in the prehospital setting, and it has been shown to be a useful airway rescue device in the event of a failed intubation. However, like the LMA, it does not provide optimum protection against aspiration (although aspiration is uncommon), and its merit relative to the LMA Fastrach is unknown. Complications are rare and mostly related to upper airway and esophageal hematomas, mucosal lacerations on insertion, pyriform sinus perforation, and perforation of the esophagus.

Increased cuff volumes are required at times to achieve a seal sufficient to permit adequate ventilation. As cuff volume is increased, the pressure transmitted to the mucosa is increased to the point, where mucosal perfusion may be compromised, particularly where the cuff is adjacent to rigid anatomical structures such as the cervical spine (pharyngeal balloon) and the larynx (esophageal balloon). Over time, this may lead to ischemic mucosal injury. A high rate of success with few complications has been reported in prehospital use for cardiac arrest victims.

Finally, it should be noted that the pharyngeal balloon on the Combitube (as opposed to the Rusch EasyTube or the King LT airway) is made of latex.

The King LT Airway

The King LT airway (also known as the laryngeal tube airway, predominantly in Europe) (Fig. 11-2) is a more recently developed multiuse (King LT) and disposable (King LT-D), latex-free, single-lumen silicon laryngeal tube with oropharyngeal and esophageal low-pressure cuffs, with a ventilation port located between the two cuffs. It is supplied in blind distal tip (King LT, LT-D) and open distal tip (King LTS, LTS-D) variants to permit gastric decompression. A single pilot balloon port is used to inflate both balloons simultaneously, which is technically easier to use than the two-step Combitube inflation system. However, this single inflation technique also allows the King LT's airway seal to sometimes be lost following insertion, requiring deflation of the balloons and repositioning, an occurrence that is not common with the Combitube.

The King LT is inserted similarly to the Combitube, although there is usually less resistance on insertion. The distal segment of the tube is straight instead of slightly curved like the Combitube, so the King LT is designed to go only into the esophagus, with no reported tracheal placements. It is advanced until definitive resistance is felt, or the colored, 15/22-mm bag connector flange touches the incisors. When seated, it works in a fashion that is very similar to that of the Combitube, with ventilation through the ports between the two cuff balloons. Because there is only one ventilation bag adaptor and one pilot balloon inflation port, and the device never enters the glottis or trachea, troubleshooting is rarely needed. If the first attempt at ventilation after insertion results in no air movement and high resistance to ventilation, the tube is too deep and can be slowly withdrawn with continued pressure on the ventilation bag, until ventilations are free flowing. Ventilation and oxygenation capabilities seem to be similar to the LMA and Combitube.

As is the case with the Combitube, sizing of the King LT airways is height based. The King LT is available for pediatric and adult patients from 35 in (90 cm) to more than 6 ft (>180 cm) tall. Approximate interdental distance of 20 mm is required for insertion, comparable to the Combitube.

Although it is possible to intubate using the King LT, caution is required as complications have been reported in a cadaver model. The 10 mm inner diameter of the ventilation lumen can accommodate a gum-elastic bougie, which can then exit the ventilation port at the distal end of the lumen. Ideally, this ventilation port lines up with the glottic opening, allowing the bougie to enter the trachea with the typical confirmatory "clicks" on the tracheal rings and "hard stop" with advancement into a small bronchus. The King LT can then be removed and a standard ETT advanced over the bougie into the trachea. Although this procedure can sometimes be accomplished in manikins, there is potential for bougie perforation of glottic structures during advancement through the King LT in human tissue. Therefore, if this procedure is attempted, extreme care must be exercised.

Rusch EasyTube

The Rusch EasyTube (Fig. 11-3) is a dual-lumen tube designed for difficult or emergency airway intubation and ventilation. Like the Combitube, the EasyTube can be placed either in the trachea or in the esophagus, and creates a viable airway in either position. When placed in the esophagus, the EasyTube allows the passage of a flexible endoscope, a suction catheter, or a tracheal tube introducer through the proximally terminating ventilation lumen. This distinguishes it from the Combitube, which does not permit passage of a tube exchanger to potentially establish a definitive airway through the device. If placed in the trachea, the size and shape of the distal tip are similar to a standard ETT. It is suggested by the manufacturer that the risk of tracheal trauma relative to the Combitube is reduced because of the smaller diameter of EasyTube device at the distal tip.

The EasyTube is supplied in two sizes, 28F and 41F. As for the Combitube, the manufacturer claims that the smaller size can be used in older children. The EasyTube is latex free.

There is minimal evidence from human studies to demonstrate the relative success rate of the EasyTube versus the LMA, Combitube, or King LT, although initial data appear promising. Multiple manikin studies show that it is similar to a Combitube in speed of insertion, successful ventilations, and skill retention. More data are needed to determine its role in emergency airway management.

EVIDENCE

- **What is the role of the Combitube as a rescue airway device?** The Combitube has been identified as a rescue airway device for the failed airway by authoritative bodies in the United States and Canada.[1,2] Its use is well described in the anesthesia, resuscitation, emergency medicine, and emergency medical services (EMS) literature both as a first-line device and as a device to be used in the face of a difficult or failed airway.[3–9] Several authors have identified the Combitube as a valuable adjunct in cardiopulmonary resuscitation,[10–12] performing as well as or better than the LMA and bag-mask ventilation.

- **What kind of airway management success rates have been reported with the Combitube?** Success rates of 98% to 100% are regularly reported in these studies. The ease of insertion[13–17] and adequacy of ventilation by physicians and nonphysician providers is well established.[18–20]

- **Has the Combitube been successful in the management of the difficult or failed airway?** The device is useful in the management of the difficult airway[21] and in rescuing a failed airway[22–24] while one prepares to undertake a cricothyrotomy.

- **Has the Combitube been used in any unusual situations?** It has been demonstrated to protect the airway, control bleeding, and permit ventilation in a case of craniofacial trauma associated with severe bleeding[25] and to secure an airway in a case of severe facial burns preventing intubation.[26]

- **What precautions should I be aware of with this device?** It is unclear whether the Combitube provides protection against the aspiration of gastric contents.[27] The downside of the Combitube includes reports of potentially serious complications related to its use, particularly pyriform sinus perforation[28–32] and esophageal perforation.[33–37] A word of caution: Mucosal pressures exerted by the inflated balloons may exceed mucosal perfusion pressure, leading to mucosal ischemia.[38]

- **Has the King LT airway been demonstrated to be similarly effective in nonemergency airway management as the LMA and Combitube?** Simple handling, possible aspiration protection, and availability in newborn to adult sizes are considered to be advantages of this airway device.[39–42]

- **Does the King LT have a place in EMS as an airway management device?** There is some evidence that this device is easily learned by EMS personnel and provides more effective ventilation than bag-mask devices.[43–45]

- **Is the King LT airway useful as an emergency airway adjunct?** The evidence that the King LT is useful as a rescue airway or in patients where intubation has failed is limited and for the most part is based on case reports.[46–48] However, a recent publication provides compelling evidence that this device may well be of use in the difficult and failed airway.[49]

- **Are there potential problems that I ought to be aware of with this device?** As with the Combitube, mucosal compression by the inflated balloons may lead to mucosal ischemic injury.[38,50]

- **The EasyTube looks as though it would be easier to insert in an emergency than the Combitube. Is there evidence to that effect?** Perhaps, but at this point, the available evidence is relatively thin.[38,51–64] Much of the published information is from simulated patients or manikins,[51,52,58,61] an operating theater,[55,56,60] or is based on opinion.[54,57] However, there is sufficient evidence to suggest that this device is at least competitive with the Combitube and King LT to be a consideration for prehospital airway management.

REFERENCES

1. Crosby ET, Cooper RM, Douglas MJ, et al. The unanticipated difficult airway with recommendations for management. *Can J Anaesth*. 1998;45:757–776.

2. Practice guidelines for management of the difficult airway. An updated report by the American Society of Anesthesiologists Task Force on Management of the Difficult Airway. *Anesthesiology*. 2003;98:1269–1277.

3. Mercer M. The role of the Combitube in airway management. *Anaesthesia*. 2000;55:394–395.

4. Gaitini LA, Vaida SJ, Agro F. The esophageal-tracheal Combitube. *Anesthesiol Clin North Am*. 2002;20:893–906.

5. Idris AH, Gabrielli A. Advances in airway management. *Emerg Med Clin North Am*. 2002;20:843–857.

6. Agro F, Frass M, Benumof JL, et al. Current status of the Combitube: a review of the literature. *J Clin Anesth*. 2002;14:307–314.

7. Keller C, Brimacombe J, Boehler M, et al. The influence of cuff volume and anatomic location on pharyngeal, esophageal, and tracheal mucosal pressures with the esophageal tracheal Combitube. *Anesthesiology*. 2002;96:1074–1077.

8. Shuster M, Nolan J, Barnes TA. Airway and ventilation management. *Cardiol Clin*. 2002;20:23–35.

9. Agro F, Frass M, Benumof J, et al. The esophageal tracheal Combitube as a non-invasive alternative to endotracheal intubation: a review. *Minerva Anesthesiol*. 2001;67:863–874.

10. Grayling M, Wilson IH, Thomas B. The use of the laryngeal mask airway and Combitube in cardiopulmonary resuscitation: a national survey. *Resuscitation*. 2002;52:183–186.

11. Gabrielli A, Layon AJ, Wenzel V, et al. Alternative ventilation strategies in cardiopulmonary resuscitation. *Curr Opin Crit Care*. 2002;8:199–211.

12. Frass M, Staudinger T, Losert H, et al. Airway management during cardiopulmonary resuscitation—a comparative study of bag-valve-mask, laryngeal mask airway and Combitube in a bench model. *Resuscitation*. 1999;43:80–81.

13. Levitan RM, Kush S, Hollander JE. Devices for difficult airway management in academic emergency departments: results of a national survey. *Ann Emerg Med*. 1999;33:694–698.

14. Lefrancois DP, Dufour DG. Use of the esophageal tracheal Combitube by basic emergency medical technicians. *Resuscitation*. 2002;52:77–83.

15. Ochs M, Vilke GM, Chan TC, et al. Successful prehospital airway management by EMT-Ds using the Combitube. *Prehosp Emerg Care*. 2000;4:333–337.

16. Tanigawa K, Shigematsu A. Choice of airway devices for 12,020 cases of nontraumatic cardiac arrest in Japan. *Prehosp Emerg Care*. 1998;2:96–100.

17. Rumball CJ, MacDonald D. The PTL, Combitube, laryngeal mask, and oral airway: a randomized prehospital comparative study of ventilatory device effectiveness and cost-effectiveness in 470 cases of cardiorespiratory arrest. *Prehosp Emerg Care*. 1997;1:1–10.

18. Calkins MD, Robinson TD. Combat trauma airway management: endotracheal intubation versus laryngeal mask airway versus Combitube use by Navy SEAL and Reconnaissance Combat Corpsmen. *J Trauma*. 1999;46:927–932.

19. Yardy N, Hancox D, Strang T. A comparison of two airway aids for emergency use by unskilled personnel: the Combitube and laryngeal mask. *Anaesthesia*. 1999;54:181–183.

20. Dorges V, Ocker H, Wenzel V, et al. Emergency airway management by non-anaesthesia house officers—a comparison of three strategies. *Emerg Med J*. 2001;18:90–94.

21. Staudinger T, Tesinsky P, Klappacher G, et al. Emergency intubation with the Combitube in two cases of difficult airway management. *Eur J Anaesthesiol*. 1995;12:189–193.

22. Blostein PA, Koestner AJ, Hoak S. Failed rapid sequence intubation in trauma patients: esophageal tracheal Combitube is a useful adjunct. *J Trauma*. 1998;44:534–537.

23. Enlund M, Miregard M, Wennmalm K. The Combitube for failed intubation—instructions for use. *Acta Anaesthesiol Scand*. 2001;45:127–128.

24. Della Puppa A, Pittoni G, Frass M. Tracheal esophageal Combitube: a useful airway for morbidly obese patients who cannot intubate or ventilate. *Acta Anaesthesiol Scand*. 2002;46:911–913.

25. Morimoto F, Yoshioka T, Ikeuchi H, et al. Use of esophageal tracheal Combitube to control severe oronasal bleeding associated with craniofacial injury: case report. *J Trauma*. 2001;51:168–169.

26. Wagner A, Roeggla M, Roeggla G, et al. Emergency intubation with the Combitube in a case of severe facial burn. *Am J Emerg Med*. 1995;13:681–683.

27. Mercer MH. An assessment of protection of the airway from aspiration of oropharyngeal contents using the Combitube airway. *Resuscitation*. 2001;51:135–138.

28. Urtubia RM, Gazmuri RR. Is the Combitube traumatic? *Anesthesiology*. 2003;98:1021–1022.

29. Urtubia RM, Carcamo CR, Montes JM. Complications following the use of the Combitube, tracheal tube and laryngeal mask airway. *Anaesthesia*. 2000;55:597–599.

30. Oczenski W, Krenn H, Dahaba AA, et al. Complications following the use of the Combitube, tracheal tube and laryngeal mask airway. *Anaesthesia*. 1999;54:1161–1165.

31. Moser MS. Piriform sinus perforation during esophageal-tracheal Combitube placement. *J Emerg Med*. 1999;17:129.

32. Richards CF. Piriform sinus perforation during esophageal-tracheal Combitube placement. *J Emerg Med*. 1998;16:37–39.

33. Krafft P, Nikolic A, Frass M. Esophageal rupture associated with the use of the Combitube. *Anesth Analg*. 1998;87:1457.

34. Krafft P, Frass M, Reed AP. Complications with the Combitube. *Can J Anaesth*. 1998;45:823–824.

35. Walz R, Bund M, Meier PN, et al. Esophageal rupture associated with the use of the Combitube. *Anesth Analg*. 1998;87:228.

36. Vezina D, Lessard MR, Bussieres J, et al. Complications associated with the use of the esophageal-tracheal Combitube. *Can J Anaesth*. 1998;45:76–80.

37. Klein H, Williamson M, Sue-Ling HM, et al. Esophageal rupture associated with the use of the Combitube. *Anesth Analg*. 1997;85:937–939.

38. Ulrich-Pur H, Hrska F, Krafft P, et al. Comparison of mucosal pressures induced by cuffs of different airway devices. *Anesthesiology*. 2006;104(5):933–938.

39. Dorges V, Ocker H, Wenzel V, et al. The laryngeal tube S: a modified simple airway device. *Anesth Analg*. 2003;96:618–621.

40. Genzwuerker HV, Hilker T, Hohner E, et al. The laryngeal tube: a new adjunct for airway management. *Prehosp Emerg Care*. 2000;4:168–172.

41. Dorges V, Ocker H, Wenzel V, et al. The laryngeal tube: a new simple airway device. *Anesth Analg*. 2000;90:1220–1222.

42. Agro F, Cataldo R, Alfano A, et al. A new prototype for airway management in an emergency: the laryngeal tube. *Resuscitation*. 1999;41:284–286.

43. Kette F, Reffo I, Giordani G, et al. The use of laryngeal tube by nurses in out-of-hospital emergencies: preliminary experience. *Resuscitation*. 2005;66:21–25.

44. Kurola J, Harve H, Kettunen T, et al. Airway management in cardiac arrest—comparison of the laryngeal tube, tracheal intubation and bag-mask-ventilation in emergency medical training. *Resuscitation*. 2004;61:149–153.

45. Asai T, Hidaka I, Kawachi S. Efficacy of the laryngeal tube by inexperienced personnel. *Resuscitation*. 2002;55:171–175.

46. Asai T. Use of the laryngeal tube for difficult fiberoptic tracheal intubation. *Anaesthesia*. 2005;60:826.

47. Matioc A, Olson J. Use of the laryngeal tube in two unexpected difficult airway situations: lingual tonsillar hyperplasia and morbid obesity. *Can J Anaesth*. 2004;51:1018–1021.

48. Genzwuerker H, Dhonau S, Ellinger K. Use of the laryngeal tube for out-of-hospital resuscitation. *Resuscitation*. 2002;52:221–224.

49. Winterhalter M, Kirchhoff K, Groschel W, et al. The laryngeal tube for difficult airway management: a prospective investigation in patients with pharyngeal and laryngeal tumours. *Eur J Anaesthesiol*. 2005;22:678–682.

50. Keller C, Brimacombe J, Kleinsasser A, et al. Pharyngeal mucosal pressures with the laryngeal tube airway versus ProSeal laryngeal mask airway. *Anasthesiol Intensivmed Notfallmed Schmerzther*. 2003;38:393–396.

51. Ruetzler K, Gruber C, Nabecker S, et al. Hands-off time during insertion of six airway devices during cardiopulmonary resuscitation: a randomised manikin trial. *Resuscitation*. 2011;82:1060–1063.

52. Ruetzler K, Roessler B, Potura L, et al. Performance and skill retention of intubation by paramedics using seven different airway devices—a manikin study. *Resuscitation*. 2011;82:593–597.

53. Chenaitia H, Soulleihet V, Massa H, et al. The Easytube for airway management in prehospital emergency medicine. *Resuscitation*. 2010;81:1516–1520.

54. Bollig G. The EasyTube and users' preferences: implications for prehospital medicine and research. *Eur J Anaesthesiol*. 2010;27:843–844.

55. Lorenz V, Rich JM, Schebesta K, et al. Comparison of the EasyTube and endotracheal tube during general anesthesia in fasted adult patients. *J Clin Anesth*. 2009;21:341–347.

56. Cavus E, Deitmer W, Francksen H, et al. Laryngeal tube S II, ProSeal laryngeal mask, and Easy-Tube during elective surgery: a randomized controlled comparison with the endotracheal tube in nontrained professionals. *Eur J Anaesthesiol*. 2009;26:730–735.

57. Bollig G. Combitube and Easytube should be included in the Scandinavian guidelines for prehospital airway management. *Acta Anaesthesiol Scand*. 2009;53:139–140.

58. Trabold B, Schmidt C, Schneider B, et al. Application of three airway devices during emergency medical training by health care providers—a manikin study. *Am J Emerg Med*. 2008;26:783–788.

59. Bercker S, Schmidbauer W, Volk T, et al. A comparison of seal in seven supraglottic airway devices using a cadaver model of elevated esophageal pressure. *Anesth Analg*. 2008;106:445–448.

60. Urtubia RM, Leyton P. Successful use of the EasyTube for facial surgery in a patient with glottic and subglottic stenosis. *J Clin Anesth*. 2007;19:77–78.

61. Bollig G, Lovhaug SW, Sagen O, et al. Airway management by paramedics using endotracheal intubation with a laryngoscope versus the oesophageal tracheal Combitube and EasyTube on manikins: a randomized experimental trial. *Resuscitation*. 2006;71:107–111.

62. Thierbach AR, Werner C. Infraglottic airway devices and techniques. *Best Pract Res Clin Anaesthesiol*. 2005;19:595–609.

63. Thierbach AR, Piepho T, Maybauer M. The EasyTube for airway management in emergencies. *Prehosp Emerg Care*. 2005;9:445–448.

64. Thierbach AR, Piepho T, Maybauer MO. A new device for emergency airway management: the EasyTube. *Resuscitation*. 2004;60:347.

12

Direct Laryngoscopy

Robert F. Reardon • Steven C. Carleton • Calvin A. Brown III

DIRECT LARYNGOSCOPY

Direct laryngoscopy (DL) is the most common technique for tracheal intubation in the emergency setting. In experienced hands, DL has a very high success rate, and the equipment is inexpensive, reliable, and widely available. However, DL requires significant experience to gain proficiency and has inherent limitations that manifest when factors such as decreased cervical mobility, a large tongue, a receding chin or prominent incisors are present.

BASICS OF DIRECT LARYNGOSCOPY

The concept of DL is simple—to create a straight line of site from the mouth to the larynx in order to visualize the vocal cords. The tongue is the greatest obstacle to laryngoscopy. The laryngoscope is used to control the tongue and displace it out of the line of sight. A laryngoscope consists of a handle, a blade, and a light source. It is a left-handed instrument despite the operator's handedness. In general, DL blades are either curved (Macintosh) or straight (Miller) (Fig. 12-1). Both blades come in a variety of sizes from newborn to large adult, and sizes 3 and 4 are commonly used in adults. Macintosh blades have a gentle curve, a vertical flange for displacing the tongue and a relatively wide square tip with an obvious knob. Variations of the original Macintosh blade design, which include a smaller vertical flange and a shorter light-to-tip distance have also been manufactured. The vertical flange height of the size 3 and 4 blades is similar making it reasonable to start with the longer size 4 blade in all adults. Curved blades are intended to be advanced into the vallecula and when the knob on the tip makes contact and depresses the hyoepiglottic ligament, the epiglottis elevates exposing the vocal cords (Fig. 12-2).

Miller blades have a narrower and shorter flange and a slightly curved tip without a knob. The smaller flange may be advantageous when there is less mouth opening, but makes tongue control more difficult and decreases the area of displacement for visualization and tube placement. Size 3 and 4 Miller blades are nearly identical except for length, so it may be reasonable to start with the longer size 4 blade in most adults. Miller blades are intended to be passed posterior to the epiglottis, to lift it directly

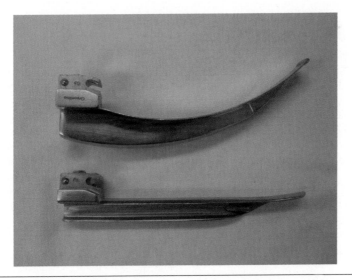

Figure 12-1 ● Macintosh (top) and Miller (bottom) Laryngoscope Blades. The curved blade is a size 4 German Macintosh, which is a good blade for routine use in adults, unlike the American design, which has a taller flange height. The straight blade is a size 3 Miller, for normal size adults. Most Miller blades have the light on the left side (as shown here), which can embed in the tongue, but better designs place the light on the right side of the blade.

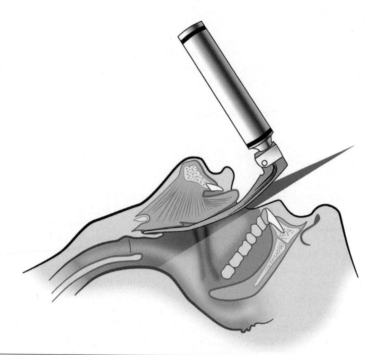

Figure 12-2 ● Direct Laryngoscopy with a Macintosh Blade. Note that the tip of the blade is properly placed into the base of the vallecula and elevates the epiglottis by pushing against the hyoepiglottic ligament.

in order to expose the vocal cords (Fig. 12-3). Most operators prefer the curved Macintosh blade because it is wider and allows better control of the tongue; however, the straight Miller blade may provide better visualization of the glottis when there is limited cervical movement, prominent upper incisors, a large tongue, limited mouth opening, or a floppy epiglottis, so it is important to master both techniques.

ANATOMY FOR DIRECT LARYNGOSCOPY

Recognition of anatomic landmarks is critical to DL success (See Figs 12-4 and 4-5 pages 124 and 41, respectively.) For laryngoscopy the most important laryngeal structures are the epiglottis, the posterior arytenoid cartilages and interarytenoid notch, and the vocal cords. Tracheal intubation is accomplished by passing the endotracheal tube (ETT) through the vocal cords. Success is more likely if the vocal cords are well visualized; however, tracheal intubation does not always require visualization of the vocal cords. If only the posterior cartilages are visible, the tube can be passed anterior to these structures in the midline and will usually enter the trachea (Fig. 12-4B). Furthermore, intubation can often be accomplished when the only visible structure is the epiglottis (Fig. 12-4C), especially if an endotracheal tube introducer (ETI or "bougie") is used. If the epiglottis cannot be identified, the likelihood of successful tracheal intubation is very low (Fig. 12-4D).

PREPARATION AND ASSISTANCE

Before embarking on the intubation attempt, the airway manager must ensure that the following are available:

- Established IV and monitoring systems.
  - Oxygen saturation and cardiac monitoring.

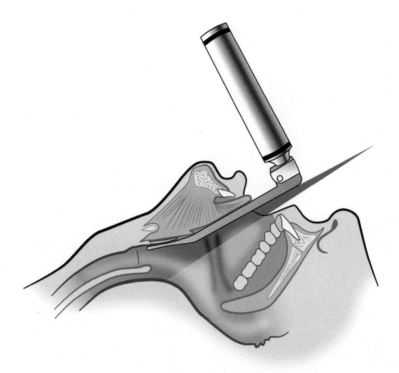

Figure 12-3 ● Direct Laryngoscopy with a Miller Blade. The tip of the blade is used to lift the epiglottis directly.

- All required equipment and medications.
  - Laryngoscope blade and handle, ETT and backup ETT of a smaller size, 10-cc syringe, lubrication, working suction, and rapid sequence intubation drugs.
  - ETI (disposable or reusable bougie, see page 131.)
- Adequate suction.
- Trained assistant standing on the patient's right.

The assistant should be prepared to do the following:

- Pass equipment as needed to the airway manager.
- Hold the head in a position as stipulated.
- Perform laryngeal manipulation as instructed.
- Retract the corner of the mouth during intubation.

PREINTUBATION ASSESSMENT AND EQUIPMENT CHOICE

Preintubation assessment of the patient's airway is essential and must be performed on every patient before administration of neuromuscular blockers. In the mnemonic LEMON, discussed in Chapter 2, the *M* stands for Mallampati, serving as a reminder to examine the oral cavity to assess the relative size of the tongue in relationship to the oropharynx and the mandibular space (see Chapter 4). The laryngoscope blade is the tool that controls and maneuvers the tongue. Fundamental to successful laryngoscopy is the selection of a blade, curved or straight, that will be wide and long enough to capture the tongue during laryngoscopy, sweep it leftward and inferiorly into the mandibular space out of the visual field, and permit direct visualization of the airway. The larger flange of the curved Macintosh blade usually provides better tongue control than the thinner blade of the straight Miller

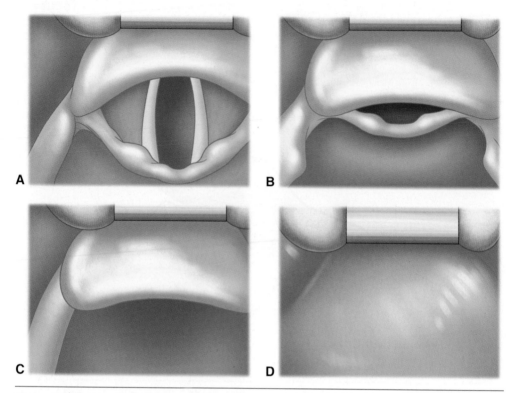

Figure 12-4 ● **A–D:** Laryngoscopic views (correlating with the Cormack–Lehane system). **A:** Full view of the vocal cords (grade I). **B:** Only the posterior glottic structures/cartilages are visible (grade II). **C:** Only the epiglottis is visible (grade III). **D:** Neither the epiglottis nor glottic structures are visible, only the soft palate (grade IV).

blade. Many laryngoscopists prefer a size 4 Macintosh blade for most emergency airways to assure adequate blade length. However, choice of a laryngoscope blade and the technique used to facilitate intubation is best guided by personal choice and experience. The literature suggests that straight blades improve laryngoscopic view (increased exposure of the vocal cords), whereas curved blades provide better intubating conditions (continuous visualization of the vocal cords during ETT passage). Using an ETI (bougie) improves intubation success rates with the straight-blade technique.

HANDLING THE LARYNGOSCOPE AND POSTURE OF THE OPERATOR

The laryngoscope should be held low on the handle, so the proximal end of the blade pushes into the thenar or hypothenar eminence of the left hand. This grip will encourage lifting from the shoulder, keeping the elbow low, and keeping the wrist stiff during laryngoscopy. The operator should be in an upright position with his or her arms and hands at a comfortable working height, rather than stooping or straining to reach the patient. The patient's bed should be elevated and the operator should step back from the patient so that his or her back is relatively straight during laryngoscopy.

PATIENT POSITIONING

Optimal head and neck positioning for DL is often described as the "sniffing position"; lower cervical flexion and atlanto-occipital extension. The sniffing position attempts to align the oral, pharyngeal, and laryngeal axes of the upper airway (Fig. 12-5). Absent contraindications, alignment of these axes is important for optimizing the laryngoscopic view. The appropriate degree of lower cervical flexion brings the external auditory meatus to the level of the sternal angle of Louis or anterior surface of the shoulder. In adult patients of normal body habitus, a 4- to 6-cm pad beneath the occiput usually suffices for this purpose. Alternatively, the operator can extend

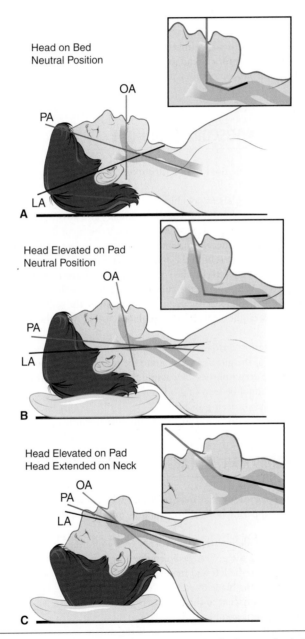

Figure 12-5 ● **A:** Anatomical neutral position. The oral axis (OA), pharyngeal axis (PA), and laryngeal axis (LA) are not aligned. **B:** Head, still in neutral position, has been lifted by a pillow flexing the lower cervical spine and aligning the PA and LA. **C:** The head has been extended on the cervical spine, aligning the OA with the PA and LA, creating the optimum sniffing position for intubation.

and lift the head with his or her right hand during laryngoscopy to determine the optimal position empirically. The head can then be supported by an assistant standing on the right side of the patient while the operator intubates or performs external laryngeal manipulation. In morbidly obese patients, optimal positioning will often require a ramp to be constructed from linens or pads placed beneath the upper torso, shoulders, neck, and occiput in order to align the ear canal with the sternal angle of Louis (see Chapter 39, Fig. 39-1). Airway ramps are also commercially available for this purpose. In small children with a protuberant occiput, the torso may need to be raised to allow the external meatus to fall back to the desired plane (see Chapter 25, Fig. 25-2). Because of individual variations in anatomy, the optimal head and neck position is often unpredictable, and may require empiric adjustment during the intubation attempt. It is critically important that some means of adjusting the patient's position be available before initiating the procedure. Understanding optimal head and neck positioning will help operators appreciate the difficulty of performing DL on trauma patients and others who must be intubated in a fixed position.

STANDARD DIRECT LARYNGOSCOPY TECHNIQUE

This is the standard technique used with both curved and straight blades.

- Open the mouth as widely as possible.
- Insert the blade along the right mandibular molars and sweep the tongue to the left.
- Use a "look as you go" approach—that is, advance the tip of the blade down the tongue in a careful step-by-step manner, lifting intermittently to ascertain the location of the tip in relation to anatomic structures, until the epiglottis is located. The epiglottis is the main anatomic landmark because the glottis can be consistently found just posterior and inferior to it.
- Lift the epiglottis. When using the curved blade, displace the epiglottis indirectly by pressing against the hyoepiglottic ligament at the base of the vallecula (Figs. 12-2 and 12-6). When using the straight blade, lift the epiglottis directly with the tip of the blade (Figs. 12-3 and 12-7).
- Identify the posterior cartilages and interarytenoid notch. These structures make up the posterior border of the glottis and separate the tracheal inlet from the esophagus. Tracheal intubation can be accomplished by passing the tube anterior to these structures, even when the vocal cords cannot be seen.
- Visualize the vocal cords, if possible.
- Pass the tube through the vocal cords and into the trachea.

PARAGLOSSAL (RETROMOLAR) STRAIGHT-BLADE TECHNIQUE

This is an alternative technique that may be useful when standard DL is unexpectedly difficult because of prominent upper incisors, a large tongue, or limited mouth opening.

- Insert the Miller blade into the right corner of the mouth.
- Pass the blade along the groove between the tongue and the tonsil.
- Sweep the tongue to the left and maintain it to the left of the blade.
- Advance the tip of the blade toward the midline, keeping the back of the blade to the right side of the mouth adjacent to the molars (Fig. 12-8).
- Identify the epiglottis and lift its tip to expose the vocal cords.
- Have an assistant retract the right corner of the mouth.
- Pass the tube through the vocal cords and into the trachea. Often one needs to use an ETI down the channel of the scope with this approach because of limited space preventing ETT advancement. The ETI was specifically designed for this purpose.

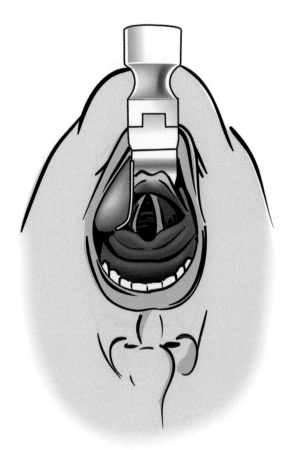

Figure 12-6 ● **Direct Laryngoscopy with a Macintosh Blade.** The mouth is opened widely and the tongue is well controlled and kept entirely to the left by the large flange of the Macintosh blade. The epiglottis is visualized and the tip of the blade is pushed into the vallecula to elevate the epiglottis and expose the vocal cords. Force is applied by lifting the entire blade upward, not by tilting the butt of the blade toward the upper incisors.

BLIND INSERTION TECHNIQUE FOR THE STRAIGHT BLADE

This is an alternative technique often used in neonates, infants, and small children using a straight blade, or in adults when other techniques are predicted to be difficult or have failed. There are two phases to this method: (1) Blind insertion of the tip of the laryngoscope blade into the esophagus, and (2) visualization of the glottis during withdrawal. The potential for esophageal and tracheal injury or regurgitation resulting from opening the upper esophageal sphincter during blind insertion of the blade has not been studied.

- Place the blade into the right side of the mouth and maintain the tongue to the left.
- Hold the laryngoscope with the fingertips and gently advance the entire length of the blade blindly toward the midline, past the base of the tongue, posterior to the glottis, and into the proximal esophagus. If there is any resistance stop and withdraw slightly, then realign and advance completely.
- While looking into the airway, lift the blade and then slowly and deliberately withdraw until the glottis drops down into view. If the epiglottis also drops into view, lift it with the tip of the blade to expose the vocal cords.
- Pass the tube through the vocal cords and into the trachea.

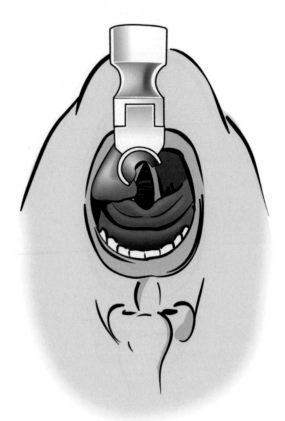

Figure 12-7 ● Direct Laryngoscopy with a Miller Blade. The mouth is opened widely and the tongue is difficult to control with the small flange of the Miller blade, but it is kept entirely to the left. The epiglottis is identified and then lifted with the tip of the blade (so it is no longer visible here) to expose the vocal cords. Force is applied by lifting the entire blade upward, not by tilting the butt of the blade toward the upper incisors.

INTUBATING THE TRACHEA

If the glottis is directly visualized, it is usually easy to pass a tube into the trachea. However, even with excellent glottic exposure, it is possible to block the line of sight with the ETT during the intubation attempt. This possibility can be minimized by inserting the tube from the extreme right-hand corner of the mouth while an assistant retracts the lip, and by keeping the tube below the line of site while advancing it toward the glottis, raising it over the posterior landmarks only during the terminal phase of insertion. Tube shape can also influence the ease of visualization during intubation. Using a malleable stylet to produce a straight tube with a single "hockey-stick" bend of <35° just proximal to the balloon facilitates cord visualization during passage, by keeping the tube out of the line of sight until it passes the cords (Fig. 12-9). As the tube approaches the depth of the glottis, it is raised up over the posterior landmarks and passed through the vocal cords. A banana-shaped tube tends to cross the visual axis twice in the course of insertion and may interfere with visual guidance during placement.

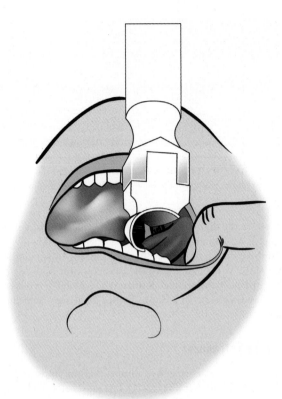

Figure 12-8 ● Paraglossal (Retromolar) Straight-blade Technique. The Miller blade enters the right corner of the mouth and the tip advances toward the midline while the proximal blade remains in the right side of the mouth. Note that the tongue is entirely to the left of the blade. This technique may improve glottic visualization in difficult situations but does not leave much room for passage of the ETT. Have an assistant retract the lip to create more room as shown.

TROUBLESHOOTING DIFFICULT DIRECT LARYNGOSCOPY

Paralysis

Chemical paralysis greatly facilitates DL. The reflexes and muscle tone of the upper airway are difficult to overcome in patients who are sedated but not paralyzed. Airway managers should understand the indications for, and use of, neuromuscular blocking agents (see chapters 2, 3, and 22).

Bimanual Laryngoscopy

Bimanual laryngoscopy involves external manipulation of the thyroid cartilage with the laryngoscopist's right hand (Fig. 12-10). Backward, upward (cephalad), and rightward pressure (referred to as BURP) on the thyroid cartilage, by an assistant, has been shown to significantly improve glottic visualization during laryngoscopy. However, external laryngeal manipulation by the laryngoscopist is better than BURP by an assistant because the operator gets immediate feedback and can quickly determine which movements provide an optimal view. These movements might include BURP, but can also involve any movement that improves visualization of the glottis. Firm

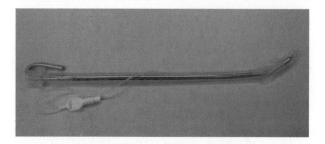

Figure 12-9 ● **Optimal ETT/Stylet Shape.** A relatively straight ETT with a "hockey stick" shape, with a bend angle <35°. This shape allows passage of the ETT without blocking the line of site.

downward pressure on the thyroid cartilage moves the vocal cords posteriorly into the line of sight of the laryngoscopist. Also, during curved blade laryngoscopy, downward pressure on the thyroid cartilage helps to drive the tip of the laryngoscope into the hyoepiglottic ligament, further lifting the epiglottis out of the visual axis. When the laryngoscopist finds the best view, an assistant can hold the thyroid cartilage in the optimal position while the ETT is placed. Bimanual laryngoscopy should not be confused with cricoid pressure (Sellick maneuver), which is performed during BMV to avoid regurgitation.

Endotracheal Tube Introducer

An ETI or bougie is a simple, inexpensive adjunct that can improve intubation success when visualization of the glottis is difficult (Fig. 12-11). It is most helpful when the epiglottis is visualized, but the vocal cords and posterior cartilages cannot be seen. The ETI is a long (60 cm), narrow

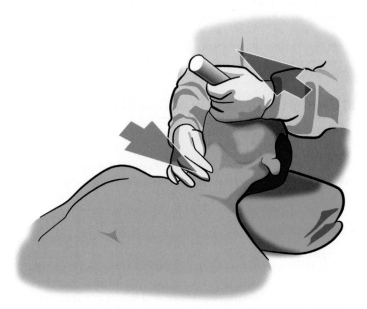

Figure 12-10 ● **Bimanual Laryngoscopy.** The laryngoscopist uses his/her right hand to manipulate the thyroid cartilage. Optimal external manipulation often involves firm pressure on the thyroid cartilage and movement to the right (backward, upward [cephalad], and rightward pressure). The advantage of the laryngoscopist performing this maneuver (not an assistant) is that he/she gets immediate visual feedback and can quickly determine what constitutes optimal external manipulation.

(5 mm), flexible plastic (SunMed Bougie, Largo, FL) or spun nylon (Eschmann Bougie/Guide, Smiths Medical-Portex, St. Paul, MN) device with a fixed 40° bend at the distal end (Coudé tip). Insertion is often facilitated by making a 60° anterior bend approximately 10 to 15 cm from the distal tip (Fig. 12-11, inset). The EI is held with the tip pointing upward. Under visual guidance with a laryngoscope, it is passed just under the epiglottis and upward into the tracheal inlet (Fig. 12-12). Tracheal placement results in palpable vibrations of the introducer as the Coudé tip bumps against the tracheal rings during insertion. Alternatively, tracheal placement can be confirmed by a hard stop at about 40 cm of insertion. Placement in the esophagus provides no such hard stop. The ETT is placed over the ETI by an assistant until the proximal end of the ETI is grasped while the operator keeps the laryngoscope in place. This is a critical, and often neglected, point. The operator then passes the ETT distally. As the tip of the ETT passes the glottis, the laryngoscopist should rotate it counterclockwise to facilitate passage through the vocal cords (Fig. 12-13A–C).

Failed Laryngoscopy and Intubation

When tracheal intubation is unsuccessful, the patient should be ventilated with BMV and high-flow oxygen if the saturations are <90%. During this reoxygenation time, the laryngoscopist should systematically analyze the likely causes of failure (Table 12-1). It makes no sense to attempt a second laryngoscopy without changing something in the procedure to improve chances for success. The following questions should be addressed:

- Is the patient in the optimum position for laryngoscopy and intubation? If the patient was placed in the sniffing position initially and the larynx still appears quite anterior, reducing the degree of head extension could be helpful. It may occasionally help to elevate and flex the patient's head and neck with the laryngoscopist's free right hand while performing laryngoscopy to create a better view of a true anterior airway.

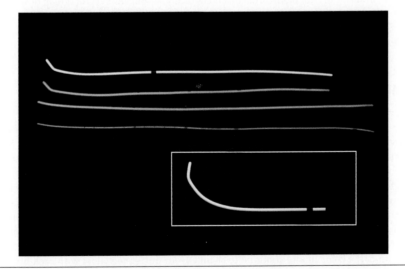

Figure 12-11 ● Endotracheal Tube Introducers (Bougies).   The classic gum elastic bougies (yellow) are reusable, 60 to 70 cm long, and available with straight and Coudé tip designs. A reusable (blue) polyethylene introducer is available with a Coudé tip and is 60 cm in length. Adult tracheal tube introducers are 5 mm in diameter. A thinner pediatric introducer can accommodate a 4.0-mm ETT. The lower right inset demonstrates the 60° optimal curve for attempting intubation when none of the glottic structures (only the epiglottis) can be visualized with laryngoscopy.

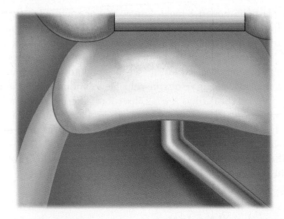

Figure 12-12 ● Endotracheal tube introducer (bougie) facilitating intubation with difficult (grade III—"epiglottis only" view) laryngoscopy. The disposable blue introducer is passed beneath the epiglottis and then anteriorly and caudally through the glottic inlet. The operator can immediately confirm tracheal placement by feeling the introducer against the tracheal rings or feeling a hard stop as the introducer enters a bronchus.

- Would a different blade provide a better view? If the initial attempt at laryngoscopy was done with a curved blade, it may be advisable to change to a straight blade, and vice versa. Alternatively, a different size blade of either type might be helpful.
- Is the patient adequately paralyzed? Appropriate paralysis can improve the view of laryngoscopy one full Cormack–Lehane grade. Laryngoscopy may have been attempted too soon after administering succinylcholine, or an inadequate dose of succinylcholine may have been administered. If the total time of paralysis has been such that the effect of succinylcholine is dissipating, then administration of a second full paralyzing dose of succinylcholine is advisable. Atropine should be available to treat bradycardia that occasionally accompanies repeat dosing of succinylcholine.
- Would external laryngeal manipulation be helpful? Manipulation of the thyroid cartilage by the laryngoscopist or the assistant often improves the laryngeal view by one full Cormack–Lehane grade.
- Is a more experienced laryngoscopist available? If so, a call for help may be in order.

CONFIRMING INTUBATION OF THE TRACHEA

Once the ETT has been placed, it is imperative to confirm that it is in the trachea. The current standard is the detection of end-tidal carbon dioxide ($ETCO_2$). Both qualitative colorimetric detectors and quantitative capnography are nearly 100% accurate for confirming tracheal tube placement in patients who are not in cardiac arrest. In the setting of cardiac arrest, continuous waveform capnography is the most reliable method for confirming correct ETT placement. Colorimetric $ETCO_2$ detectors quickly change from purple ("poor") to yellow ("yes") when $ETCO_2$ is detected. This color change should occur within a few breaths after tracheal intubation, and a lack of color change indicates an esophageal intubation. Uncommonly, CO2 from the stomach can create a color change to yellow, but this will revert to purple within 4-6 breaths, With proper tracheal intubation, the color should continue to change from purple to yellow with each breath. A color change to tan, rather than bright yellow, may indicate esophageal or supraglottic misplacement. In cardiac arrest, colorimetric detectors are of limited value because the $ETCO_2$ may be less than the detectable limit for color change (usually 5% CO_2 in exhaled gas), so capnography or suction esophageal detection devices (see below) should be used. When waveform capnography is used, tracheal intubation is confirmed by visualization of a square waveform that persists for at least six breaths. Absence of a waveform confirms esophageal placement. In cardiac arrest, the presence

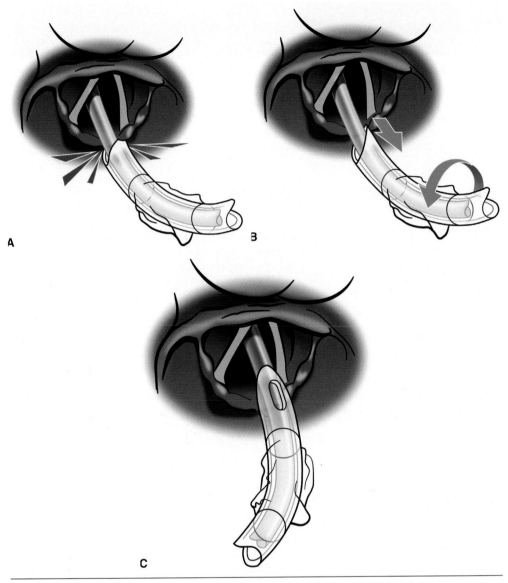

Figure 12-13 ● **A–C:** Counterclockwise rotation of the endotracheal tube (ETT) during insertion over an introducer. **A:** The tip of the ETT is hung up on the glottis, which is common. **B:** The ETT is withdrawn 1 to 2 cm and then rotated 90° counterclockwise. **C:** With the bevel facing posteriorly, the ETT passes smoothly through the glottis.

of a waveform confirms endotracheal intubation, whereas the lack of a waveform is ambiguous, requiring use of an alternative detection method. There are two types of suction esophageal detecting devices (EDDs): the piston syringe and the self-inflating bulb. Studies have shown that the sensitivity of the self-inflating bulb is greater than that of the piston syringe. The principle behind these devices is simple; releasing the deflated bulb or pulling back on the piston creates a negative pressure at the tip of the device. The negative pressure causes the esophagus to collapse around the tip of the device in an esophageal intubation, preventing the bulb from reinflating or the syringe plunger from being pulled back easily. The trachea does not collapse with negative pressure, so tracheal placement is confirmed if the bulb reinflates or the piston is easily pulled

<table>
<tr><td colspan="2">

TABLE 12-1
Errors Associated with Failed Laryngoscopy

</td></tr>
<tr><td>Rushed/frantic laryngoscopy</td><td>If the patient is rapidly desaturating, do not try to intubate hurriedly. Use BMV to improve oxygenation and then perform relaxed, methodical laryngoscopy</td></tr>
<tr><td>Laryngoscopy without a plan</td><td>Do not just insert the blade and hope that the vocal cords appear. This will usually result in advancing the blade too deeply missing anatomic landmarks. Use a methodical approach with progressive visualization of anatomic structures—follow the tongue to the epiglottis and then the epiglottis to the vocal cords</td></tr>
<tr><td>Poor tongue control</td><td>No tongue should be visible on the right side of the blade during properly performed laryngoscopy. This will prevent good visualization of the glottis and passage of the ETT</td></tr>
<tr><td>Poor ergonomics</td><td>Holding the laryngoscope incorrectly, bending over in an awkward position, resting your elbow on the patient or the bed, and positioning your eyes too close to the procedure are recipes for failure</td></tr>
</table>

back. These devices are quite sensitive and specific, but are not perfect, so they should be used in combination with other confirmation methods, such as visualizing the ETT passing through the vocal cords. Bronchoscopic confirmation of tracheal intubation is helpful when other methods of confirmation are confusing, especially in cardiac arrest. Auscultation is important for detecting mainstem intubation and pulmonary pathology but is unreliable for confirming tracheal tube placement. Chest X-rays should not be used to differentiate whether the ETT is in the trachea or the esophagus, but only to assess proper ETT depth and to evaluate for mainstem intubation. Fogging (condensation) of the ETT is a *completely unreliable* method of confirming tracheal intubation and should not be used.

EVIDENCE

- **How should the head and neck be best positioned for laryngoscopy?** Cormack and Lehane devised the most widely accepted system of categorizing the view of the larynx achieved with an orally placed laryngoscope.[1] More recently, Levitan et al.[2] devised a scoring system to quantitate the percentage of glottic opening visible, which is becoming used more frequently in the literature. The sniffing position (head extension and neck flexion) has been widely accepted as the optimum position for orotracheal intubation. However, there is conflicting evidence that increased head elevation (increased neck flexion) or just simple extension (head extension and neck extension) may be better than the sniffing position.[3,4] For difficult intubations, there is even literature to support simple flexion (head flexion and neck flexion) to optimize visualization.[5,6] Although the question of optimal head positioning remains, it is likely that it will vary from patient to patient. This highlights the importance of a two-handed technique for intubation, allowing for individualized adjustments during laryngoscopy. Morbidly obese patients should be placed in a "ramped" position, with significant elevation of the shoulders, neck, and head such that a horizontal line can be drawn from the external auditory meatus to the sternal angle of Louis.[7–9]
- **Is thyroid cartilage manipulation during laryngoscopy really necessary?** It has clearly been shown that external laryngeal manipulation, one example of which is BURP, improves

laryngeal view grade by one full grade, on average.[10–12] In addition, one recent study demonstrated the importance of operator-directed laryngeal manipulation (as opposed to assistant-directed manipulation) in maximizing visualization of the glottic structures.[13] The importance of laryngoscopy being a bimanual technique is emphasized regardless of which direction the thyroid cartilage is displaced.

- **Is an ETI or bougie truly helpful?** The literature clearly supports the use of ETIs to enhance success rates of intubation, particularly with grade 3 views.[14–18] In one study, the success rate improved from 66% to 96% when an ETI was used.[15] When using an ETI, it is important to continue laryngoscopy while the ETT is placed over the ETI and rotate the ETT counterclockwise as it passes through the larynx. Also, it may help to release cricoid pressure as the ETT is passed over the ETI.[19] Pathogenic bacteria may colonize ETIs and their containers, so it may be best to use disposable ETIs.[20] Bronchial perforation is a rare complication of using an ETI.[21]

- **Does it matter which laryngoscopic blade I use?** It is generally believed that one's choice of a laryngoscope blade and the technique used to facilitate intubation is best guided by personal choice and experience.[10,22,23] The literature suggests that straight blades improve laryngoscopic view (increased exposure of the vocal cords), whereas curved blades provide better intubating conditions (continuous visualization of the vocal cords during ETT passage).[23] Using an EI improves intubation success rates with the straight-blade technique.[15]

- **What are the best methods for confirming correct ETT placement?** No confirmation method is perfect, so providers should always use a combination of clinical assessment and detection devices. Continuous waveform capnography is recommended by the American Heart Association as the most reliable method for confirming and monitoring correct placement of an ETT.[24] Waveform capnographers provide a quantitative measure of $ETCO_2$ as well as a distinct repeating waveform that facilitates continuous monitoring of ETT position, even in most cases of cardiac arrest.[24–29] An $ETCO_2$ waveform may be absent in cases of prolonged cardiac arrest or monitor malfunction, but good chest compressions and a viable patient will usually produce a detectible waveform. Colorimetric and non-waveform exhaled CO_2 detectors are not as useful in cardiac arrest but are nearly 100% accurate for confirming correct ETT placement in patients who are not in cardiac arrest.[30–35] Soft drinks in the stomach containing CO_2 may mimic the exhaled CO_2 from the lungs for a few breaths, the so-called Cola complication; this confounding result ought not to persist beyond six breaths.[26,36]

There are several types of EDDs that detect esophageal intubation by creating negative pressure in the ETT, causing the walls of the esophagus to collapse around the tip of the ETT. Although these devices detect about 99% of esophageal intubations, and are better in cases of prolonged cardiac arrest, they are generally less accurate than $ETCO_2$ devices.[29,31,37–44] EDDs can give false-positive results (indicating an esophageal intubation when the ETT is correctly placed in the trachea) in morbidly obese patients and those with copious airway secretions.

It would be reasonable to believe that visualization of the ETT entering the larynx is a reliable method of verifying correct ETT position, but large studies have shown that additional confirmation methods are necessary, even when experienced providers place the ETT.[45] Flexible bronchoscopy is a reliable method for verifying correct ETT placement by permitting the direct visualization of tracheal rings.[46] However, this equipment is not available in many emergency settings and identification of the airway may be confusing for providers who do not perform bronchoscopy regularly. Auscultation of the chest for breath sounds and of the epigastrium for absence of air entry into the stomach and observation of chest motion during ventilation are common but notoriously inaccurate methods of confirming correct ETT placement.[45,47] Looking for condensation inside the ETT is a completely unreliable method for confirming correct placement.[48]

None of these techniques alone guarantee correct placement, and as many of them as possible should be used in every case.

REFERENCES

1. Cormack RS, Lehane J. Difficult tracheal intubation in obstetrics. *Anaesthesia*. 1984;39:1105–1111.

2. Levitan RM, Ochroch EA, Kush S, et al. Assessment of airway visualization: validation of the percentage of glottic opening (POGO) scale. *Acad Emerg Med*. 1998;5:919–923.

3. Adnet F, Baillard C, Borron SW, et al. Randomized study comparing the "sniffing position" with simple head extension for laryngoscopic view in elective surgery patients. *Anesthesiology*. 2001;95:836–841.

4. Levitan RM, Mechem CC, Ochroch EA, et al. Head-elevated laryngoscopy position: improving laryngeal exposure during laryngoscopy by increasing head elevation. *Ann Emerg Med*. 2003;41:322–330.

5. Hochman II, Zeitels SM, Heaton JT. Analysis of the forces and position required for direct laryngoscopic exposure of the anterior vocal folds. *Ann Otol Rhinol Laryngol*. 1999;108:715–724.

6. Zeitels SM. Universal modular glottiscope system: the evolution of a century of design and technique for direct laryngoscopy. *Ann Otol Rhinol Laryngol Suppl*. 1999;179:2–24.

7. Brodsky JB, Lemmens HJ, Brock-Utne JG, et al. Anesthetic considerations for bariatric surgery: proper positioning is important for laryngoscopy. *Anesth Analg*. 2003;96:1841–1842; author reply 1842.

8. Brodsky JB, Lemmens HJ, Brock-Utne JG, et al. Morbid obesity and tracheal intubation. *Anesth Analg*. 2002;94:732–736; table of contents.

9. Collins JS, Lemmens HJ, Brodsky JB, et al. Laryngoscopy and morbid obesity: a comparison of the "sniff" and "ramped" positions. *Obes Surg*. 2004;14:1171–1175.

10. Benumof JL, Cooper SD. Quantitative improvement in laryngoscopic view by optimal external laryngeal manipulation. *J Clin Anesth*. 1996;8:136–140.

11. Knill RL. Difficult laryngoscopy made easy with a "BURP." *Can J Anaesth*. 1993;40:279–282.

12. Takahata O, Kubota M, Mamiya K, et al. The efficacy of the "BURP" maneuver during a difficult laryngoscopy. *Anesth Analg*. 1997;84:419–421.

13. Levitan RM, Kinkle WC, Levin WJ, et al. Laryngeal view during laryngoscopy: a randomized trial comparing cricoid pressure, backward-upward-rightward pressure, and bimanual laryngoscopy. *Ann Emerg Med*. 2006;47:548–555.

14. Combes X, Le Roux B, Suen P, et al. Unanticipated difficult airway in anesthetized patients: prospective validation of a management algorithm. *Anesthesiology*. 2004;100:1146–1150.

15. Gataure PS, Vaughan RS, Latto IP. Simulated difficult intubation. Comparison of the gum elastic bougie and the stylet. *Anaesthesia*. 1996;51:935–938.

16. Green DW. Gum elastic bougie and simulated difficult intubation. *Anaesthesia*. 2003;58:391–392.

17. Henderson JJ. Development of the "gum-elastic bougie." *Anaesthesia*. 2003;58:103–104.

18. Noguchi T, Koga K, Shiga Y, et al. The gum elastic bougie eases tracheal intubation while applying cricoid pressure compared to a stylet. *Can J Anaesth*. 2003;50:712–717.

19. McNelis U, Syndercombe A, Harper I, et al. The effect of cricoid pressure on intubation facilitated by the gum elastic bougie. *Anaesthesia*. 2007;62:456–459.

20. Cupitt JM. Microbial contamination of gum elastic bougies. *Anaesthesia*. 2000;55:466–468.

21. Viswanathan S, Campbell C, Wood DG, et al. The Eschmann tracheal tube introducer. (Gum elastic bougie). *Anesthesiol Rev*. 1992;19:29–34.

22. Practice guidelines for management of the difficult airway: an updated report by the American Society of Anesthesiologists Task Force on Management of the Difficult Airway. *Anesthesiology*. 2003;98:1269–1277.

23. Arino JJ, Velasco JM, Gasco C, et al. Straight blades improve visualization of the larynx while curved blades increase ease of intubation: a comparison of the Macintosh, Miller, McCoy, Belscope and Lee-Fiberview blades. *Can J Anaesth*. 2003;50:501–506.

24. Neumar RW, Otto CW, Link MS, et al. Part 8: adult advanced cardiovascular life support: 2010 American Heart Association Guidelines for Cardiopulmonary Resuscitation and Emergency Cardiovascular Care. *Circulation*. 2010;122:S729–S767.

25. Grmec S. Comparison of three different methods to confirm tracheal tube placement in emergency intubation. *Intensive Care Med*. 2002;28:701–704.

26. Ko FY, Hsieh KS, Yu CK. Detection of airway CO2 partial pressure to avoid esophageal intubation. *Zhonghua Min Guo Xiao Er Ke Yi Xue Hui Za Zhi*. 1993;34:91–97.

27. Linko K, Paloheimo M, Tammisto T. Capnography for detection of accidental oesophageal intubation. *Acta Anaesthesiol Scand*. 1983;27:199–202.

28. Silvestri S, Ralls GA, Krauss B, et al. The effectiveness of out-of-hospital use of continuous end-tidal carbon dioxide monitoring on the rate of unrecognized misplaced intubation within a regional emergency medical services system. *Ann Emerg Med*. 2005;45:497–503.

29. Tanigawa K, Takeda T, Goto E, et al. The efficacy of esophageal detector devices in verifying tracheal tube placement: a randomized cross-over study of out-of-hospital cardiac arrest patients. *Anesth Analg*. 2001;92:375–378.

30. Bhende MS, LaCovey DC. End-tidal carbon dioxide monitoring in the prehospital setting. *Prehosp Emerg Care*. 2001;5:208–213.

31. Bozeman WP, Hexter D, Liang HK, et al. Esophageal detector device versus detection of end-tidal carbon dioxide level in emergency intubation. *Ann Emerg Med*. 1996;27:595–599.

32. Li J. Capnography alone is imperfect for endotracheal tube placement confirmation during emergency intubation. *J Emerg Med*. 2001;20:223–229.

33. MacLeod BA, Heller MB, Gerard J, et al. Verification of endotracheal tube placement with colorimetric end-tidal CO2 detection. *Ann Emerg Med*. 1991;20:267–270.

34. Ornato JP, Shipley JB, Racht EM, et al. Multicenter study of a portable, hand-size, colorimetric end-tidal carbon dioxide detection device. *Ann Emerg Med*. 1992;21:518–523.

35. Varon AJ, Morrina J, Civetta JM. Clinical utility of a colorimetric end-tidal CO2 detector in cardiopulmonary resuscitation and emergency intubation. *J Clin Monit*. 1991;7:289–293.

36. Zbinden S, Schupfer G. Detection of oesophageal intubation: the cola complication. *Anaesthesia*. 1989;44:81.

37. Baraka A, Khoury PJ, Siddik SS, et al. Efficacy of the self-inflating bulb in differentiating esophageal from tracheal intubation in the parturient undergoing cesarean section. *Anesth Analg*. 1997;84:533–537.

38. Baraka A, Siddik S, Sfeir M, et al. The self-inflating bulb versus end-tidal capnography for confirming tracheal intubation in the parturient undergoing cesarean section. *Anesth Analg*. 1997;85:944.

39. Davis DP, Stephen KA, Vilke GM. Inaccuracy in endotracheal tube verification using a Toomey syringe. *J Emerg Med*. 1999;17:35–38.

40. Hendey GW, Shubert GS, Shalit M, et al. The esophageal detector bulb in the aeromedical setting. *J Emerg Med*. 2002;23:51–55.

41. Takeda T, Tanigawa K, Tanaka H, et al. The assessment of three methods to verify tracheal tube placement in the emergency setting. *Resuscitation*. 2003;56:153–157.

42. Tanigawa K, Takeda T, Goto E, et al. Accuracy and reliability of the self-inflating bulb to verify tracheal intubation in out-of-hospital cardiac arrest patients. *Anesthesiology*. 2000;93:1432–1436.

43. Tong YL, Sun M, Tang WH, et al. The tracheal detecting-bulb: a new device to distinguish tracheal from esophageal intubation. *Acta Anaesthesiol Sin*. 2002;40:159–163.

44. Wee MY. The oesophageal detector device. Assessment of a new method to distinguish oesophageal from tracheal intubation. *Anaesthesia*. 1988;43:27–29.

45. Holland R, Webb RK, Runciman WB. The Australian Incident Monitoring Study. Oesophageal intubation: an analysis of 2000 incident reports. *Anaesth Intensive Care*. 1993;21:608–610.

46. Hutton KC, Verdile VP, Yealy DM, et al. Prehospital and emergency department verification of endotracheal tube position using a portable, non-directable, fiberoptic bronchoscope. *Prehosp Disaster Med*. 1990;5:131–136.

47. Katz SH, Falk JL. Misplaced endotracheal tubes by paramedics in an urban emergency medical services system. *Ann Emerg Med*. 2001;37:32–37.

48. Kelly JJ, Eynon CA, Kaplan JL, et al. Use of tube condensation as an indicator of endotracheal tube placement. *Ann Emerg Med*. 1998;31:575–578.

13

Video Laryngoscopy

John C. Sakles • Calvin A. Brown III • Aaron E. Bair

INTRODUCTION

When the concept of orotracheal intubation was developed, more than 100 years ago, the procedure was performed blindly using palpation to identify the laryngeal inlet and guide the tube into the trachea. Shortly thereafter, laryngoscopes were invented, allowing for direct visualization of the larynx. These early laryngoscopes consisted of a metal spatula with a light bulb on the tip. The blade lifted the tongue out of the way, and the light bulb illuminated the glottic structures. The straight blade, or Miller blade, was introduced by Robert Miller in 1941, and 2 years later, Macintosh introduced the curved or Macintosh blade. Interestingly, little changed over the next five decades, and intubations largely were performed with Miller and Macintosh blades until the advent of video laryngoscopy from 2002 onward. This new approach to laryngoscopy involves placement of a micro-video camera along the laryngoscope blade to transmit glottic images to an external monitor, allowing the operator to perform tracheal intubation while watching the video screen instead of looking directly through the mouth. Video laryngoscopy has several important advantages over traditional direct laryngoscopy. First, fundamentally, video laryngoscopy transforms intubation from a technique requiring a straight line of sight from outside the patient's mouth to the glottic aperture to one in which the image is acquired by the video camera, placed beyond the tongue, and requiring no such straight line of sight. Second, video laryngoscopy magnifies the view of the airway and allows the operator to see the airway in greater detail. Third, some video laryngoscopes have an exaggerated anterior angulation of the blade and this, along with the placement of the video camera, allows the operator to see structures that would be difficult or impossible to see under direct vision. Furthermore, video laryngoscopy can enhance education by allowing other health care providers to visualize the anatomy, and perhaps guide and offer assistance during the process of intubation. The use of a video laryngoscope also makes it possible to record the procedure to provide an excellent teaching resource and documentation for the medical record. There have been several video laryngoscopes introduced over the past few years. This chapter reviews the most important and well-studied video laryngoscopes currently available on the market.

DEVICES

GlideScope Video Laryngoscope

Device components

GlideScope system

The original GlideScope video laryngoscope (GVL) consists of a micro-video camera encased within a sharply angulated blade, a rechargeable video liquid crystal display (LCD) monitor and a video cable that transmits the image. There are three system configurations for the GVL system and two mounting options. The monitor can be mounted on a mobile stand or attached to any available pole with a C-clamp. An alternative configuration of the GVL is associated with a hard shell case with foam compartments housing the monitor, cable, and room for all three blades. This configuration may be ideal for mobile or remote field emergency applications.

The laryngoscope portion of the GVL consists of a combined handle and laryngoscope blade that are made from durable medical-grade plastic. The video camera is placed in a recess midway along the undersurface of the laryngoscope blade, partially protecting it from contamination from bodily secretions. In addition, the GVL incorporates an antifog mechanism that heats the lens around the video camera, thereby eliminating fogging during laryngoscopy. There are four blade sizes for the GVL (GVL-2 through GVL-5). The GVL-2 is designed for small children (2 to 10 kg), whereas the GVL-5 is meant to overcome anatomic challenges seen with morbidly obese patients. The GVL size 3 and 4 blades are appropriate for small adults and large adults, respectively. Additionally, neonatal sizes are available with the single-use, Cobalt version. Because the GVL does not incorporate an endotracheal tube (ETT) guide or stylet connected to the device, ETTs of any size can be used.

The laryngoscope attaches to a portable LCD monitor through a video cable that also carries power to light-emitting diodes (LEDs) mounted alongside the video camera. The monitor has a video-out port that requires a proprietary cable to connect to the composite video input, allowing the image to be transmitted to another monitor or recording device. The monitor can be rotated to the optimal viewing angle, and the cradle rests on a mobile telescoping pole that allows easy adjustment of the height of the monitor. The unit is powered by standard alternating current or backup rechargeable lithium battery. The battery can provide 90 minutes of continuous use and has a low-battery indicator light to warn the operator that the unit must be plugged in.

GlideScope Cobalt/Cobalt AVL

The GlideScope Cobalt is a disposable one-time use version of the original design. The Cobalt consists of a flexible video baton housing the micro-video camera that inserts into a disposable clear plastic protective blade, called the Stat. The Cobalt video baton may connect to either of two different video displays. The original Cobalt uses the same color video LCD monitor as the GVL and is used in identical fashion as the original GlideScope. A new version, the Cobalt Advanced Video Laryngoscope (AVL), uses a high-definition video baton and digital video display (Fig. 13-1A). The monitor has similar dimensions to the original unit but has the benefit of a built-in tutorial as well as image and video clip acquisition that can be stored on a removable memory card. Currently, there are two baton sizes and four blade sizes available (GVL Stat sizes 1 to 4). The small baton works with Stat sizes 0, 1, and 2, and the large baton works with size 3 and 4 blades. The Cobalt blade is angled slightly more steeply than the original design. The primary advantage of the Cobalt is its single-use design—eliminating the logistical problems, costs, and downtime associated with high-level disinfection of the traditional GlideScope.

GlideScope Ranger

The GlideScope Ranger is a rugged, portable, battery-operated GlideScope unit designed for field use (Fig. 13-1B). It is operational in a wide variety of temperatures, humidity, and altitudes and weighs roughly 2 lb (0.9 kg), making it very portable. It uses a 3.5-in (9 cm) LCD screen that allows good image clarity even when used outdoors. The Ranger has two available blade sizes (Ranger GVL 3 and 4) both with a 60° viewing angle suitable for visualizing anterior airways. It also incorporates the antifogging system to maintain a clear view of the airway at all times. The video camera is positioned approximately halfway along the blade to protect the lens from contamination, including secretions, blood, and vomitus. The rechargeable lithium polymer battery provides 90 minutes of continuous use. The GlideScope Ranger is contained within a soft-sided case with belt attachments for ease of use and mobility. The manufacturer recently has developed the Ranger Single Use, which incorporates the Cobalt design within the Ranger system. Similar to the Cobalt, the Ranger Single Use has two different-sized batons and variably sized Stats.

Use of device

The GlideScope is intended as an everyday device for routine intubation and can also be considered an alternative airway device for difficult or failed airways. The device's distal angulation makes it ideally suited to visualize and intubate an anterior larynx where direct laryngoscopy has proven unsuccessful. Because the handle has a narrow profile and does not require direct visualization of the larynx through the mouth, it is useful when cervical mobility or mouth opening is limited. Patients in whom it is desirable to minimize movement of the neck are excellent candidates because little force is needed to expose the glottis with the laryngoscope blade. The GlideScope generally performs well in the presence of secretions, blood, and vomitus, and thus is a good choice even in these circumstances.

The GlideScope is used in the following manner to perform tracheal intubation (Box 13-1 and Fig. 13-2). The handle is grasped with the left hand, in the same fashion as a conventional laryngoscope, and the tip of the laryngoscope blade is gently inserted into the mouth, in the midline, under direct vision. The critical point here is to keep the handle in the midline as you enter further into the mouth, noting key midline structures, such as the uvula, as you advance. There is no sweeping

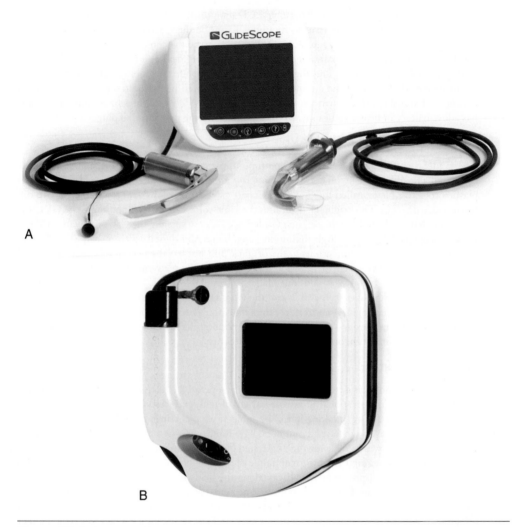

Figure 13-1 ● **A:** The GlideScope AVL showing the video baton inside the transparent Cobalt Stat blade **(right)** and the newly introduced GlideScope Direct Intubation Trainer **(left).** The high-resolution digital screen is able to record still images, video clips, and has a built-in tutorial. (Photo courtesy of Kevin Reilly, MD.) **B:** The GlideScope Ranger. The cord wraps around the device, and the blade locks in place on the left-hand side. The blade and cord detach from the monitor and can be sent for sterilization. The "working light" on the handle is helpful when using the device in low-light conditions such as in the prehospital setting. (Photo courtesy of Kevin Reilly, MD.)

of the tongue to the left as is done with conventional laryngoscopy. It is difficult to identify landmarks if the blade is off the midline. As soon as the tip of the laryngoscope blade passes the teeth, the operator should direct his or her attention to the video monitor and use the landmarks on the video screen to navigate to the glottic aperture. As mentioned above, the uvula will be seen if the blade is correctly situated in the midline. The operator should then continue to gently advance the blade down the tongue and past the uvula, with a slight elevating motion until the epiglottis is seen. At that point, it is best to continue advancing the blade into the vallecula, with some gentle upward force, to lift the epiglottis out of the way. The blade should ultimately be seated in the vallecula, much in the same way that a Macintosh blade is used. If the glottic view is insufficient, often a gentle tilt of the handle will expose it fully, in contrast to the lifting motion with a conventional

Box 13-1 The Four-step Method for GlideScope Intubation

1. Look into the mouth to introduce the blade
2. Look at the monitor to obtain the best view of the glottis
3. Look into the mouth to introduce the tube
4. Look at the monitor to guide the tube through the glottis

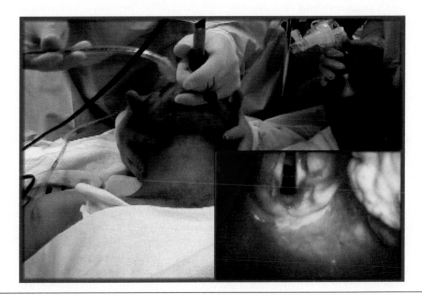

Figure 13-2 ● Intubation Using the Standard GlideScope. Note that the operator has the GlideScope placed directly in the midline and is inserting the tube from the right side of the mouth. The inset photo demonstrates what the operator sees on the GlideScope monitor. Note that the larynx appears in the upper half of the view. This is by design so the operator can see and direct the "approach" of the tube to the airway. A small amount of blood is present on the interarytenoid notch and right vocal cord.

laryngoscope. If the glottic aperture still cannot be exposed, the blade can be withdrawn slightly, placed under the epiglottis, and used like a Miller blade to physically displace the epiglottis up and out of the way. This motion can tilt the larynx more sharply, making advancement of the tube into the trachea technically more challenging. When an optimal glottic view (almost 100% of GVL views are either grade I or grade II) is obtained, the operator again looks into the mouth, to insert the ETT, with a stylet curved to match the curve of the GVL blade, alongside the blade. When the tube is placed where desired, the operator again views the video monitor to guide advancement of the tube to the glottis. Thus, intubation with the GlideScope can be thought of in four steps. For two of these steps, the operator is viewing the video monitor; for the other two, the operator is looking into the patient's mouth (see Box 13-1).

Identifying and exposing the glottis generally is easy using the GlideScope. However, advancing the ETT toward the image of the glottis displayed on the video screen can still be challenging. Negotiating the oropharynx and traversing the glottis with an acutely shaped ETT can be somewhat technically difficult for two reasons. First, the GlideScope blade is angulated at 60°, and thus, the angle of attack of the tube is quite steep. The second issue is that using the screen to navigate to the glottis requires a form of hand–eye coordination that is different from traditional direct laryngoscopy. The critical factor in getting the tube to enter the trachea is configuring the ETT into a shape that conforms to that of the GlideScope blade so that the ETT is able to follow the same trajectory as the blade. Under direct vision, the operator places the tip of the ETT in the corner of the right side of the patient's mouth with the tube nearly parallel to the ground (operator's hand at the 2- to 3-o'clock position) and advances the tube into position alongside the GVL blade. When the tube is felt to be well positioned, that is, proximate and parallel to the blade, the operator looks at the screen and advances the tube along its curved axis to guide it to the laryngeal inlet with the curvature heading anteriorly toward the airway. The manufacturer has developed a preformed rigid reusable ETT stylet (GlideRite Rigid Stylet) that is intended to provide an optimal curve and angle of approach to the glottis. If this stylet is not available, a malleable stylet can be shaped into a similar 60° curve. When the glottis is entered, the stylet is withdrawn 2 cm to reduce the rigidity of the sharply angulated distal tip of the tube, facilitating advancement into the trachea. Withdrawal of the stylet may be done by an assistant or by the intubator, particularly if using the proprietary stylet as it has a flange designed to be actuated by the operator's thumb. The manufacturer of the GVL has recently released the GlideRite Auto Stylet, which has a mechanism to withdraw the stylet and advance the ETT with the simple push of a button on the stylet. If the tube continues to impinge on the anterior trachea, the GlideScope can be withdrawn about 2 cm, causing the larynx to drop down, lessening the angle of approach and thus greatly facilitating further advancement of the tube. Additionally, the ETT can sometimes become engaged on the arytenoids or the anterior tracheal wall because of the steep anterior angle through the glottis. Using a soft tapered tip ETT, such as the proprietary Parker ETT, can help overcome this issue and facilitate intubation by easing entry of the tube through the glottic inlet.

The only absolute contraindication to use of the GlideScope is restricted mouth opening of <16 mm because this is the width of the widest portion of the blade.

The GlideScope GVL version laryngoscope blade/handle unit must be cleaned and disinfected after each use. Gross contaminants and large debris can be scrubbed off with a surgical scrub brush or enzymatically removed with a proteolytic compound such as Medzyme. Laryngoscope blades must undergo high-level disinfection. This can be accomplished with STERIS, STERRAD, ethylene oxide, or Cidex solutions, containing glutaraldehyde. The electrical connector cap should be placed over the contact port on the laryngoscope handle to prevent corrosion of the contacts. The only method of sterilization that is absolutely contraindicated is autoclaving, which involves exposure of the device to very high temperatures that will damage the electronic components of the video camera. In fact, the GlideScope has a silver temperature indicator on the side of the handle that turns black if the device is exposed to temperatures exceeding 80°C.

GlideScope Cobalt systems

Intubation is performed with the GlideScope Cobalt system in a manner analogous to that described above for the GVL. The major difference between this and the original version is the development of a disposable blade that attaches to a newly designed flexible video baton. The disposable blade slides easily over the flexible baton and locks in place with a notched mechanism. This combination provides a similar view to the original GlideScope, and the user can follow the previous recommendations for use. After the intubation is complete, the Stat can be removed, discarded, and returned to readiness by simply replacing the Stat. This design allows a more rapid turnaround time than sterilization. If necessary, the video baton can be cleaned and sterilized by using a nonautoclavable method such as STERRAD or STERIS.

GlideScope Direct Intubation Trainer

The GlideScope Direct Intubation Trainer (GVL Direct) is the newest addition to the GlideScope family of video laryngoscopes. Although clinical use of video laryngoscopy has been growing rapidly, health care providers continue to learn and maintain skills in direct laryngoscopy. To that end, the GVL Direct was developed (Fig. 13-1A). The GVL Direct is a metal blade that has the same look and feel of a standard Macintosh blade (roughly equivalent to a Macintosh "3.5"), except that it has a video camera on the undersurface of the blade. This allows the operator to perform a conventional direct laryngoscopy while an instructor monitors the procedure on the GlideScope monitor. Alternatively, if the operator has difficulty visualizing the airway during direct laryngoscopy, the video monitor can be used to facilitate visualization and complete the intubation videoscopically. The GVL Direct can be used in the same fashion as the other GVL blades or in a manner used for direct laryngoscopy. If intended for use as a video laryngoscope, the blade is inserted down the midline, and when used as a direct laryngoscope, it should be inserted in the right-hand corner of the mouth so that the tongue can be swept to the left, as for direct laryngoscopy (see Chapter 12). At the time of this writing, there have been no studies using the GVL Direct, but preliminary clinical experience demonstrates a very high rate of success with this device for emergency intubations. The GVL Direct thus shows promise both for use as a direct laryngoscope (particularly in a training setting) and as a video laryngoscope, either primarily or when intubation through direct visualization is not possible.

At the time of this writing, the manufacturer of the GlideScope announced some new GlideScope products that are on the near horizon. One version of the GVL will have a tube guide on the anterior surface of the blade to direct the tube through the glottis inlet without the need for a stylet. The channel blade will be available in a reusable version, as well as a disposable stat blade that covers the handle as well as the blade to mimimize infection transmission. The GlideScope Direct trainer system is to be expanded to include a disposable blade. A new pediatric Cobalt blade, size 2.5, will allow for intubation of children up to 5 years of age. A novel apneic oxygenation stylet will deliver oxygen at up to 15 L per minute. This has the potential to reduce periods of hypoxia during the intubation.

Summary

The GlideScope is a rugged, well-designed device designed for both routine and difficult intubation. There are multiple configurations and blade sizes that allow the devices to be used in a variety of clinical situations. Because of its anterior video angulation, antifog capabilities, and capacity to maintain an adequate view despite secretions, the GlideScope is particularly useful for anticipated or identified difficult emergency intubations.

C-MAC Video Laryngoscope

Device components

The C-MAC video laryngoscope system (Karl Storz, Tuttlingen, Germany) replaces earlier versions of hybrid video-fiberoptic systems. The C-MAC system uses a CMOS micro-video camera, which provides an enhanced field of view and resists fogging. The device also incorporates a video recording system, with controls on the handle, which supports both teaching and quality management. The C-MAC is powered by a rechargeable lithium battery, permitting 90 minutes of operation without a power source. The system comprises a variety of blades that accommodate the video camera, which connects through a single cable to a 7-in (17.8 cm) video screen, with straightforward controls (Fig. 13-3). One series of the C-MAC blades maintains standard Macintosh geometry and can be used for direct laryngoscopy as well as video laryngoscopy. Because more traditional laryngoscopic mechanics are used, the trajectory from the mouth to the glottic opening is almost straight and a rigid preformed stylet is not required. Tube insertion tends to be easier with the C-MAC than with the GlideScope because the stylet is shaped as for conventional laryngoscopy, thus permitting more direct insertion and avoiding the impingement on the anterior trachea that occurs with the GlideScope. In fact, when using the C-MAC, the operator can direct the tube along the curvature of the blade, using the right angle flange as a guide, without obstructing the view of the airway. Currently, there are several blades available. The standard C-MAC blades are available in sizes 2, 3, and 4, which compare to standard Macintosh 2, 3, and 4 blades. In addition, straight Miller blades have just been introduced for use in pediatric patients. Other configurations include the D-Blade, which is more sharply curved, resembling that of the GlideScope. This is intended to improve glottic visualization when the larynx is high in the neck (anterior) or in other difficult laryngoscopy situations where there are limitations with the standard geometry of Macintosh-based curvatures. The C-MAC monitor is portable and can be placed on any flat surface near the bedside but is likely most useful when mounted to a pole and used in conjunction with a mobile stand. The newest version

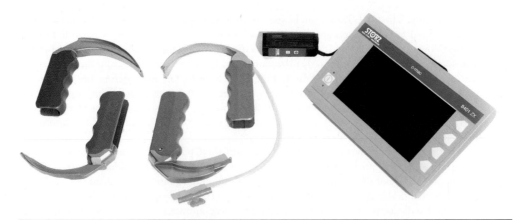

Figure 13-3 ● **The C-MAC Video Laryngoscope.** Shown are the monitor and four blades. The three blades on the left are the standard Mac 2, 3, and 4 blades. The blade to the far right is the newly introduced D-blade with a sharply angulated curve and a suction channel on the side. (Photo courtesy of Kevin Reilly, MD.)

of the C-MAC has a 2.4 inch monitor directly attached to the handle, thus eliminating cables and external viewers.

As is the case for other video laryngoscopes, the C-MAC blades cannot be autoclaved because this will damage the electronic circuitry of the micro-video camera. However, most other types of high-level disinfection such as STERIS, STERRAD, and Cidex are acceptable.

Use of device

The C-MAC can be plugged into any wall outlet, or is cordless if it is fully charged. The video cartridge slides into the laryngoscope handle and the video cable plugs into the back of the monitor. There is a single power switch. The image autofocuses and image clarity is automatically maximized. Antifog is not required once the device has warmed for 90 seconds. The blade can

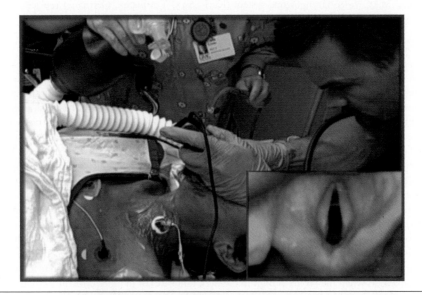

Figure 13-4 ● **Intubation Using the C-MAC.** The glottic image is shown in the lower right. Note that the operator is using the C-MAC to perform direct laryngoscopy while a supervising physician is monitoring the procedure by watching the video screen of the C-MAC.

be inserted like a traditional Macintosh blade when being used as a teaching device, but for video laryngoscopy, it is inserted in the midline because the placement of the video camera makes the traditional tongue sweep unnecessary. The operator inserts the blade until the distal tip is past the uvula, and then advances in the midline while observing the screen until the epiglottis comes into view. The blade tip is placed within the vallecula (usual) or under the epiglottis (alternative) to provide visualization of the glottic inlet (Fig. 13-4). The angle of attack is less acute than with the GlideScope, and the tube is curved in a similar shape that is used for conventional direct laryngoscopy.

As of this writing, the manufacturer plans to release an expanded range of blades of the Miller type, including sizes 0 and 1, permitting use in small children. A disposable blade system also is planned, as is a camera adaptor for standard eyepieces of flexible and rigid fiberoptic scopes allowing display on the C-MAC video screen.

Summary

As is the case for the GlideScope, the Storz C-MAC is another dramatic improvement over direct laryngoscopy. The system is simple to learn and use, has autofocus and antifogging capabilities, and provides a wide field of view for intubation. The system is useful as a primary video laryngoscope for routine and difficult intubations, the latter being facilitated by the D-blade, and also as a training aid, with the trainee performing a conventional direct laryngoscopy and the instructor viewing the image on the screen.

McGRATH Video Laryngoscope Series 5

Device components

The McGRATH video laryngoscope (MVL) (Fig. 13-5) consists of three main parts. First, the handle of the video laryngoscope is made of latex-free medical-grade rubber and stainless steel, housing a single AA battery to power the device and an attached 1.7-in (4.3 cm) color LCD monitor. The power button is placed at the top of the handle. Second is the camera stick, a module that incorporates a light source and a micro-video camera to illuminate and provide a view of the glottis. The last component is a disposable laryngoscope blade made of medical-grade optical polymer that slides over and attaches to the camera stick. The blade can be adjusted into three different positions, purportedly to create the desired length to facilitate intubation for various anatomical and patient differences. However, in practice, the working portion of the blade tends to remain the same, regardless of the blade position on the handle, and there is not a locking mechanism for the three blade positions, and thus, the potential exists for the blade to slip when force is applied during intubation. A locking pin keeps the blade from disengaging completely from the handle. The MVL neither incorporates antifog technology nor incorporates a channel guide within the blade, so any ETT size can be used using a standard stylet.

The LCD screen is attached to the proximal portion of the handle module and can be adjusted for an optimal viewing angle. Placement of the screen at the top of the handle improves operator comfort by allowing visualization of the device and patient simultaneously. The LCD screen can be rotated to a variety of positions to optimize clarity and can be rotated along the axis of the handle, so the device can lay completely flat when not in use. The camera, display, and light are powered by a single AA 1.5-V battery providing approximately 60 minutes of operating time. A battery-warning indicator begins to flash when little operating time remains. The MVL does not incorporate an auto-off feature, so the device will exhaust the battery if inadvertently left on.

The MVL is constructed of durable materials and demonstrates a solid feel in the operator's hand. It is one of the most portable of all the video laryngoscopes because the screen is integrated into the end of the handle and it is void of cables. However, its ultraportable nature may also make it susceptible to loss and theft. The screen size is small, so visualization is not as good as with the larger monitors incorporated into the GlideScope and C-MAC systems. In addition, a protective carrying case is not included with the MVL, increasing the risk of damage during storage and transport.

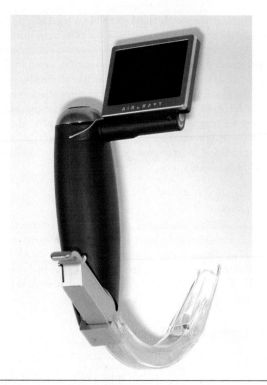

Figure 13-5 ● McGRATH Video Laryngoscope.   The disposable plastic blade is engaged on the camera stick. The camera stick is in the midposition. Sliding the camera stick forward one notch will lengthen the blade, allowing it to be used for larger patients, while retracting it one notch will shorten it, allowing it to be used for smaller patients. The video monitor is attached to the upper aspect of the handle and can be rotated to the optimal position for viewing. (Photo courtesy of Kevin Reilly, MD.)

Use of device

The shape and size of the blade of the MVL are almost identical fashion to those of the GlideScope, and the device is used in much the same manner. There is little setup needed for the MVL, and once a disposable blade is placed on the camera stick and the device turned on, it is ready for use (Fig. 13-6). Similar to the other video laryngoscopes, the MVL is inserted into the patient's mouth in the midline. The tip of the blade is then guided into the vallecula and tilted to lift the epiglottis anteriorly, similar to a conventional Macintosh blade. As with the GlideScope and C-MAC, the blade tip can be placed in the vallecula or under the surface of the epiglottis. Once a clear view of the airway appears on the LCD screen, the operator looks back into the mouth to insert and align the acutely curved or shaped ETT as for the GlideScope. The tube is advanced into the trachea while visualizing the process on the video screen. The manufacturer recommends the ETT be bent sharply at a point roughly 5 cm from the tip of the tube. This facilitates advancement of the tip of the tube through the glottic inlet. Use of the GlideRite proprietary stylet can also facilitate directing the tube through the laryngeal inlet. In either case, impingement of the tube on the anterior wall of the trachea can occur, and is mitigated by withdrawing the stylet 2 cm when the glottis is entered.

After intubation, the disposable blade is removed and discarded while the handle is cleaned with an antiseptic towelette. The disposable blade does not protect the handle or proximal portion of the device; therefore, it is susceptible to contamination, and the rubber handle can be difficult to clean and sterilize. The original MVL could not undergo any immersion sterilization processes or hydrogen peroxide sterilization process (STERIS or STERRAD), but a new version of the MVL (MVL Series 5 HLDi) can undergo complete high-level disinfection.

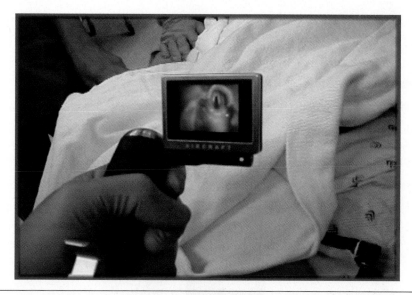

Figure 13-6 • Intubation Using the McGRATH Video Laryngoscope. As with other video laryngoscopes, the device is inserted in the midline and can be used with either a straight-blade approach or a curved blade approach. The picture shows the view of the glottis as seen with a curved blade approach, which tends to cause less distortion of the laryngeal anatomy and facilitates tube passage. This view was the initial view attained during laryngoscopy. As the blade was left in the patient's mouth during laryngoscopy, the lens became increasingly fogged, making visualization of the structures much more difficult. It is highly recommended that antifog solution be applied to the tip of the blade before insertion.

McGRATH MAC Video Laryngoscope

A newer version of the McGRATH video laryngoscope, called the McGRATH MAC, is based on the original McGRATH Series 5, but has several important differences. Foremost, rather than using a highly angulated blade, the McGRATH MAC, as its name implies, uses a standard curved Macintosh blade. The McGRATH MAC, therefore, can be used to perform or teach direct laryngoscopy, in a manner comparable to that of the Storz C-MAC video laryngoscope. Use as a direct laryngoscope might serve as a fallback technique if the lens becomes contaminated and the video view is compromised. As for the Series 5, the McGRATH MAC uses a CameraStick, onto which plastic disposable blades, which are provided in sizes 2, 3, and 4, are placed. There is no heat-based antifogging system on the McGRATH MAC, but the manufacturer claims that the blades have a hydrophilic polymer optical surface that resists condensation. The screen on the McGRATH MAC is a 2.5-in (6.3 cm), vertically oriented monitor, and the system uses a proprietary 3.6-V lithium disposable battery. The battery has a runtime of 250 continuous minutes, and an indicator on the bottom of the video monitor image counts down the exact number of minutes left on the battery. There is very limited clinical experience with the McGRATH MAC to date, and no published reports at the time of this writing, but the new design looks promising. Although portability is an advantage, the small screen size, lack of a heat-based antifogging system, and lack of a video out option will likely limit the usefulness of the device in emergency situations.

Summary

The McGRATH is a compact, easy-to-use, intuitive device. The device is comfortable in the operator's hand and does not require prolonged setup time. However, the blade is narrower than the other devices, and for patients with large tongues, this can hinder the operator's view. Without the application of antifogging solution, the blade fogs quickly. The delicate nature of the device and lack of an included case make it less suitable for prehospital use. Although there are few studies comparing the McGRATH to conventional laryngoscopy, performance should be superior as for other video laryngoscopes. The new McGRATH MAC video laryngoscope may overcome some of the problems evident with the series 5.

Pentax Airway Scope

Device components

The Pentax Airway Scope (AWS) consists of two components (Fig. 13-7). The first, an unconventional handle with a more linear design that encompasses a monitor screen, power button, battery compartment, video-out port, locking connection ring for the disposable blade, and a flexible cable

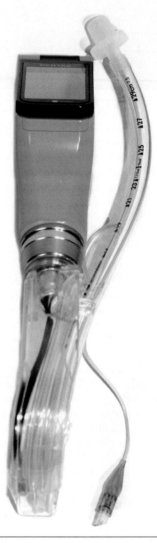

Figure 13-7 ● **Pentax Airway Scope.** The disposable blade is attached to the rigid handle. On the side of the blade, the tube guide that holds the endotracheal tube in place can be seen. The video monitor is on the upper posterior aspect of the handle and can flip up for easier viewing or for viewing when intubating the patient face to face. An optional disposable clear plastic sleeve can be placed on the handle to protect it from gross contamination by body fluids. (Photo courtesy of Kevin Reilly, MD.)

that houses the light source and CCD micro-video camera that provides 90° of visualization. The AWS has a disposable sleeve that covers and protects the reusable handle from contamination. The second component is a polycarbonate Lexan disposable blade (PBlade) that incorporates an ETT channel and 12F suction port. The blade does not feature an antifog mechanism; however, the Lexan plastic technology used in the blade resists fogging and contamination. As of this writing, only a single adult-size blade is available that will accept ETT sizes between 6.0 and 8.5 mm internal diameter. The ETT can be preloaded alongside the disposable blade with clips that hold the tube in place. The AWS has a green targeting reticle that can be displayed on the LCD screen to guide the user into the correct position for ETT placement. This targeting reticle is sometimes helpful as the side-mounted ETT does not advance into the true center of the field of view. The 2.4-in (6.1 cm) color LCD monitor is attached to the handle and can be tilted into various positions to allow easier viewing. The AWS has video output capabilities, allowing the image to be transmitted to an external video monitor or recording device. The AWS is powered by two AA 1.5-V batteries that provide approximately 60 minutes of continuous operation. A low-battery indicator flashes to alert the operator when 5 minutes of battery life remain. The AWS has a protective soft carrying case with preformed foam compartments to house the scope, video cables, and extra batteries. The case does not include space to carry blades.

The AWS is solidly built of strong plastic and stainless steel. It is somewhat larger and more awkward to hold than the three devices discussed earlier in this chapter. The unit is water resistant and portable, making it a reasonable option for prehospital use.

Use of device

There is little setup necessary for the AWS. A disposable blade is locked onto the video cable, a lubricated ETT is loaded, the optional plastic sheath is secured, and the device is turned on and ready for use (Fig. 13-8). The operator may activate the targeting reticle on the LCD by pressing the on–off button. Antifog solution is recommended for use because the Lexan plastic resists fogging but does not eliminate it. The device is inserted into the mouth and advanced in the midline

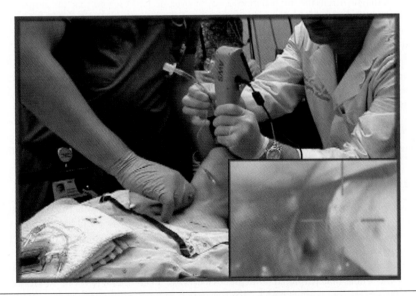

Figure 13-8 ● **Intubation Using the Pentax Airway Scope.** The operator is guiding the tube into the airway by advancing it through the tube guide. No stylet is necessary. The inset photo shows the view of the glottis seen on the attached monitor by the operator. The scope must be positioned so the green targeting reticle is centered over the glottic inlet. Note, the reticle is to the right of the glottic inlet. Also, the tip of the blade must lift the epiglottis out of the way so the tube can pass unobstructed into the airway.

along the posterior pharyngeal wall, resulting in elevation of the epiglottis. Unlike the earlier three devices, the AWS must be used to lift the epiglottis directly. If the tip of the blade is placed in the vallecula, the tube will engage the epiglottis as it emerges from the channel and the intubation will not be successful. The reticle is "aimed" at the vocal cords for appropriate position. The reduction in ETT maneuverability requires the AWS to be positioned correctly in front of the glottic inlet and decreases the operator flexibility to manipulate the ETT and the laryngoscope independently. Therefore, the operator does not use a stylet or provide manual control over the distal portion of the ETT. The ETT is advanced from the channel through the vocal cords. The AWS has the option of recording the intubation through the video output port and a proprietary RCA cable. This feature allows recording of the entire intubation for later viewing and teaching purposes. The AWS can be rinsed in water without submersion and wiped clean. The protective sheath and disposable blade make the AWS easy to clean and quickly ready for another intubation.

Summary

The AWS is a well-built video laryngoscope with outstanding optics. However, the lack of an anti-fog mechanism can impair the quality of the image and make successful intubation more difficult. A more significant issue with the design of the AWS is tendency of the optical elements of the device to pass through secretions or blood that may be pooled in the posterior pharynx. This can contaminate the optics of the AWS and make visualization of the airway very difficult or impossible, and is different from most other video laryngoscopes, which are advanced along the tongue, clear of most secretions or blood that might be pooling in the (supine) patient's oral pharynx.

King Vision Video Laryngoscope

Device components and setup

The King Vision video laryngoscope (KVL) from King Systems is a relative newcomer to the video laryngoscope field (Fig. 13-9). This is a unique integrated blade and display device with a 2.4-in (6.1 cm) diagonal reusable high-definition color organic LED screen that sits atop a plastic staff, onto which a variety of single-use blades can be mounted. The screen has antiglare properties, a high-refresh rate for smooth image motion, provides autowhite balancing, and offers a 160° field of view. Blades with and without an integrated tube channel are available and are made of high-quality polycarbonate plastic. Both house a complementary metal oxide semi-conductor (CMOS) micro camera and LED light source and are disposable. The device is battery operated, lightweight, water resistant, and ultraportable. With three fresh alkaline AAA batteries, it can operate for 90 minutes, and a warning light informs the operator that power is low. Additionally an integrated power management system with auto-shutoff helps preserve battery life. There is a video-out port on the device that can be connected to a proprietary video cable that terminates in a composite plug. Thus the display can be output to a larger video monitor or recorded on a video recording device.

Use of device

The intubator should select a blade, either with or without a tube channel, and plug the reusable screen into the top. The KVL is rather long, and in some patients it will be difficult to insert the device into the mouth because the video screen impinges on the chest wall. There are two options to overcome this problem. One is to insert only the blade into the mouth initially, and then plug the video screen into it after the insertion. The other option is to insert the KVL into the mouth while the whole unit is rotated 90 degrees clockwise. Then after insertion, the device is rotated back 90 degrees counterclockwise so that it is in the patient's midline. If a blade with tube channel is used, a lubricated ETT should be preloaded into the device before insertion. After power up, the KVL is inserted into the midline of the mouth, similar to others in this class of devices, and advanced gently with only slight lifting force used to visualize the laryngeal inlet (Fig. 13-10). Once the vocal cords are visualized, the tube is advanced forward, down the channel and into the airway.

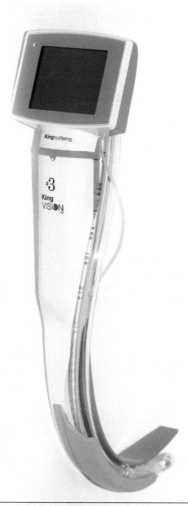

Figure 13-9 ● The King Vision Video Laryngoscope.   The video monitor attaches to the disposable blade at the purple interface line. Shown is the channeled King Vision with an endotracheal tube preloaded to the right of the blade. Blades are available without the channel and these require standard tube guidance with a stylet. (Photo courtesy of Kevin Reilly, MD.)

It is critical to rotate the ETT counterclockwise in the channel as you advance it toward the glottic inlet. This will prevent the ETT from engaging and getting blocked by the right arytenoid. If a nonchanneled blade is used, then a standard ETT with a preformed curved, malleable stylet should be used. Again, when inserting the tube into the mouth, the operator should be looking at the patient, not at the video screen. The tube should enter the right corner of the patient's mouth and is rotated counterclockwise until it is well proximated to the scope. The operator then looks to the video screen to identify the tip of the tube, and the tube is advanced through the glottis. Once the intubation is complete, the blade is discarded and the reusable screen can be cleaned with an aseptic wipe.

Summary

The new KVL is a novel, lightweight, integrated device that incorporates CMOS chip technology into a disposable blade design. The two blade configurations (channeled and unchanneled) give the

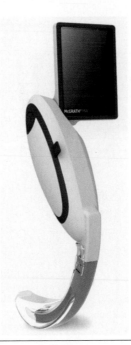

Figure 13-10 ● Intubation Using the King Vision Video Laryngoscope. This intubation is being performed with the channeled blade. Note that the assistant is preparing to hand the endotracheal tube to the operator. The device is being used in a curved blade fashion with the epiglottis being indirectly elevated to expose the glottis inlet.

device a great deal of flexibility as operators with different skill levels can choose the blade that works best for them. The cost of this device is considerably less than the other video laryngoscopes on the market. At the time of this writing, the device is newly released, so there is no clinical or research experience yet available. Initial clinical evaluation reveals that the device has significant potential.

CONCLUSION

The technology fundamental to video laryngoscopy is progressing at a rapid pace, and video laryngoscopy provides a superior glottic view with less effort than does direct laryngoscopy. Video laryngoscopy is a first-line technique both for routine and difficult airways. The video-assisted laryngoscopes outperform conventional laryngoscopy, especially in those patients with reduced mouth opening, cervical spine immobility, and head and facial trauma. Most users report only a handful of video laryngoscopies are necessary before they adopt the video laryngoscope as their everyday device, relegating direct laryngoscopy to a backup role. Several models have disposable versions that greatly reduce cleaning time and the potential spread of infectious agents. We have also discovered additional areas where these devices are particularly helpful: confirmation of ETT placement for patients in whom tube location is in question, visualization of upper airway obstructions and foreign material, and aiding in difficult tube exchanges. Most important, all video-assisted laryngoscopes allow real-time feedback for assistance or airway management education. The instructor can provide advice for successful intubation while allowing the operator to maintain control of the scope.

Direct laryngoscopy for the purpose of endotracheal intubation was introduced into clinical medicine almost a century ago. Since then, little has changed in its application and performance. The development of video laryngoscopes over the last decade, typified by the Glidescope, is a significant advancement in the field of laryngoscopy and intubation. As users become familiar with the distinct advantages conferred by the video laryngoscope, direct laryngoscopy largely will be abandoned as the primary method of airway management, both in emergency and in routine situations.

EVIDENCE

- **What is known about the GlideScope in clinical practice?** The GVL was the first video laryngoscope introduced into clinical practice and thus is the most extensively studied device. Several studies have looked at its performance both in routine intubations and in difficult airway scenarios. There is enough evidence currently to say, unequivocally, that the GlideScope provides better glottic visualization than direct laryngoscopy. Agro et al.[1] compared the glottic exposure achieved with the GlideScope to the view obtained with a Macintosh blade in 15 patients with cervical immobilization. They found that the GlideScope improved the Cormack–Lehane (C–L) view of the glottis by one grade in 14 out of 15 patients. In one patient, who was a grade III airway, the GlideScope did not improve the view of the glottis, so the patient was intubated with the aid of a bougie. The glottic views in this series of patients were poor during conventional laryngoscopy, when compared with a routine operating room (OR) population or with earlier intubation studies, suggesting a difficult airway cohort, although the author did not report this. For example, using a standard Macintosh blade, one patient was a grade 4, nine patients were grade 3, five patients were grade 2, and no patients were grade 1. Thus, in this small series, the vocal cords could be identified by conventional laryngoscopy in only 5 out of 15 patients (33%), compared with 95% in routine OR series. In an abstract by Sakles et al.,[2] the GlideScope (GVL) was compared with two fiberoptic airway devices, the UpsherScope (US) and the Shikani optical stylet (SOS; see Chapter 16). Emergency medicine residents with no earlier experience with these devices were asked to intubate manikins, and the success rate for each device and the time needed to perform the intubation were evaluated. The GVL was successful 100% of the time and, on average, required one attempt and 65 seconds to perform the intubation. The US had a success rate of 71% and, on average, required 1.4 attempts and 65 seconds. The SOS was successful in only 43% of the cases and, on average, required 2.2 attempts and 128 seconds. Sun et al.[3] performed a randomized clinical trial comparing the GlideScope to direct laryngoscopy. Two hundred healthy preoperative patients were randomly assigned to laryngoscopy with either a conventional Macintosh 3 blade or GlideScope. All patients were initially assigned a C–L grade by a separate anesthetist using a Mac 3. In most patients with C–L grade >1 (28/41), the laryngoscopic view was improved using the GlideScope, and nearly all patients with a C–L grade 3 or higher view had improvement in glottic exposure. However, time to ETT placement took an average of 16 seconds longer in the GlideScope group. In 2005, Cooper et al.[4] published a multicenter trial with 728 consecutive patients evaluated with both direct laryngoscopy and the GlideScope. Nearly all patients (99%) had a C–L grade of 1 or 2 using the GlideScope, which significantly improved a poor direct laryngoscopic view in the majority of cases. Intubation success was 96%, and failed intubations occurred despite adequate visualization, again suggesting that difficulty with ETT manipulation can impair intubation success. A 90° angle placed proximal to the cuff has been suggested as the optimal ETT shape to help facilitate tracheal intubation.[5,6] A smaller performance assessment in 50 preoperative surgical patients again showed laryngoscopic superiority of one to two C–L grades using the GlideScope compared with direct laryngoscopy.[7] In simulated difficult airway scenarios, the GlideScope also seems to perform equal to or better than direct laryngoscopy. A recent manikin study evaluated 30 anesthetists using a Macintosh laryngoscope versus the GlideScope in three simulated difficult airways: cervical rigidity, pharyngeal obstruction, and tongue edema.[8] Although numbers were small, the GlideScope was superior to direct laryngoscopy in the pharyngeal obstruction scenario. There was no significant advantage in the other settings. Other smaller studies have shown similar results with the GlideScope significantly outperforming conventional Macintosh laryngoscopes both in preoperative patients and in selected difficult airways such as ankylosing spondylitis.[9,10] In a compelling study, Tremblay et al.[11] evaluated 400 patients undergoing general anesthesia. All patients had direct laryngoscopy followed by GlideScope laryngoscopy. All 400 patients had a grade I or II video view and all but one were successfully intubated using GVL. The GlideScope has also made its way into mainstream practice. A large review of >70,000 OR intubations between 2007 and 2009 showed that the GlideScope was used in nearly 3% of all intubations. The majority (>80%) were either obese or had markers of potential airway management difficulty. Ultimate intubation success was 97%.[12] The GlideScope has successfully been integrated in at least one emergency medical services system with high intubation success rates and fewer attempts required compared with direct laryngoscopy.[13] Overall, the GlideScope is superior to direct laryngoscopy in providing optimal visualization of the laryngeal inlet and vocal cords in both routine and difficult airways. However, the data suggest a slightly longer time to tube placement, especially for routine (i.e., not anticipated difficult airways). An ETT configuration that includes a 90° angle may expedite intubation. Specialized, preformed ETTs with angled tips and easily retractable stylets are now available.

- **What are the advantages of the Video Macintosh Laryngoscope (V-MAC) or C-MAC video laryngoscope intubating systems?** Kaplan et al.[14] reported a large prospective multicenter trial of 865 patients undergoing general anesthesia with paralysis. Using the V-MAC, an earlier fiberoptic/video hybrid scope made by Storz, the operator would obtain the best view with direct visualization, and then record the best view by the video monitor. Intubation was then performed using the video monitor. Visualization was considered easy when a C–L grade 1 or 2 was obtained by either method and was significantly easier using the video monitor when compared with direct visualization. In addition, maneuvers such as external laryngeal manipulation and Backward, Upward, Rightward Pressure were less often needed for adequate visualization with video assistance. In addition to improving glottic exposure, the video laryngoscope will likely become an effective teaching tool for airway managers in training.[15] Brown et al.[16] looked at glottic exposure during emergency department intubations using the V-MAC. All patients enrolled underwent simultaneous direct and video laryngoscopy using the video Macintosh system. A best DL and best VL view were recorded for each patient. There were statistically higher proportions of "good glottic views" (C–L grade I or II) with VL and of 14 patient with a grade IV C–L direct view, 11 were converted to a grade I or II view using video technology. In one of the only C-MAC studies available to date, early OR experience has been reassuring. Cavus et al.[17] reviewed 60 C-MAC intubations in patients undergoing general anesthesia. All patients had a grade I or II video glottic view and were intubated successfully. We anticipate that the C-MAC will be a substantial improvement over the VMAC as the newer imaging technology provides a much greater field of view and is far less prone to fogging than its predecessor.
- **What evidence supports use of the McGRATH Video Laryngoscope (MVL)?** There are few studies evaluating the MVL. Shippey et al.[18] described their initial experience in 75 patients being electively intubated, all with normal airway anatomy. This small prospective single-center study recorded intubation success rates, laryngoscopic view, and time to ETT placement, and found that in nearly all patients (99%), a C–L grade 1 or 2 was obtained with an average time of 6.3 seconds needed for optimal visualization. Overall success rate was 98%. In a recent OR study, the MVL was found to be effective at intubation rescue when DL failed because of poor glottic visualization.[19] More emergency department experience is needed before a firm recommendation can be made.
- **What evidence exists regarding the use of the AWS?** There is little published about this device. Suzuki et al.[20] published their experience with 100 patients undergoing elective surgery and compared the C–L grade obtained with the Macintosh laryngoscope with that of the AWS. They were able to obtain grade 1 views on every patient using the AWS and in 65% of patients using a conventional laryngoscope. Any recommendation about this device is premature, and its performance in difficult or emergency airway situations has not been adequately studied.
- **Are there any data supporting the use of the KVL?** No studies are published as of this writing.

REFERENCES

1. Agro F, Barzoi G, Montecchia F. Tracheal intubation using a Macintosh laryngoscope or Glide-Scope in 15 patients with cervical spine immobilization [letter]. *Br J Anaesth*. 2003;90:705–706.

2. Sakles JC, Tolby N, VanderHeyden TC, et al. Ability of emergency medicine residents to use alternative optical airway devices. Paper presented at the Western Meeting of the Society for Academic Emergency Medicine; April 2003; Phoenix, AZ.

3. Sun DA, Warriner CB, Parsons DG, et al. The GlideScope video laryngoscope: randomized clinical trial in 200 patients. *Br J Anaesth*. 2005;94(3):381–384.

4. Cooper RM, Pacey JA, Bishop MJ, et al. Early clinical experience with a new video laryngoscope (GlideScope) in 728 patients. *Can J Anaesth*. 2005;52(2):191–198.

5. Dupanovic M, Diachun CA, Isaacson SA, et al. Intubation the GlideScope videolaryngoscope using the "gearstick technique." *Can J Anaesth*. 2006;53(2):213–214.

6. Jones PM, Turkstra TP, Armstrong KP, et al. Effect of stylet angulation and endotracheal tube camber on time to intubation with the GlideScope. *Can J Anaesth*. 2007;54(1):21–27.

7. Rai MR, Dering A, Verghese C. The GlideScope system: a clinical assessment of performance. *Anaesthesia*. 2005;60(1):60–64.

8. Benjamin FJ, Boon D, French RA. An evaluation of the GlideScope, a new video laryngoscope for difficult airways: a manikin study. *Eur J Anaesthesiol*. 2006;23(6):517–521.

9. Hsiao WT, Lin YH, Wu HS, et al. Does a new video laryngoscope (GlideScope) provide better glottic exposure? *Acta Anaesthesiol Taiwan*. 2005;43(3):147–151.

10. Lai HY, Chen IH, Chen A, et al. The use of the GlideScope for tracheal intubation in patients with ankylosing spondylitis. *Br J Anaesth*. 2007;98(3):408–409.

11. Tremblay MH, Williams S, Robitaille A, et al. Poor visualization during direct laryngoscopy and high upper lip bite test score are predictors of difficult intubation with the GlideScope videolaryngoscope. *Anesth Analg*. 2008;106:1495–1500.

12. Aziz MF, Healy D, Kheterpal S, et al. Routine clinical practice effectiveness of the Glidescope in difficult airway management: an analysis of 2,004 Glidescope intubations, complications, and failures from two institutions. *Anesthesiology*. 2011;114:34–41.

13. Wayne MA, McDonnell M. Comparison of traditional versus video laryngoscopy in out-of-hospital tracheal intubation. *Prehosp Emerg Care*. 2010;14:278–282.

14. Kaplan MB, Hagberg CA, Ward DS, et al. Comparison of direct and video-assisted views of the larynx during routine intubations. *J Clin Anesth*. 2006;18(5):357–362.

15. Kaplan MB, Ward DS, Berci G. A new video laryngoscope—an aid to intubation and teaching. *J Clin Anesth*. 2002;14(8):620–626.

16. Brown CA III, Bair AE, Pallin DJ, et al. Improved glottic exposure with the Video Macintosh Laryngoscope in adult emergency department tracheal intubations. *Ann Emerg Med*. 2010;56(2):83–88. Epub 2010 Mar 3.

17. Cavus E, Kieckhaefer J, Doerges V, et al. The C-MAC videolaryngoscope: first experiences with a new device for videolaryngoscopy-guided intubation. *Anesth Analg*. 2010;110:473–477.

18. Shippey B, Ray D, McKeown D. Case series: the McGrath videolaryngoscope—an initial clinical evaluation. *Can J Anaesth*. 2007;54(4):307–313.

19. Noppens RR, Möbus S, Heid F, et al. Evaluation of the McGrath® Series 5 videolaryngoscope after failed direct laryngoscopy. *Anaesthesia*. 2010;65:716–720.

20. Suzuki A, Toyama Y, Katsumi N, et al. Pentax-AWS improves laryngeal view compared with Macintosh blade during laryngoscopy and facilitates easier intubation. *Masui*. 2007;56(4):464–468.

14

Optical and Light-Guided Devices

John C. Sakles • Julie A. Slick

INTRODUCTION

Traditional laryngoscopes require the operator to achieve a direct line of site of the glottis by aligning the oral, pharyngeal, and laryngeal axes (Chapter 12). Video laryngoscopes capitalize on a video camera or chip, which is mounted on a specially designed blade, to circumvent the need for a straight line of sight, while providing superior views of the glottis and surrounding spaces (Chapter 13). Optically enhanced devices are those laryngoscopes that allow the operator to visualize the glottis without creating a straight line of sight, but without using video or fiberoptic technology. The glottic view is obtained by the use of inexpensive optics consisting of combinations of prisms, mirrors, and lenses. The relatively inexpensive cost of the technology is one of the major benefits of these devices when compared with the more expensive fiberoptic and video devices. The manufacturers of these devices also offer video capability through attachable video cameras, which are customized for use with individual optically enhanced laryngoscopes. The addition of video capability provides a magnified view of the glottis, and enhances education by allowing other providers to visualize what the airway manager is observing. There are only two true optical devices of relevance to emergency airway management, the Airtraq and the Truview.

DEVICES

Airtraq

Components

The Airtraq is a single-use, disposable laryngoscope that provides the operator with a magnified view of the glottic structures (Fig. 14-1). The Airtraq is now available in four sizes for orotracheal intubation. The orotracheal devices have an endotracheal tube (ETT) channel in which the ETT is preloaded before insertion. Airtraq also offers two devices that lack the ETT channel and are intended for use during nasotracheal intubation. These devices are intended for insertion through the mouth to facilitate nasotracheal intubations with the assistance of glottic visualization. They also offer a device with a larger channel that will accommodate double lumen endobronchial tubes. The Airtraq devices have a relatively narrow profile. The minimal mouth opening required is 18 mm for the the regular Airtraq (size 3) and 16 mm for the small Airtraq (size 2).

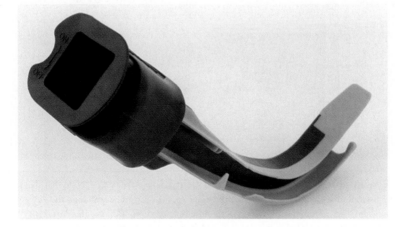

Figure 14-1 ● **Airtraq Optical Laryngoscope.**   Note the black rubber eyepiece atop the viewing channel and blue endotracheal tube guide. Shown is the standard adult Airtraq, size 3.

All of the Airtraq devices are made of plastic and are designed for single use. They cannot be cleaned or sterilized, and they will not function properly if this is attempted. This single use attribute makes the Airtraq particularly suitable for use in field settings for both emergency medical services (EMS) and military applications. The devices are powered by three AAA batteries, which will provide approximately 90 minutes of operating time. The shelf life is approximately 2 years. The Airtraq is turned on by pressing a button on the top of the unit that illuminates a low-heat light-emitting diode (LED). The device has a built-in antifog mechanism. A rubber eyepiece is connected to the optical channel. This rubber eyepiece can be removed and replaced with an optional video composite unit that will allow transmission of the optical image to a wired or wireless video monitor.

Operation

The Airtraq requires little setup time and is self-contained within its protective packaging. The Airtraq's antifogging mechanism requires the device be turned on for approximately 30 seconds to maximize this benefit. The LED will flash when the device is turned on and become constant when the heating element has reached the appropriate antifog temperature and the device is therefore ready for use. The ETT should be lightly lubricated and preloaded into the ETT channel. No stylet is used. The anterior surface of the Airtraq blade, which will come in contact with the tongue, can be lubricated to help facilitate passing the device around the tongue. The Airtraq should be placed into the mouth using a midline approach. Gentle outward traction may be applied to the tongue using the operator's free hand, if necessary, to ensure that the tongue is not pushed into the hypopharynx. As the Airtraq is advanced, the operator visualizes the epiglottis through the eyepiece and continues to move the device forward into the vallecula. When the vallecula is entered, the Airtraq is lifted in the vertical plane to elevate the epiglottis and align the vocal cords within the center of the optical field (Fig. 14-2). The ETT is slowly advanced through the vocal cords, and then disengaged from the device and the Airtraq is removed. If the ETT is obstructed by the epiglottis or arytenoids, the entire device is manipulated to better align the ETT position with the

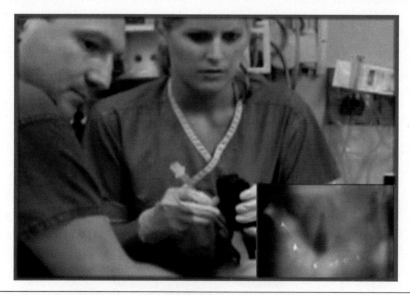

Figure 14-2 ● Intubation being performed using the Airtraq. Note that the optional camera adapter is being used. Rather than looking through the eyepiece, the operator is watching the video screen, as is the supervising physician. The glottic view is shown in the inset of the photo. Because the Airtraq contains a built-in tube guide, the tube (without a stylet) is simply advanced into the airway. If the tube does not enter the laryngeal inlet because it is off center, then the *whole* device, *not just* the endotracheal tube, is manipulated to achieve better alignment and successful intubation.

glottic entrance. The Airtraq can be pulled back slightly and rotated along its longitudinal axis to help align the glottic structures. Alternatively, the epiglottis can be lifted directly by the Airtraq blade through a straight blade approach to appropriately align the glottic structures. However, this technique can somewhat distort the anatomy and is not the recommended approach.

If the proprietary composite video system is to be used, the rubber optical eyepiece is removed and the video adaptor is snapped onto the Airtraq before insertion. The operator then visualizes the entire procedure on the external monitor. This approach allows the operator to maintain a safe distance from the patient and provides a larger view of the anatomical structures.

Summary

The Airtraq optical laryngoscope is a lightweight, inexpensive single-use device that may have very practical applications in emergency airway management. Multiple sizes of this device are now offered for orotracheal, nasotracheal, and endobronchial tube placement. This self-contained device requires very little setup making it extremely portable, offering added benefits for field and other "out of the department" applications. The optical device alone offers a clear image of the glottis. The addition of the video capability provides a magnified image with greater detail for improved visualization and obvious educational benefits. Although significantly different from standard direct laryngoscopes, the device is reasonably easy to learn and use in the emergency and difficult airway settings.

Truview PCD

Components

The Truview Picture Capture Device (PCD) is a third-generation optical laryngoscope manufactured by Truphatek (Fig. 14-3). The latest edition was introduced in 2010, and it now also includes video laryngoscopy capabilities. The Truview uses a conventional laryngoscope handle, which gives the device a familiar feel. The blades are the more unique parts of these devices. The blades are markedly angled near their midpoint and incorporate a telescope-like device with an angulated, prism-like, distal lens to provide the view of the difficult anterior airway. The blades are available in five sizes, allowing intubation from the 800-g neonate to the morbidly obese adult. The low-profile blades require minimal mouth opening. They are made of stainless steel and can be easily cleaned and sterilized.

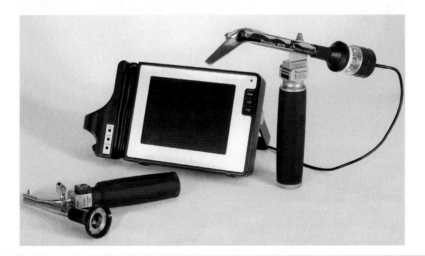

Figure 14-3 ● The newly released Truview PCD optical laryngoscope with video camera attached to the eyepiece of one of the blades.

The device can be awkward to use, as the eyepiece is designed to be viewed with the operator's eye at a distance of 2 ft (0.6 m) from the lens. Although this can provide a clear view of the glottic structures, the image appears small and distant when viewed in this manner. The system is much more capable when an optional video camera is affixed to the proximal lens of the telescope. A proprietary high definition camera feeds to a 5-in (12.7 cm) digital liquid crystal display screen. Additionally, the eyepiece will also accept universal 32-mm endoscopic camera heads to be viewed on a nonproprietary external monitor. Either of the methods provides a significantly better image than is obtained without video enhancement, and allows for other providers to see what the operator sees.

The Truview blades also incorporate oxygen ports through which oxygen can be delivered at 10 L per minute. The oxygen flow is directed at the distal portion of the optical system to potentially clear secretions from the lens and to prevent fogging. This apneic diffusion oxygenation may provide for longer time to desaturation in the truly difficult airway (see Chapters 5 and 19). Patients who may experience rapid desaturation such as young children, pregnant women, obese patients, and those with acute or chronic respiratory illness might benefit from this feature. The device also comes with a preformed OptiShape stylet that mimics the blade shape to facilitate ETT placement, but a standard stylet also may be used.

Operation

The setup time is for the device is minimal. The blade is connected to the handle, and oxygen tubing is connected to the oxygen port. Oxygen flow rate should be set at 10 L per minute. Antifog solution may be applied to the distal lens to minimize fogging. The operator should either use the preformed OptiShape stylet or configure the standard stylet to the shape of the Truview blade. The blade is placed in the midline of the patient's mouth and advanced until the handle is 2 to 3 cm from the patient's lips. Very little or no neck manipulation is required. The operator then looks through the eyepiece at a comfortable standing position to visualize the glottic structures (Fig. 14-4). Small adjustments may be made to optimize the view. If the video attachment is used, the operator will look at the monitor to visualize the magnified glottic inlet. The technique for

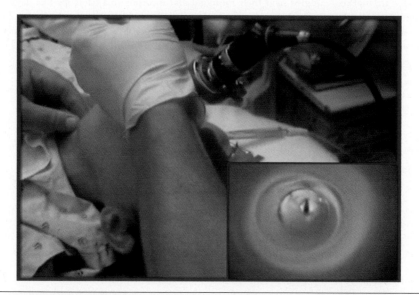

Figure 14-4 ● **Clinical use of the original Truview. (Truview EVO) with optional camera attachment and oxygen delivery at 10 L per minute.** The insert in the right lower corner shows the glottic inlet surrounded by reflection within the metal eyepiece. Notice the V-shaped clearing of the upper portion of the lens provided by the oxygen flow that is surrounded by fogging. This view is similar to that obtained when the operator looks through the optical channel.

insertion of the ETT is similar to that for the GlideScope. The ETT is inserted at the right corner of the patient's mouth in a horizontal plane. It is then rotated clockwise 90° toward midline during advancement to place the tip of the ETT at the glottic inlet. The ETT is advanced through the vocal cords. The stylet and the laryngoscope are then removed, and tube placement is confirmed.

Summary

The Truview PCD provides a unique, inexpensive option for difficult airway management. This third-generation optical laryngoscope offers definite improvements over its predecessors, particularly with the addition of improved video capabilities. Visualization can be difficult without the optional video camera, but magnified video images eliminate the difficulty navigating toward the glottic structures with such a small field of view. The addition of the oxygen port may add benefit to this device for those patients prone to rapid desaturation.

Conclusion

Both the Airtraq and the Truview PCD offer good glottic views without the need to obtain a direct line of sight. They do so more economically than their video or fiberoptic competitors do by using simple optics with prisms and mirrors, but do so at the cost of some reduction in performance and image quality. The Airtraq device functions very well without the need for video enhancement, but the Truview PCD is difficult to use without the attached video system.

CONCLUSION

These two devices both capitalize on optics to improve glottic view without requiring a direct line of sight from outside the patient's mouth, and so share many of the advantages of the more expensive video and fiberoptic systems. Both devices have been subjected to several clinical trials (see evidence below), and have fared well in these limited studies. From the visualization perspective, the Airtraq provides generally better images than the Truview PCD, but each has strengths and weaknesses. Further study is required to clarify the roles for these devices in routine and difficult airway management.

EVIDENCE

- **Is the Airtraq device better than a direct laryngoscope for patients predicted to be difficult intubations?** There have been several trials over the past few years that have evaluated success of intubations in elective surgical patients using the Airtraq device versus the conventional Macintosh laryngoscope. A study by Koh et al.[1] placed surgical patients into Philadelphia cervical collars to simulate patients with cervical spine injury. The patients were randomized to the Airtraq group or the Macintosh group and compared regarding the ease of intubation and hemodynamic stability. The Airtraq proved to be superior with a 96% success rate on first intubation attempt versus 40% in the Macintosh group.

  A study by Ndoko et al.[2] looked at intubation success rates in morbidly obese surgical patient in a similar comparison of the two devices. This study showed less time to intubation with the Airtraq than with the Macintosh laryngoscope at 24 and 56 seconds, respectively. Consequently, SpO_2 was better maintained in the Airtraq group than in the Macintosh laryngoscope group with one and nine patients, respectively, demonstrating decline of SpO_2 to 92% or less ($p < .05$).[2]

- **Is it easy to learn how to use the Airtraq?** In a study by DiMarco et al.,[3] first-year residents with no earlier intubating experience attempted intubation on at least six patients with the Airtraq and an equal number of patients with the Macintosh. A more rapid acquisition of skills was observed in the Airtraq group as evidenced by time to intubation. The device was also judged to be easier to use by the residents.

- **How does the Airtraq perform in the prehospital setting?** Trimmel et al.[4] studied 212 patients requiring intubation in a prehospital setting. Anesthesiologists or emergency physicians responding with EMS intubated the patients. When the Airtraq was used as first-line airway device (n = 106) versus direct laryngoscopy (n = 106), success rate was 47% versus 99%, respectively ($p < .001$). The reasons for failed Airtraq intubation were related to the optical characteristic of the device (i.e., impaired sight resulting from blood and vomitus, n = 11) or to presumed handling problems (i.e., cuff damage, tube misplacement, or inappropriate visualization of the glottis, n = 24). This European study stands alone in its finding of a high-failure rate using the Airtraq.

- **Does the Truview improve glottic view as compared to the Macintosh laryngoscope?** In a random crossover study by Li et al.,[5] 120 elective surgical patients in China underwent laryngoscopy with either a Macintosh or the Truview and were given a Cormack–Lehane (C–L) grade. They then underwent laryngoscopy with the other device and were intubated. Time to intubation was recorded for the second device used. The results showed that the Truview improved the glottic view of 87.5% of patients with a C–L view grade >1 by direct laryngoscopy. Another study by Miceli et al.[6] using mannequins to simulate patients with tongue swelling and neck stiffness also showed that a better C–L view was obtained with the Truview.

- **How does the time to intubation with the Truview compare to times seen with the Macintosh laryngoscope?** The study by Li et al.[5] showed that the time to intubation in the Truview group was longer by an average of 17 seconds, which probably is of no clinical significance. The mannequin study by Miceli et al.[6] also showed no significant difference in time to intubation or ease of tracheal tube placement.

REFERENCES

1. Koh JC, Lee JS, Lee YW, et al. Comparison of the laryngeal view during intubation using Airtraq and Macintosh laryngoscopes in patients with cervical spine immobilization and mouth opening limitation. *Korean J Anesthesiol*. 2010;59(5):314–318.

2. Ndoko SK, Amathieu R, Tual L, et al. Tracheal intubation of morbidly obese patients: a randomized trial comparing performance of Macintosh and Airtraq laryngoscopes. *Br J Anaesth*. 2008;100(2):263–268.

3. DiMarco P, Scattoni L, Spinoglio A, et al. Learning curves of the Airtraq and the Macintosh laryngoscopes for tracheal intubation by novice laryngoscopists: a clinical study. *Anesth Analg*. 2011;112(1):122–125.

4. Trimmel H, Kreutziger J, Fertsak G, et al. Use of the Airtraq laryngoscope for emergency intubation in the prehospital setting: a randomized control trial. *Crit Care Med*. 2011;39(3):489–493.

5. Li JB, Xiong YC, Wang XL, et al. An evaluation of the Truview EVO2 laryngoscope. *Anaesthesia*. 2007;62:940–943.

6. Miceli L, Cecconi M, Tripi G, et al. Evaluation of new laryngoscope blade for tracheal intubation, Truview EVO2: a manikin study. *Eur J Anaesthesiol*. 2008;25(6):446–449.

15

Flexible Endoscopic Intubation

Michael F. Murphy • Peter M.C. DeBlieux

DESCRIPTION

Tracheal intubation over a flexible endoscope is an invaluable technique in airway management, particularly in patients for whom standard laryngoscopy and orotracheal intubation have failed, or are anticipated to be difficult or impossible. Endoscopic devices are used both for diagnostic evaluation of the upper airway and for tracheal intubation.

INDICATIONS AND CONTRAINDICATIONS

Indications for endoscopic intubation in emergency airway management generally are identified during the LEMON evaluation for the difficult airway (see Chapter 2) and include the following:

- The patient with distorted upper airway anatomy, such as angioedema, oropharyngeal abscess, hematoma (or other trauma), or Ludwig's angina, or those with slowly progressive laryngeal lesions, such as lingual and laryngeal cancers.
- The patient with laryngeal trauma or tracheal disruption. In these cases, intubation with continuous visualization is recommended. The endoscope meets this indication.
- The patient for whom cervical spine immobility is required, particularly if the airway is predicted to be difficult.
- The patient who fails the 3-3-2 rule (restricted mouth opening, small mandible, or high larynx) or has a grade 4 Mallampati score.
- The patient with morbid obesity.
- Failed intubation in the "can't intubate, can oxygenate" scenario, when continuing deterioration of the airway is not anticipated.

Contraindications to endoscopic intubation are mostly relative and may include the following:

- Excessive blood and secretions in the upper airway, which have the great potential to obscure the view and reduce the success rate with the endoscopic technique. Some experienced bronchoscopists use the endoscope to transilluminate their way into the trachea, only then looking through the scope to verify the position of the endoscope in the trachea, but this is highly operator dependent.
- High-grade upper airway obstruction (resulting from foreign bodies or other lesions), where the procedure may precipitate total airway obstruction. If a patient has a high-grade supraglottic airway obstruction, with impending complete airway closure, the delays and risks of precipitating complete airway obstruction or laryngospasm argue strongly against endoscopic intubation and in favor of cricothyrotomy.
- Inadequate oxygenation by bag and mask does not permit endoscopic intubation because of the time required (can't intubate, can't oxygenate).

TECHNIQUE

Overview

Endoscopic intubation is a technical challenge that requires initial training, and then skill maintenance activities to maintain speed and success. Manual dexterity in manipulating the endoscope is essential to performing endoscopic intubation in a timely fashion. This skill is best learned by attending endoscopic intubation workshops with expert instruction, and then practicing on intubation manikins or high-fidelity human patient simulators before one attempts to intubate a patient. This is particularly true in patients with difficult airways. The manufacturers of endoscopes can usually provide training videos, product support personnel, and manikins to support this endeavor.

The requisite psychomotor skills cannot be developed without dedicated practice, and lack of training, practice, and experience constitute the most common cause of failed endoscopic intubation. A reasonable level of dexterity in bronchoscopic manipulation can be achieved within 3 to 4 hours of independent practice using an intubation model. Recent studies have shown that the technique can also be learned in real-life situations by the performance of upper airway endoscopy when diagnostic opportunities, such as searching for foreign bodies and evaluating the causes of hoarseness, severe sore throat, and other upper airway conditions, present themselves. As is the case with many of the specialized airway techniques, the patient who requires semi-emergent, but controlled, intubation, such as an overdose victim without an anticipated difficult airway and patients who are easily ventilated with normal oxygen saturation, may be appropriate candidates for endoscopic intubation. Because success depends on familiarity and skill in using the device, gaining experience in routine cases is invaluable before one is required to perform a difficult endoscopic intubation in a crisis.

Preparation

Although the emergency difficult or failed airway situation often does not permit lengthy preparation and a methodical approach, maximal success with this technique requires both psychological

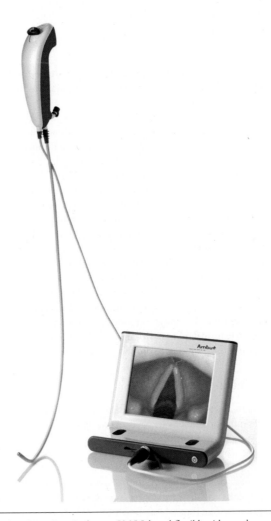

Figure 15-1 ● The Ambu aScope is a single use, CMOS-based flexible video endoscope.

and pharmacologic patient preparation. When the procedure is to be done "awake" (see Chapter 23), optimizing the chances for success includes the following:

- Explain to the patient what to expect.
- Administer an antisialogogue, such as glycopyrrolate 0.01 mg per kg IM or IV, at least 10 minutes (20 minutes if possible) in advance of the procedure to reduce secretions, enhancing both the visualization and the effect of topically applied local anesthesia.
- Achieve profound local anesthesia of the airway. An endoscopic intubation may require as much sedation and topical anesthesia as is necessary for awake direct laryngoscopy.
- Administer adequate sedation (see Chapter 23).

Scope Selection

Instrument selection for the emergency department (ED) is an important issue. Affordable and durable scopes are easily available from a variety of manufacturers. Selection of a manufacturer may be guided by existing service contracts in your specific institution. These instruments, although expensive, find several uses in the ED to justify such an expenditure:

- Tracheal intubation, both nasal and oral.
- Diagnostic laryngoscopy.
- Oropharyngeal foreign body location and extraction.

Recently, at least one manufacturer has introduced a single-use flexible endoscope, using complementary metal-oxide semiconductor (CMOS) video, making flexible endoscopy much less expensive. (Fig. 15-1)

The scope should be of sufficient caliber and stiffness to guide the passage of an endotracheal tube (ETT) over itself through the angles of the airway without kinking and resist being flipped out of the trachea, while maintaining flexibility and ease of manipulation. Most endoscope manufacturers produce intubation-specific devices that have the added stiffness of the fiber bundle to allow ETTs to be guided into the trachea over the scope. This feature allows scopes that are small enough (3- to 4-mm tip diameter) to be painlessly and atraumatically passed through a topically anesthetized nose for diagnostic work also to be used for endoscopic intubation. Neonatal and pediatric endoscopes (2- to 3-mm tip diameter) are also available.

The endoscopic bundle should be long enough (600 mm) to allow bronchoscopy and airway toilet in the ED. Standard bronchoscopes are 600 mm in length. Some manufacturers produce 400-mm intubating endoscopes that are not long enough for pulmonary care if this is planned. A separate channel for the injection of local anesthetic or saline and suctioning is essential, although the smaller neonatal and pediatric endoscopes may not have them owing to their small size. A formerly recommended practice, the insufflation of oxygen through the suction working channel to maintain saturations and blow secretions out of the way, is now contraindicated following several cases of gastric insufflation, perforation, and death. Endoscopes with battery-powered, portable, self-contained light sources are compact and may be preferable for ED applications.

Care of the Instrument

Some general precautions are necessary to prevent damage to the relatively delicate fiberoptic bundles in a fiberoptic scope and similar precautions are prudent even with the less damage-prone video endoscopes:

- Do not drop the scope.
- Use a bite-block (e.g., oral airway) to protect the scope. Most oral endoscopic intubation guides incorporate this feature (e.g., the Berman intubating/pharyngeal airway, also called the "Berman breakaway airway") and are invaluable aids to successful oral endoscopic intubation (Fig. 15-2). The Rapid Oral Tracheal Intubation Guidance System (ROTIGS) airway has the advantage of keeping one above the tongue and away from the gag-producing glossopharyngeal nerve territory (Fig. 15-3).

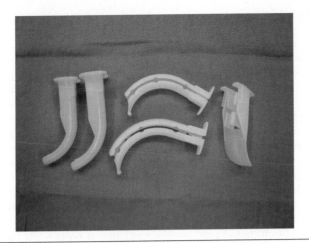

Figure 15-2 ● Three Oral Endoscopic Intubation Aids are on The Market:the Williams (left), the Berman intubating/pharyngeal airway (center), and the Ovassapian guide (right). The Williams and the Berman also serve a "bite-block" function.

- Avoid acute bending or kinking of the endoscope, especially when advancing the ETT over the scope into the trachea.
- If rotation of the ETT during intubation is necessary, rotate both the ETT and the scope to avoid damage to the fibers.
- Lubricate the ETT by spraying local anesthetic agent or other water-soluble material down the tube to allow easy removal of the scope after the ETT is in place. Lubricating the scope makes it slippery and difficult to manipulate.
- Clean the device, including the working channel, immediately after use. The best routine is to suction 1 L of saline through the device immediately after use. Manufacturers and endoscopy units will provide instructions for acceptable cleaning routines.
- Do not flex the tip against undue resistance to manipulate the direction of an ETT or use it to move tissue out of the way.

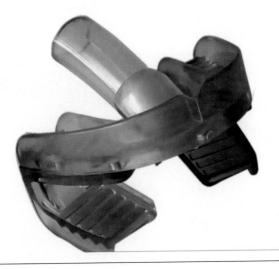

Figure 15-3 ● ROTIGS.

Technique of Endoscopic Intubation

The endoscope has two main components: a body (handpiece) housing the controls and accessories and a longitudinal flexible tube, containing video or fiberoptic components (Fig. 15-4). Scope tip control is simple: flexion forward and backward is achieved with the thumb toggle on the body of the endoscope, whereas rotation clockwise and counterclockwise is done by rotating the wrist of the hand that is holding the body of the endoscope in a manner somewhat reminiscent of the "Royal Wave".

The scope can be used with or without a video screen. Many EDs do not have a video-capable system, so this description assumes the operator is holding the eyepiece to the eye. When looking through the eyepiece of the endoscope, select visual targets and center these in the field of view as you advance the scope using the hand holding the fiber bundle to pull the hand holding the body of the scope along. Move toward these targets slowly, but steadily using small manipulations forward and back (toggle) and left and right (wrist flexion and extension) to keep successive targets in the center of the visual image. The hand–eye coordination needed for successful endoscopic intubation has been likened to the kind of hand–eye coordination used to play a video game.

Preparation for the task depends on how much time is available. At the first thought of performing a flexible endoscopic intubation, consider giving the intravenous dose of glycopyrrolate to allow maximal time for effect. Generally, most things should be in a state of rapid readiness on the difficult and failed airway cart:

1. Gather all equipment (usually preassembled on a tray):
   a. Topical airway anesthesia supplies and equipment, including three 5-ml syringes loaded with 4% lidocaine to inject into the airway through the scope as needed
   b. Endoscope, ETTs, airways, bite-blocks
   c. Tonsil suction
   d. Lubricant and antifog solution
   e. Additional airway management equipment as indicated in case of patient deterioration and need for rapid intervention
2. Obtain an able and knowledgeable assistant.
3. Prepare the patient:
   a. Antisialogogue, such as glycopyrrolate 0.01 mg per kg intramuscularly or intravenously, allowing sufficient time for this to work (minimum 10 minutes) if possible
   b. Vasoconstrictor for the nose (if nasal route is chosen)
   c. Local, topical airway anesthesia
   d. Sedation as appropriate
   e. Preoxygenate the patient as for rapid sequence intubation (see Chapter 19) as much as possible

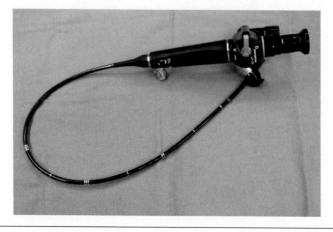

Figure 15-4 ● **A Flexible Endoscopic Bronchoscope.** Note the white marks denoting 10, 15, 20, 25, 30, 35 and 40 cms on the wand portion of the scope.

4. Lubricate the inside and outside of the endotracheal tube because lubricating the scope makes it slippery and too hard to manipulate.
5. Put a drop of silicone liquid (antifog solution) on the tip of the scope or place the tip of the fiber bundle in a bottle of warmed saline (usually available in the warming cabinets of most EDs) or in a warmed blanket for 1 minute to prevent fogging.
6. Insert a bite-block if the oral route is chosen, or, preferably, use an intubating guide such as a Berman intubating/pharyngeal airway. If a Berman guide is used, mount the ETT in the guide, ensuring that the tip of the ETT is at the end of the tubular portion of the airway before inserting the guide into the mouth, and then insert the endoscope through the ETT.
7. Stand up straight, either at the head of, the side of, or facing the patient. Operator positioning is mostly a matter of personal preference and patient tolerance.
8. Oral technique: Stay in the midline, stay in the midline, stay in the midline! The best way is to place the long or ring finger in the middle of the upper lip to maintain a reference point and hold the fiber bundle with the index finger and thumb. Gentle traction on the tongue by an assistant using a gauze bandage helps open the airway and prevent the patient from using the tongue to obstruct access to the airway. If the patient is supine, placing the patient in the upright sitting position (if possible) also makes the tongue less of an issue. Custom made airways, such as the Berman intubating/pharyngeal airway and the ROTIGS, are helpful in keeping the scope in the midline and obviate the need for the tongue traction maneuver. If such an adjunct is used, insert the ETT into the airway and then insert the scope through the airway/ETT combination, obviating the need to jam or tape the ETT connector onto the scope handpiece. Nasal technique: Soften the nasotracheal tube by placing the ETT in a bottle of warmed saline or sterile water from the warming closet for 3 to 5 minutes before inserting the ETT through the nostril. It may be is helpful to dilate the chosen anesthetized nostril by gently and slowly inserting increasingly large nasopharyngeal airways or a lubricated and gloved small finger into the nostril as far as possible immediately before inserting the ETT. This allows the operator to choose the most patent nare. Advance the lubricated nasal tube to the level of the uvula in the nasopharynx, and then pass the scope through the tube.
9. Hold the body of the endoscope in the same hand as your dominant eye. This allows one to turn slightly to the side when using the scope, an important detail in keeping the fiber bundle of the scope straight during the procedure for reasons described later. Some advocate holding the body of the scope in the left hand to facilitate clearance of the light source cable and suction tubing, which exit the body of the scope on its left side (Fig. 15-3). Use your thumb to toggle the tip control lever up and down. The index finger can be used to depress and activate the suction feature. Flexing and extending the wrist moves the tip of the fiber bundle left and right, although the fiber bundle must be held straight with mild tension between the two hands to optimize this maneuver. Slackness in the fiber bundle will not permit wrist motion to rotate its tip. The nondominant hand advances, withdraws, and manipulates the fiber bundle, and maintains a midline oral position if the oral route is chosen. The operator should move the hands and arms, not the whole torso, to manipulate the fiber bundle into the airway.
10. The assistant should have tonsil suction available to aspirate oral secretions and blood. The working channel of the scope may provide insufficient suction to clear the volume of secretions that may be present during the procedure. If the tip becomes soiled or fogged and obscures clear vision, bouncing the tip gently against the mucosa may be sufficient to clear it.
11. Get your bearings. At the head of the bed, the base of the tongue is up; beside or in front of the patient, it is down. Advance slowly while flexing the tip up to pass over the back of the tongue. The epiglottis comes into view. Keep it above you. You will see the white cords opening and closing with respiration.
12. It may be challenging to coordinate, but attempt to advance the scope through the vocal cords during inspiration, when the cords are open. It may be necessary to inject 1-2 ml of 4% lidocaine through the working channel onto the larynx to obtund the cough or closure reflex and permit entry into the trachea.
13. If you get lost, withdraw to the oropharynx and find a landmark.
14. Once the tip of the fiber bundle is through the vocal cords, advance the scope almost to the carina. Then slowly advance the ETT over the scope into the trachea, being careful not to kink

the scope. A conventional laryngoscope may be useful to straighten out the angle of approach to the glottis, but rarely is required, except in the supine patient. Gentle rotation of the scope/tube unit through 180° may be necessary if the ETT catches on the cords (usually on the arytenoids). Newer ETT tip designs may facilitate passage of the ETT through the cords (e.g., Parker tube).

15. If coughing is a persistent problem, inject 5 ml of 2% aqueous lidocaine through the scope.
16. After the ETT has been successfully passed into the trachea, the scope can be used to correctly position the ETT in the midportion of the trachea. Push the tip of the scope through the ETT until it is just distal to the end of the ETT and flex it gently forward. Grasp both the endoscope and the ETT, and move them together until light transilluminates the sternal notch. The light is shining forward immediately beyond the tip of the ETT, so this corresponds to the midtracheal position. Straighten the tip and remove the entire endoscope.

COMPLICATIONS

Patient complications with this technique are uncommon and include mucosal damage to the airway and epistaxis. As with all techniques, damage to the vocal apparatus is possible, but rare. The most frequent complication is damage to the scope from biting, twisting, kinking, or dropping. In the past, it was taught that oxygen ought to be insufflated down the working channel of the scope to blow secretions out of the way and provide an element of oxygenation for the patient. This practice has been associated with gastric insufflation and rupture leading to death, and thus is no longer recommended.

EVIDENCE

- Intubating over an endoscope, nasally and orally, is a well-established technique for managing difficult airways.[1–4] It has been demonstrated that the technique is relatively easily learned and the skill maintained,[5] and that nonhuman models are useful in teaching the manipulative skills that are key to successful intubation.[6] It is recognized as a skill important to the training of residents in emergency medicine.[7] Levitan et al.[8] surveyed academic EDs in 1999, attempting to determine what alternative airway management devices were available for difficult airway management. Sixty-four percent of them had bronchoscopes. Several studies have demonstrated a success rate for ED endoscopic intubation by emergency physicians in the 70% to 99% range, depending on training and frequency of use.[9–13] Both endoscopic nasal (adults and children) and oral intubation in the ED have been described in the literature.[14,15] Emergency endoscopic intubation has been used in blunt and penetrating head and neck trauma, laryngeal malignancies, tracheal stenosis, and other difficult airway situations.[16–20] As mentioned in the Complications section, the practice of insufflating oxygen down the working channel of the scope has been associated with gastric insufflation and rupture leading to death[21] and is no longer recommended.[22]

  Finally, no discussion of endoscopic intubation would be complete without at least mentioning the uncommon, but real risk of sudden and total airway obstruction in patients undergoing topical anesthesia for awake endoscopic intubation[23–26] (see Chapter 23). This factor simply serves to reinforce the need for preparedness for any eventuality when one is managing an airway in an emergency.

REFERENCES

1. Morris IR. Fibreoptic intubation. *Can J Anaesth*. 1994;41:996–1008.
2. Messeter KH, Pettersson KI. Endotracheal intubation with the fibre-optic bronchoscope. *Anaesthesia*. 1980;35:294–298.

3. Dellinger RP. Fiberoptic bronchoscopy in adult airway management. *Crit Care Med*. 1990;18:882–887.

4. Patel VU. Oral and nasal fiberoptic intubation with a single lumen tube. *Anesthesiol Clin North America*. 1991;9:83–95.

5. Ovassapian A, Yelich SJ. Learning fiberoptic intubation. *Anesthesiol Clin North America*. 1991;9:175–185.

6. Naik VN, Matsumoto ED, Houston PL, et al. Fiberoptic orotracheal intubation on anesthetized patients. *Anesthesiology*. 2001;95:343–348.

7. Gallagher EJ, Coffey J, Lombardi G, et al. Emergency procedures important to the training of emergency medicine residents: who performs them in the emergency department? *Acad Emerg Med*. 1995;2:630–633.

8. Levitan RM, Kush S, Hollander JE. Devices for difficult airway management in academic emergency departments: results of a national survey. *Ann Emerg Med*. 1999;33:694–698.

9. Afilalo M, Guttman A, Stern E, et al. Fiberoptic intubation in the emergency department: a case series. *J Emerg Med*. 1993;11:387–391.

10. Mlinek EJ Jr, Clinton JE, Plummer D, et al. Fiberoptic intubation in the emergency department. *Ann Emerg Med*. 1990;19:359–362.

11. Schafermeyer RW. Fiberoptic laryngoscopy in the emergency department. *Am J Emerg Med*. 1984;2:160–163.

12. Blanda M, Gallo UE. Emergency airway management. *Emerg Med Clin North Am*. 2003;21:1–26.

13. Hamilton PH, Kang JJ. Emergency airway management. *Mt Sinai J Med*. 1997;64:292–301.

14. Delaney KA, Hessler R. Emergency flexible fiberoptic nasotracheal intubation: a report of 60 cases. *Ann Emerg Med*. 1988;17:919–926.

15. Rucker RW, Silva WJ, Worcester CC. Fiberoptic bronchoscopic nasotracheal intubation in children. *Chest*. 1979;76:56–58.

16. Mulder DS, Wallace DH, Woolhouse FM. The use of the fiberoptic bronchoscope to facilitate endotracheal intubation following head and neck trauma. *J Trauma*. 1975;15:638–640.

17. Wei WI, Siu KF, Lau WF, et al. Emergency endotracheal intubation under fiberoptic endoscopic guidance for malignant laryngeal obstruction. *Otolaryngol Head Neck Surg*. 1988;98:10–13.

18. Wei WI, Siu KF, Lau WF, et al. Emergency endotracheal intubation under fiberoptic endoscopic guidance for stenosis of the trachea. *Surg Gynecol Obstet*. 1987;165:547–548.

19. Mandavia DP, Qualls S, Rokos I. Emergency airway management in penetrating neck injury. *Ann Emerg Med*. 2000;35:221–225.

20. Edens ET, Sia RL. Flexible fiberoptic endoscopy in difficult intubations. *Ann Otol Rhinol Laryngol*. 1981;90:307–309.

21. Hershey MD, Hannenberg AA. Gastric distention and rupture from oxygen insufflation during fiberoptic intubation. *Anesthesiology*. 1996;85:1479–1480.

22. Ovassapian A, Mesnick PS, Oxygen insufflation through the fiberscope to assist intubation is not recommended. *Anesthesiology*. 1997;87:183–184.

23. Ho AM, Chung DC, To EW, et al. Total airway obstruction during local anesthesia in a non-sedated patient with a compromised airway. *Can J Anaesth*. 2004;51:838–841.

24. Shaw IC, Welchew EA, Harrison BJ, et al. Complete airway obstruction during awake fibreoptic intubation. *Anaesthesia*. 1997;52:582–585.

25. McGuire G, el-Beheiry H. Complete upper airway obstruction during awake fibreoptic intubation in patients with unstable cervical spine fractures. *Can J Anaesth*. 1999;46:176–178.

26. Donlon JV Jr. Anesthetic management of patients with compromised airways. *Anesth Rev*. 1980;7:22–31.

16

Fiberoptic and Video Intubating Stylets

Valerie A. Dobiesz • Calvin A. Brown III • John C. Sakles

INTRODUCTION

Fiberoptic and video intubating stylets are novel intubating devices that permit visualization of the glottis by way of an image conveyed to an eyepiece or video screen from a distally positioned video or fiberoptic image source. Therefore, they do not require a direct line of sight from the operator's eye to the glottis, as must occur for successful direct laryngoscopy. Distinct from the video laryngoscopes (see Chapter 13) and optical devices (Chapter 14), the fiberoptic and video stylets are intended to have the endotracheal tube (ETT) mounted directly over them, as for any conventional stylet, and are used to guide the tube through the cords and into the trachea under continuous visualization. Unlike flexible fiberoptic devices, these devices are rigid or semirigid and include a fiberoptic bundle or video apparatus enclosed in a preformed, curved steel stylet designed to navigate around the tongue and traverse the hypopharynx to visualize laryngeal structures, often with minimal mouth opening or neck mobility. This carries significant advantages; anatomical impediments to direct laryngoscopy, such as a high larynx, cervical spine immobility, or limited mouth opening often create little or no difficulty. Also, rigid stylets do not have any control mechanisms like their flexible fiberoptic counterparts and thus typically are easier to maneuver, especially for nonexperts. Rigid stylets have nonmalleable curved metal sheaths, the shape of which cannot be altered, whereas semirigid devices, although not flexible, can be bent slightly to alter their angulation and thus fit the particular airway geometry of each patient.

Semirigid fiberoptic stylets include the Shikani optical stylet (SOS) and the Levitan/"first pass success" (FPS) scope (Clarus Medical, Minneapolis, MN). The predominant semirigid video stylet is the Clarus Video System (CVS). Rigid stylets include the Bonfils Retromolar Intubation Fiberscope (Karl Storz Endoscopy, Tuttlingen, Germany) and the Video Rigid Flexible Laryngoscope (RIFL) (AI Medical Devices, Inc., Williamston, MI). New intubating stylets, all similar in shape and principle, are appearing on the market at regular intervals.

Although these devices are not yet a routine part of emergency airway management, they have shown significant potential as adjunctive devices for the difficult airway especially when mouth opening is limited, as a method of awake intubation, or as rescue devices for the failed airway. Their clear advantages over direct laryngoscopy suggest that they will come into increasing use as an airway management tool, even for "routine" emergency airways. They also may serve an expanding role in airway training because they all have video displays or are easily adapted for video by attachment of an eyepiece video camera adapter that transmits images to a video monitor.

The prototypical fiberoptic intubating stylet is the SOS; therefore, more time is devoted to its description, proper use, advantages, and contraindications. The other devices are similar in their core design and application, and are therefore described in less detail, highlighting specific features and differences.

SEMIRIGID STYLETS

Shikani Optical Stylet

The SOS is a semirigid stylet containing fiberoptic bundles for light and image transmission (Fig. 16-1). The stylet, rounded distally to an angle of about 70° to 80°, ends proximally in a high-resolution, fixed-focus eyepiece. The adult stylet can accommodate ETTs of 5.5-mm internal diameter (ID) or larger. A pediatric version is available and accommodates tubes of 3.0- to 5.0-mm ID. A bright halogen light is powered from the attached handle, which holds four AA batteries, but the stylet is also compatible with green-specification fiberoptic laryngoscope handles or remote light sources through a fiberoptic cable. A camera can be attached to the eyepiece and the image displayed on a video monitor for teaching purposes. A push-button power switch can be found on the top of the handle. An adjustable tube stop is mounted on the proximal portion of the stylet to hold the ETT in the desired position and prevents the tip of the stylet from protruding from the distal end of the ETT. The tube stop incorporates an oxygen port, permitting insufflation of

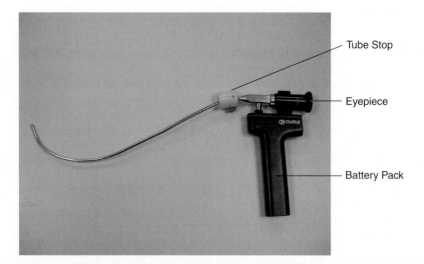

Tube Stop

Eyepiece

Battery Pack

Figure 16-1 ● Shikani Optical Stylet.

oxygen. This helps prevent contamination of the tip of the stylet and can mitigate oxygen desaturation during prolonged intubation attempts. The malleable distal section of the stylet can be adjusted by hand, increasing or decreasing the angle of the bend to conform to the patient's anatomy. The manufacturer also sells a stylet-bending guide that helps to bend the stylet in a smooth curve and helps avoid damage to the fiberoptic bundles by bending it too acutely.

To prepare the SOS, an ETT is loaded on the stylet, with the distal end of the stylet positioned just proximal to the ETT tip, and stabilized in this position by adjusting the tube stop proximally. Lubrication of the stylet will facilitate tube withdrawal when the intubation is completed, but care should be taken not to contaminate the tip of the scope, which will obscure the image. Before insertion, the stylet tip should be warmed with either warmed saline or a warm blanket. It is highly recommended that antifog solution be applied to minimize fogging during the intubation attempt. The device is held by the fingertips and thumb of the dominant hand, with the handle cradled in the web space between the thumb and index finger and the pads of all other fingers resting on the anterior part of the eyepiece and proximal stylet (Fig. 16-2). Despite its appearance, the handle should not be gripped in the hand, but is properly held in the fashion demonstrated in Figure 16-2. The ETT-stylet combination is then inserted into the mouth in the midline and advanced into the hypopharynx under direct vision, not by using the eyepiece. The entire stylet is oriented in the midline and advanced along its curve gently around the base of the tongue. A firm jaw lift/tongue pull during insertion will lift the soft tissues of the upper airway and create some anatomical space through which to navigate the scope. The operator should begin to visualize glottic structures through the eyepiece as the tip navigates the base of the tongue. The epiglottis should quickly come into view. Guide the stylet under the epiglottis to visualize the laryngeal inlet. The operator should then attempt to advance the tip of the stylet through the cords. Typically the operator can advance the scope 1 to 2 cm into the laryngeal inlet. A common error is to advance the fiberoptic tip too far into the hypopharynx as it is inserted, giving a view of the posterior aspect of the hypopharynx or upper esophagus. To avoid this, ensure that the primary motion of the scope is initially rotation around the tongue and not advancement into the hypopharynx. If no anatomical structures are recognized on the initial insertion, it is best to withdraw the stylet, ensure positioning in the midline, ensure proper elevation of the tongue and mandible, and attempt slow reinsertion, identifying the epiglottis or other laryngeal structures as the assembly is advanced. As with other intubating stylets, the instrument can be used in conjunction with direct laryngoscopy. For example, when an unanticipated grade 3 direct laryngoscopy (epiglottis only) occurs, the ETT–SOS stylet combination can be inserted under the epiglottis during direct laryngoscopy, and the glottic opening can then be located by looking through the eyepiece. With either technique, the

ETT-stylet is advanced through the cords as the operator looks through the eyepiece, and then the ETT is held in place as the stylet is withdrawn by the operator, using a large circular motion, in an arc initially upward toward the ceiling in the axis of the proximal end of the tube, and then continuing toward the patient's chest and feet, following the curve of the stylet to facilitate removal (Fig. 16-3). Tube placement confirmation is with end-tidal carbon dioxide (CO_2), auscultation, and chest radiography, as for any other methods of intubation.

The SOS is advertised as being useful for the management of difficult and routine airways, with the video capability facilitating airway management teaching. In the teaching setting, coupling the device with a video system can greatly enhance success by allowing the instructor to help guide and, if necessary, reorientate the learner.

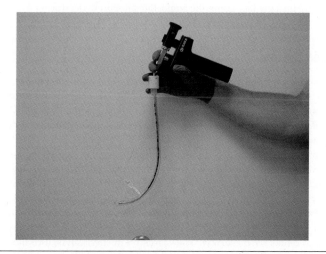

Figure 16-2 ● **Shikani Optical Stylet—in Hand.**

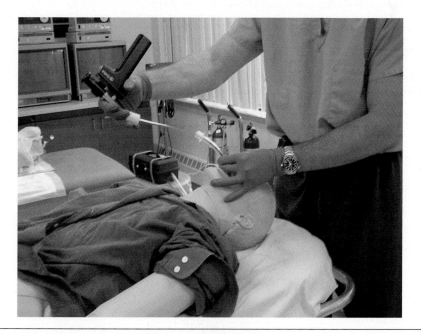

Figure 16-3 ● **Removal of a Shikani Optical Stylet.**

The primary limitation of the SOS is its inability to maintain clear vision occasionally because of fogging or the presence of secretions or blood. Fogging can be greatly reduced by warming the lens and applying antifog solution, as described previously. Although secretions, vomitus, or blood can obscure the distal lens of the scope, two key design elements come into play:

1. The patient is typically supine, and with the jaw thrust and tongue pull, most of the manipulation of the scope is occurring anterior to the location of the pooled liquids.
2. If the lens becomes obscured and cannot be cleared, it is quickly and easily removed, wiped, and reinserted in a matter of seconds.

Occasionally, the glottis cannot be visualized using the scope, and in such cases, adjustment of the scope's curvature (usually increasing the angle, but sometimes decreasing it) provides an improved "angle of attack."

Clarus Video System

The Clarus Video System (Clarus Medical, Minneapolis, MN) is the latest incarnation of the SOS (Fig. 16-4). It is the same shape and design as the SOS but has some new features that make it a superior device. Most importantly, a camera and a 4 in (10 cm) liquid crystal display (LCD) screen replace fiberoptic bundles and the eyepiece on the SOS. The stylet is more malleable at the end than the SOS, making it adjustable for individual airway anatomy. The stylet can be removed from the handle and display unit making it efficient to clean and disinfect. During intubation, the operator stands upright and looks at the screen instead of having to bend forward with the eye opposed to the eyepiece. The screen swivels, making it easy for the operator to adjust the viewing angle during the intubation. Another novel feature of the Clarus VS is the presence of a red light-emitting diode (LED) on the tip of the fiberoptic stylet. This provides transillumination through the soft tissues of the anterior neck during intubation and thus can potentially be useful as a guide or "locator" if the lens gets contaminated and the operator cannot see the airway. The Clarus VS in effect can be used like a lighted stylet, with tracheal entry being signified by a strong glow of red light through the anterior neck. The Clarus VS also has a video out port allowing the operator to display the image of the airway on a larger monitor or record the intubation using a video recorder. Instead of using disposable batteries like the SOS, the Clarus VS uses an internal rechargeable battery system that provides hours of power under typical conditions.

Levitan/FPS Scope

The Levitan/FPS scope is a small, semirigid fiberoptic stylet intended to be used in concert with a standard laryngoscope. Its preformed shape is similar to other intubating stylets but with a gentler

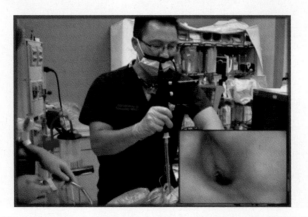

Figure 16-4 ● **Clarus Video System in Use with Screen Image in Lower Right.**

curve (approximately 45°); however, it can be gently bent to meet the unique geometry of most airways (Fig. 16-5). It has a handle with a small battery pack that powers an LED to provide illumination. A screw-down cap, rather than a push button, is used to activate the light source. The eyepiece is at the proximal end of the stylet, near the top of the battery pack. The mechanics of the Levitan/FPS are similar to that of the SOS with one important difference: the Levitan/FPS is *intended* to be used with a standard laryngoscope. The ETT should be cut to 26 cm because the stylet is shorter than a standard ETT. The ETT is held in place by inserting it into a round, nonadjustable tube stop near the body of the scope. As with all intubating fiberoptic stylets, the distal

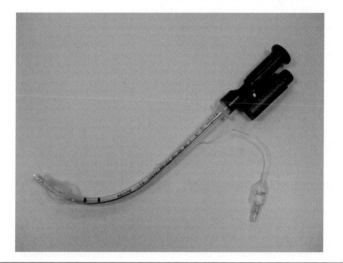

Figure 16-5 ● **Levitan/FPS Scope.**

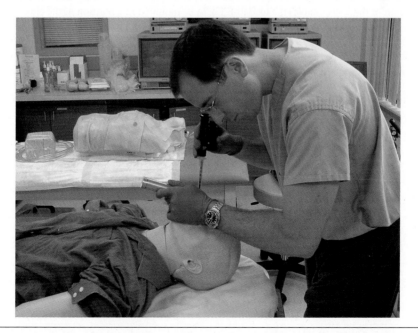

Figure 16-6 ● **Levitan/FPS Scope in Use with Standard Direct Laryngoscope.**

end of the stylet is positioned within 0.5 cm of the ETT tip because positioning more proximally in the ETT obscures the view through the lens and results in severe "tunnel vision."

Unlike the SOS, the oxygen port is on the distal part of the handle and there is no adjustable tube stop. A flow of 5 to 10 L per minute is intended to clear secretions and avoid hypoxia during laryngoscopy and tube placement. However, this practice has led to gastric insufflation and perforation during flexible fiberoptic–assisted intubation and should be used with caution.

The Levitan/FPS scope is intended to be of particular benefit in patients with Cormack–Lehane grade 3 view on direct laryngoscopy. If a poor view is obtained by direct laryngoscopy, the operator positions the Levitan/FPS scope with mounted ETT so the tip of the scope is under the proximal tip of the epiglottis. The operator then looks through the eyepiece to visualize the laryngeal inlet (Fig. 16-6). When vocal cords are seen, the entire apparatus is advanced into the trachea. The laryngoscope is then removed. The stylet is removed while the tube is well immobilized in a fashion similar to that described for the SOS. Tube confirmation is done in the standard fashion with immediate end-tidal CO_2 detection and auscultation, followed by chest radiography. In the event that laryngoscopy identifies a grade 4 view, the lack of the epiglottis as a landmark greatly impairs the utility of the scope. In such cases, the scope might be used to search for the epiglottis, which, if found, might allow repositioning of the direct laryngoscope to achieve a grade 3 view.

RIGID STYLETS

Bonfils Retromolar Intubating Fiberscope

The Bonfils fiberoptic stylet uses high-grade fiberoptic bundles for light and optical transmission in a manner analogous to that of the SOS (Fig. 16-7). Unlike the SOS, which is inserted in the midline of the mouth, the Bonfils is intended to use a right paraglossal or retromolar approach, capitalizing on the proximity of the glottis to the third (most posterior) molar and was specifically designed to permit retromolar intubation in patients with limited mouth opening. The stylet incorporates a distal bend of approximately 40° and ends proximally in an eyepiece, which can be adjusted to different angles for operator comfort and ease of use. A small movable tube holder on the shaft of the stylet enables the loaded ETT to be mounted in a position of the clinician's choice. The continuous insufflation of oxygen reduces fogging and contamination during use, but an antifog solution is advised. The earlier caveat applies regarding the risk of gastric insufflation and perforation by oxygen insufflation. The Bonfils is intended to be used as a sole intubating device, but it can also be used in conjunction with a direct laryngoscope or a video laryngoscope.

A small combination battery pack and light source affixes near the proximal end of the stylet, making the device light and easily manipulated. A conventional external fiberoptic light source

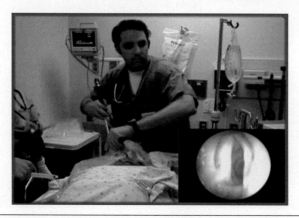

Figure 16-7 ● Bonfils Retromolar Intubation Fiberscope with Screen Image at Lower Right.

cable can be used in place of the self-contained pack, if desired. A standard camera adapter can be attached to the eyepiece, as for the SOS, and is particularly helpful for learning how to use the Bonfils.

The Bonfils has been used extensively in Europe and in various North American sites for both routine intubations and difficult airways, but as with the SOS and Levitan/FPS, there is insufficient literature to draw conclusions about its performance in large series, and there are no published head-to-head comparisons with other devices. There is, however, a growing body of literature supporting its use as an effective airway adjunct.

Video RIFL

The Video RIFL (RIgid Flexible Laryngoscope) is a hybrid intubating device with a rigid stylet that ends in a flexible tip that can be dynamically and continuously adjusted with a proximal lever up to a 135° angle (Fig. 16-8). It incorporates a complementary metal oxide sensor distal chip imaging system and a real-time articulation tip to combine features desired in flexible fiberoptic bronchoscopy as well as video laryngoscopy. The handle features a portable inline LCD, an integrated composite video output access for use with a monitor or recording device, and a self-contained power supply in addition to the lever that controls flexion of the distal tip. The manufacturer's literature states that it is intended for use in difficult airways and awake intubations, and can be used both with and without direct laryngoscopy, but clinical experience with the device is too limited to specify its role at the time of this writing. The Video RIFL uses a bright LED light source and can accommodate an ETT size of 6.5 and higher. There is no pediatric model. The RIFL can be sterilized with STERIS or Cidex OPA.

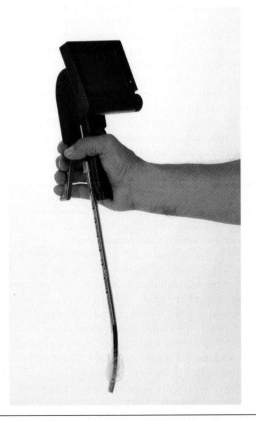

Figure 16-8 ● **Video Rigid Intubating Fiberoptic Laryngoscope.** (Courtesy of AI Medical Devices Inc.)

SUMMARY

Intubating fiberoptic stylets are useful adjunctive devices for emergency airway management. The clear design advantages offered by these thin, curved, and sometimes malleable or controllable stylets have the potential to make both routine and difficult intubations more successful and safer. The primary advantage is the elimination of the need to create a straight line of sight from outside the patient's mouth to the glottic aperture, the major barrier to successful direct laryngoscopy. By positioning the "viewing port" at the distal end of a stylet, these fiberoptic intubating stylets offer a great advantage over direct laryngoscopy, allowing the operator to "steer" the distal end of the ETT through the cords. Considerable work needs to be done to fully evaluate these devices in the emergency arena; however, it seems reasonable that many of the benefits seen in anesthesia literature would apply to patients requiring emergency airway management.

EVIDENCE

- **Do we have any proof that the SOS is superior to direct laryngoscopy?** Most existing studies are relatively small reports in the anesthesia literature using healthy elective surgical patients but studies in the Emergency Medicine literature are emerging. Shikani[1] first described use of the SOS in the management of difficult airways in adults and children undergoing elective otolaryngologic surgery. Agro et al.[2] did a performance assessment with the SOS in 20 healthy preoperative surgical patients and successfully intubated 14 out of 20 patients on the first attempt. The remaining six were successfully intubated on subsequent attempts. Consistent with the findings of a recent study comparing the SOS to the Macintosh laryngoscope,[3] Agro et al. also noted negligible effects on hemodynamics, a property that could be beneficial in emergency patients with head injury. Only a single case report describes SOS use in emergency airway management, where it was successfully used for awake intubation of an obese patient with chronic obstructive pulmonary disease.[4] Many versions of fiberoptic stylets exist; the literature to date suggests they are useful adjuncts and perform as well as or better than direct laryngoscopy in both real and simulated difficult airway scenarios.[5,6] Reports of use in pediatrics have been confined to difficult airway management.[7,8] A clear role in care of trauma patients has not been elucidated, but one study shows that the SOS causes less C-spine motion than Macintosh direct laryngoscopy.[9] In a study of simulated difficult tracheal intubation in manikins, the SOS outperformed the gum elastic bougie, achieving higher success rates and shorter intubation times.[10]
- **Are there any studies supporting the use of the Levitan/FPS stylet?** Similar to other fiberoptic devices, there is little literature besides case studies describing use of the Levitan/FPS scope in emergency airway management, although it has been suggested that it can and should be used in both difficult and routine intubations.[11] A study comparing the Levitan fiberoptic stylet and the bougie as adjuncts to direct laryngoscopy in manikin-simulated difficult airways found them both equally effective in simulated Cormack–Lehane grade 3a views but the Levitan was significantly more effective than the bougie in facilitating intubation of a Cormack–Lehane grade 3b view.[12] In a similar study on 34 elective anesthesia patients with simulated grade 3 laryngoscopy, the bougie and the Levitan FPS performed similarly. The Levitan was limited by secretions obscuring the lens; the bougie by failing to hold its shape.[13] In another human subjects study, a single operator modified the FPS into an S-shape and successfully intubated 300/301 patients with a mean intubation time of 23 seconds without using a direct laryngoscope.[14] These results likely cannot be generalized, though, and we recommend using the FPS only with conventional direct laryngoscopy.
- **What is known about the Bonfils Retromolar Intubating Fiberscope?** There have been multiple studies published involving the Bonfils fiberscope. A European case series reported on six prehospital intubations, the majority being difficult intubations, with all six patients successfully intubated on the first attempt.[15] The Bonfils appears to be highly successful in

routine airways as well. Halligan and Charters[16] published a report of 60 healthy preoperative patients and found an intubation success rate of >98%. A study of its use in predicted difficult airways identified equivalent success to the intubating laryngeal mask airway (LMA), with the Bonfils-assisted intubations being significantly more rapidly achieved than those using the LMA.[17] Overall intubation times ranged from 30 to 60 seconds across several studies. Like other intubating stylets, the Bonfils may find an expanding role in trauma airway management because similar findings of reduced cervical spine motion during intubation have been reported.[18] This was substantiated in another study of 76 normal patients placed in a cervical collar before induction with intubation successful more frequently and with a shorter intubation time when using the Bonfils compared with direct laryngoscopy.[19] The Bonfils also appears to be a successful rescue device following multiple failed direct laryngoscopic attempts by anesthetists.[20] Another study compared the Bonfils with standard direct laryngoscopy in simulated difficult pediatric intubations in manikins and found that the Bonfils was easier to use and provided a better view of the larynx than simple direct laryngoscopy. Success rate and time to intubate were comparable to direct laryngoscopy, however. The role of the Bonfils in the difficult pediatric airway is still being delineated.[21] Several studies have shown the utility of the Bonfils in awake intubations on patients with difficult airways demonstrating that it is well tolerated and highly successful (96.6%) in this setting even by inexperienced operators.[22,23] Patients should be premedicated and anesthetized in a similar fashion as awake intubations using flexible fiberoptic laryngoscopy.

- **Is there any evidence supporting use of the Video RIFL?** This device has not been subjected to comparative study. There is a limited case series reporting use of the Video RIFL in patients with limited neck mobility, historically difficult airway intubations, when direct laryngoscopy failed, and to successfully place an ETT through a supraglottic airway device.[24]
- **Is there a comprehensive analysis of the performance of fiberoptic stylets and nonstandard laryngoscopes versus direct laryngoscopy?** One study attempted a quantitative review and meta-analysis of the performance of nonstandard laryngoscopes and rigid fiberoptic intubation aids but was limited by data heterogeneity, which the authors deemed too difficult to interpret. Therefore no definitive studies comparing these alternative airway devices are available to make recommendations of success rates, ease of use, and time to intubation.[25] There have been several review articles written updating the advances and utility of these devices in airway management.[26,27] Overall, the role of fiberoptic intubating stylets in emergency airway management has yet to be clearly defined but appears to have utility especially as an adjunct in managing the difficult airway.

REFERENCES

1. Shikani AH. New "seeing" stylet-scope and method for the management of the difficult airway. *Otolaryngol Head Neck Surg*. 1999;120:113–116.

2. Agro F, Cataldo R, Carassiti M, et al. The seeing stylet: a new device for tracheal intubation. *Resuscitation*. 2000;44:177–180.

3. Zhao SB, Jia NG, Liu KP, et al. Comparison of hemodynamic responses to orotracheal intubation with shikani laryngoscope or Macintosh direct laryngoscope. *Zhongguo Yi Xue Ke Xue Yuan Xue Bao*. 2010;32(3):303–309.

4. Kovacs G, Law AJ, Petrie D. Awake fiberoptic intubation using an optical stylet in an anticipated difficult airway. *Ann Emerg Med*. 2007;49(1):81–83.

5. Liem EB, Bjoraker DG, Gravenstein D. New options for airway management: intubating fibreoptic stylets. *Br J Anaesth*. 2003;91:408–411.

6. Biro P, Weiss M, Gerber A, et al. Comparison of a new video-optical intubation stylet versus the conventional malleable stylet in simulated difficult tracheal intubation. *Anaesthesia*. 2000;55:886–889.

7. Pfitzner L, Cooper MG, Ho D. The Shikani seeing stylet for difficult intubation in children: initial experience. *Anaesth Intensive Care*. 2002;30:462–466.

8. Shukry M, Hanson RD, Koveleskie JR, et al. Management of the difficult pediatric airway with Shikani optical stylet. *Paediatr Anaesth*. 2005;15(4):342–345.

9. Turkstra TP, Pelz DM, Shaikh AA, et al. Cervical spine motion: a fluoroscopic comparison of Shikani optical stylet vs. Macintosh laryngoscope. *Can J Anaesth*. 2007;54(6):441–447.

10. Evans A, Morris S, Petterson J, et al. A comparison of the Seeing Optical Stylet and the gum elastic bougie in simulated difficult tracheal intubation: a manikin study. *Anaesthesia*. 2006;61(5):478–481.

11. Levitan RM. Design rationale and intended use of a short optical stylet for routine fiberoptic augmentation of emergency laryngoscopy. *Am J Emerg Med*. 2006;24(4):490–495.

12. Kovacs G, Law JA, McCrossin C, et al. A comparison of a fiberoptic stylet and a bougie as adjuncts to direct laryngoscopy in a manikin-simulated difficult airway. *Ann Emerg Med*. 2007;50(6):676–685.

13. Greenland KB, Liu G, Tan H, et al. Comparison of the Levitan FPS Scope and the single-use bougie for simulated difficult intubation in anaesthetised patients. *Anaesthesia*. 2007;62(5):509–515.

14. Aziz M, Metz S. Clinical evaluation of the Levitan Optical Stylet. *Anaesthesia*. 2011;66(7):579–581. Epub 2011 May 13.

15. Byhahn C, Meininger D, Walcher F, et al. Prehospital emergency endotracheal intubation using the Bonfils intubation fiberscope. *Eur J Emerg Med*. 2007;14(1):43–46.

16. Halligan M, Charters P. A clinical evaluation of the Bonfils intubation fibrescope. *Anaesthesia*. 2003;58(11):1087–1091.

17. Bein B, Worthmann F, Scholz J, et al. A comparison of the intubating laryngeal mask airway and the Bonfils intubating fibrescope in patients with predicted difficult airways. *Anaesthesia*. 2004;59(7):668–674.

18. Wahlen BM, Gercek E. Three-dimensional cervical spine movement during intubation using the MacIntosh and Bullard laryngoscopes, the bonfils fibrescope and the intubating laryngeal mask airway. *Eur J Anaesthesiol*. 2004;21(11):907–913.

19. Byhahn C, Nemetz S, Breitkreutz R, et al. Brief report: tracheal intubation using the Bonfils intubation fibrescope or direct laryngoscopy of patients with a simulated difficult airway. *Can J Anaesth*. 2008;55:232–237.

20. Bein B, Yan M, Tonner PH, et al. Tracheal intubation using the Bonfils intubation fibrescope after failed direct laryngoscopy. *Anaesthesia*. 2004;59(12):1207–1209.

21. Vlatten A, Aucoin S, Litz S, et al. A comparison of bonfils fiberscope-assisted laryngoscopy and standard direct laryngoscopy in simulated difficult pediatric intubation: a manikin study. *Paediatr Anaesth*. 2010;20(6):559–565.

22. Corbanese U, Possamai C. Awake intubation with the Bonfils fibrescope in patients with difficult airway. *Eur J Anaesthesiol*. 2009;26(10):837–841.

23. Abramson SI, Holmes AA, Hagberg CA. Awake insertion of the Bonfils Retromolar Intubation Fiberscope in five patients with anticipated difficult airways. *Anesth Analg*. 2008;106(4):1215–1217.

24. Setty H, Rawlings JL, Dubin S. Video RIFL: a rigid flexible laryngoscope to facilitate airway management. *J Clin Anesth*. 2010;22(8):642–647.

25. Mihai R, Blair R, Kay H, et al. A quantitative review and meta-analysis of performance of nonstandard laryngoscopes and rigid fibreoptic intubation aids. *Anaesthesia*. 2008;63(7):745–760.

26. Pott LM, Murray WB. Review of video laryngoscopy and rigid fiberoptic laryngoscopy. *Curr Opin Anaesthesiol*. 2008;21(6):750–758.

27. Hurford W. The video revolution: a new view of laryngoscopy. *Respir Care*. 2010;55:1036–1045.

17

Blind Intubation Techniques

Steven A. Godwin

DESCRIPTION

Blind intubation techniques are those methods of airway management that are done without visualization of the larynx or glottis. Both blind nasotracheal intubation (NTI) and digital tracheal intubation (DTI) use indirect indicators of airway identification in lieu of direct vision laryngoscopy. NTI relies on listening to and feeling air movement, whereas DTI depends on the provider's ability to use tactile senses to distinguish airway anatomy as the tube is inserted. Other methods of airway management that do not require direct visualization of the glottis, but that do require specialized equipment, such as lighted stylets and gum elastic bougies, are discussed in other chapters. Some consider flexible bronchoscopic intubation as being a "blind" technique as the actual passage of the endotracheal tube (ETT) through the vocal cords into the trachea is not visualized.

BLIND NASAL INTUBATION

Although NTI was widely used in emergency departments (EDs) in the past, it has been supplanted by superior techniques of oral intubation with neuromuscular blockade, even in the prehospital setting. In general, NTI has a number of serious drawbacks, and few advantages when compared with the other techniques that are now commonly used for emergency airway management. NTI has largely fallen out of favor in the ED because it takes longer, has a higher failure rate, has a higher complication rate, and requires smaller tube sizes than oral rapid sequence intubation (RSI). However, despite these inherent problems, NTI is still considered an important skill because it may be useful in certain difficult airway situations, particularly in departments without flexible endoscopic intubation capability.

Indications and Contraindications

As clinicians become more facile and comfortable with neuromuscular blockade and a variety of other approaches, the one remaining indication for NTI may be the spontaneously breathing patient with an identified difficult airway, for whom RSI is judged to be inadvisable (see Chapters 2 and 3). NTI is achieved by listening to the patient's spontaneous respirations through the tube and, therefore, should not be attempted in the apneic patient. It is relatively contraindicated in combative patients; in those with anatomically disrupted or distorted airways (e.g., neck hematoma, upper airway tumor, etc.); in cases of increased intracranial pressure; in the context of severe facial trauma with suspected basal skull fracture; in upper airway infection, obstruction, or abscess (e.g., Ludwig angina, epiglottitis, etc.); and in the presence of coagulopathy. NTI should be performed with great reservation on any patient who needs rapid intubation because, despite optimistic claims to the contrary, intubation usually requires several minutes to perform using this technique, and significant oxygen desaturation can occur. Therefore, it is a poor choice for patients with respiratory failure, such as the asthmatic patient in extremis, who cannot be oxygenated during a protracted nasal intubation attempt. In addition, one of the primary indications for NTI in the past, the patient with multiple injuries and potential cervical spine injury, has been discarded, and oral RSI with inline stabilization is now the recommended route (see Chapter 31).

Technique

1. If the patient is awake, explain the procedure. This is a crucial step that is often neglected. If the patient becomes combative during intubation, the attempt must cease because epistaxis, turbinate damage, or even pharyngeal perforation may ensue. A brief, reassuring explanation of the procedure, its necessity, and anticipated discomfort may avert this undesirable situation. Preoxygenate the patient with 100% oxygen as for RSI

(see Chapter 19), if possible. Try to avoid bagging with positive pressure if spontaneous ventilation is adequate.

2. Choose the nostril to be used. Inspect the interior of the naris, with particular reference to the septum and turbinates. It may help to occlude each nostril in turn and listen to the flow of air through the orifices. If there appears to be no clear favorite, the right naris should be selected because it better facilitates passage of the tube with the leading edge of the bevel laterally placed.

3. Instill two or three drops of Neo-Synephrine (phenylephrine) or oxymetazoline nasal solution into each nostril. This will vasoconstrict the nasal mucosa and may make tube passage easier. The incidence of epistaxis may also be reduced, although there is little evidence to that effect. It may also be helpful to soak two or three cotton-tipped applicators in the vasoconstrictor solution and place them gently and fully into the naris until the tip touches the nasopharynx. This provides vasoconstriction at the area that is often most difficult to negotiate blindly with the ETT. Nasal topical anesthesia may then be placed as time permits. Insertion of a 4% cocaine pack or instillation of 2% lidocaine jelly will provide anesthesia for the nose. The oral cavity can be sprayed with 4% lidocaine or a similar spray, and, if desired, the pharynx may be anesthetized similarly. An alternative is to nebulize a solution of 4 ml of 4% lidocaine with 1 ml of 0.5% Neo-Synephrine in a gas-powered nebulizer, as one would do with albuterol. This takes approximately 5 to 10 minutes but provides reasonable anesthesia and is well tolerated. Still another suggested method involves insertion of an absorbent nasal tampon (as is used for epistaxis) and application of several milliliters of 2% lidocaine with 1:100,000 epinephrine. Cricothyroid puncture with instillation of 5 to 10 ml of 1% to 2% lidocaine is often advocated. This technique is reasonably simple and effective but usually produces coughing, perhaps an undesirable result. Importantly, complete anesthesia of the glottis may not be desirable in all cases. Advancing the tube during the inspiratory phase of a cough sometimes allows immediate intubation of an otherwise elusive trachea.

4. Lubricate the tube and the nostril. The use of 2% lidocaine jelly has been advocated, but it will not normally be in contact with the nasal mucosa long enough to result in anesthesia. However, the jelly is an adequate lubricant and is not harmful, so it is a reasonable choice.

5. Select the appropriate size of ETT. In general, the tube should be the largest one that will fit through the nostril without inducing significant trauma. In most patients, a tube with an internal diameter (ID) of 6.0 to 7.5 cm will suffice. A smaller tube will fit through a difficult or tight space better than a larger tube. Test the ETT cuff for leaks.

6. Because the patient is often seated, it is probably easiest for a right-handed person to intubate from the patient's left side. This allows the right hand to be used for the intubation, while the left hand manipulates the location of the larynx and provides feedback to the right hand. By leaning slightly forward between the two hands, the operator can listen to the breath sounds and guide the tube into place. If the patient is supine, the operator will position him- or herself immediately above the patient's head. Positioning the head as for oral intubation is worthwhile, if possible. The so-called sniffing position, with the neck flexed on the body and the head extended on the neck, optimizes the alignment of the mouth and pharynx with the vocal cords and trachea (see Chapter 12). Care must be taken to avoid overextension, however, which causes the tube to pass anteriorly to the epiglottis. A small towel may be placed behind the patient's occiput to help maintain this relationship.

7. Some advise gently inserting a gloved and lubricated little finger into the chosen nostril as deeply as possible to check for patency and to dilate the nostril to accept the tube as atraumatically as possible. The intubation sequence begins by gently inserting the ETT into the nostril with the leading edge carefully avoiding the rich vascular area of the anterior septum. For consistency, the remainder of this discussion assumes a right naris intubation by a right-handed operator. The tube should be turned so that the leading edge of the bevel is "out" (i.e., away from the septum). This will minimize the chances of septum injury and epistaxis. This also orients the natural curve of the ETT tube with the natural curve of the airway.

The major nasal airway is located below the inferior turbinate and the placement of the ETT should follow the floor of the nose backward. The tip of the tube should be directed caudad at an approximately 10° angle to follow the gently downsloping floor of the nose (see Chapter 4). This entire process should be done slowly and with meticulous care. Once the nasal portion of the airway is navigated, inciting epistaxis is unlikely. When the tip of the tube approaches the posterior pharynx, resistance will often be felt, particularly if the leading edge of the ETT enters the depression in the nasopharynx where the eustachian tube enters. At this point, it is possible to penetrate the nasopharyngeal mucosa with the ETT and dissect submucosally if care is not taken (see Chapter 4). If this occurs, the ETT should be removed and the alternate nostril attempted. In the event that this anatomical structure cannot be navigated, the insertion of a stylet into the ETT with a gentle C-shaped curve and reinserting the curve will keep the ETT off the postnasopharynx and is usually successful. Often, rotating the proximal end of the ETT 90° toward the left nostril once this resistance is felt will facilitate "turning the corner" by orienting the leading edge of the ETT away from the depression. Once the oropharynx is successfully entered, restore the tube to the original orientation and proceed.

8. The tube should now be advanced until the breath sounds are best heard through it (usually approximately 3 to 5 cm). At this point, the distal tip of the tube is positioned immediately above the vocal cords. Occluding the opposite naris and closing the mouth may allow for breath sounds to become more audible.

9. Simultaneous with an inspiratory effort by the patient, advance the tube gently but firmly 3 to 4 cm while applying laryngeal pressure with the left hand. The vocal cords abduct during inspiration and are most widely separated at this time.

10. When the tube is advanced, one of three things will occur. If the trachea is entered, a series of long, wheezy coughs will usually emanate from the patient. Inflation of the cuff and a few ventilations with an end-tidal carbon dioxide (CO_2) detector will confirm intratracheal placement. If the trachea is not entered, the tube either will slide easily down the esophagus or will come to an abrupt halt as it tries to pass anterior to the vocal cords or abuts against the anterior wall of the larynx. In the former case, the patient will not cough, and ventilation through the tube will be better heard over the stomach than over the lungs. End-tidal CO_2 will not be detected. If the tube has passed down the esophagus, it is necessary to bring the distal tip of the tube further anteriorly. Withdraw the tube until the breath sounds are well heard again. Then extend the patient's head slightly and try again. If the intubation is being performed on a patient with possible cervical spine trauma, movement is impossible, and the intubation should be reattempted without any change in patient position. In the event the ETT repeatedly passes anterior to the larynx, flex the head on the neck.

11. Inflate the cuff and confirm position with an end-tidal CO_2 detection device. *Do not administer neuromuscular blocking agents to a patient who has undergone NTI unless tracheal tube placement has been confirmed by end-tidal CO_2 detection.* Breath sounds are never reliable as an indicator of tracheal placement, but this is particularly true in the spontaneously breathing patient who has undergone nasoesophageal intubation, whose own breath sounds will continue to be heard over the lungs, even when the ETT is being bag ventilated. A chest radiograph should also be obtained. If the presence of the tube or inflation of the cuff leads to prolonged coughing by the patient, administer 2 ml of 2% lidocaine solution through the ETT during an inspiration. This will often dramatically improve tube tolerance in seconds.

12. Only 60% to 70% of intubations will succeed on the first attempt. The "blind" nature of the procedure requires adjustment and attention to feedback. If the intubation is proving extremely difficult, consider the various options in Box 17-1.

Box 17-1. Nasotracheal Intubation: Techniques

- The "Endotrol" tube, which has a ringlike apparatus connected to the distal end to allow anterior deflection of the tip of the tube, may be extremely helpful in such cases.
- If the tube has met with a "dead end," it is anterior to the cords or abutted against the anterior wall of the trachea. It may be possible to ascertain by palpation with the left hand whether the tube is off to the left, off to the right, or anterior in the midline. If the tube is truly anterior, slight withdrawal of the tube until breath sounds are well heard followed by slight flexion of the head should facilitate passage. This is a common pitfall. When a first attempt fails, the operator often continues to further extend the neck in an attempt to succeed, each extension making the situation anatomically more impossible. If it is believed that the tube is off to the left or right in addition to being anterior, withdraw the tube, flex the head slightly (if possible), and turn the head slightly in the direction to which the distal tip of the tube was off the midline. For example, if the distal end of the tube was off to the right, turning the head to the right will cause the distal end of the tube to swing to the left (i.e., toward the midline), which is the desired corrective direction. Alternatively, if it is desirable to keep the patient's head in the midline, the proximal end of the ETT may be rotated to the side where the distal end was detected to achieve this effect.
- Inflation of the cuff as the tube lies in the oropharynx may aid in alignment of the ETT with the glottic opening. The tube is then advanced until it meets resistance at the cords, and then the cuff is deflated before being pushed through the cords during inspiration. Inflation of the cuff is felt to lift the end of the tube away from the esophagus and into alignment with the vocal cords.
- Use of a guide such as a nasogastric tube or ETT changer in combination with the previously described inflated cuff technique may improve success rates. With this method, after the ETT has been advanced with the cuff inflated to meet resistance at the laryngeal opening, the nasogastric tube is inserted through the ETT. The inflated cuff allows for alignment of the outlet of the ETT with the vocal cords, and the nasogastric tube will slide through the outlet, through the glottis, and into the trachea. As the nasogastric tube slides through the glottis, coughing may occur, suggesting proper placement. The cuff can then be deflated and guided into the trachea over the nasogastric tube, which is then withdrawn from the ETT.
- Pass a flexible endoscopic laryngoscope or bronchoscope through the tube into the trachea (see Chapter 15).
- Change to a new tube, perhaps one that is 0.5 to 1.0 mm ID smaller. The tube often becomes warm and soft during the intubation attempt and is no longer capable of being appropriately manipulated.
- Use a laryngoscope and Magill forceps. This may require conditions that are not present (i.e., the ability to insert a laryngoscope into the mouth and visualize the vocal cords).
- Grasp the tongue with a piece of gauze and pull it forward, or sit the patient up (if possible). This may improve the angle at the back of the tongue.
- Abandon the attempt. Prolonged attempts are associated with hypoxemia and glottic edema caused by local trauma. Either condition can worsen the situation substantially. Repeated attempts are not significantly more successful than the first. In 10% to 20% of cases, NTI will simply not be possible.
- In an unconscious patient, the nasal passage may be dilated with a nasopharyngeal airway or a gloved small finger if problems are encountered trying to get the tube through the naris. Again, a smaller tube may be advisable.

DIGITAL TRACHEAL INTUBATION

DTI is a tactile intubation technique in which the intubator uses his or her fingers to direct an ETT into the larynx. The technique has gained limited utility in clinical practice. It is neither easy to perform, especially if the intubator has small hands or short fingers, nor is it aesthetically pleasing. However, in certain failed airway circumstances in an austere environment, DTI may be an option.

Indications and Contraindications

DTI may be indicated:

1. In situations with poor lighting, difficult patient position, disrupted airway anatomy, or potential C-spine instability. Many of these situations are more likely in the prehospital setting (e.g., a patient trapped in an automobile).
2. If laryngoscopy equipment is unavailable or not working.
3. When visualization of the larynx is impossible (e.g., blood secretions) and no alternative devices or techniques are possible.
4. In failed intubation in an austere environment without rescue airway devices.

The patient must be sufficiently obtunded to prevent a biting injury to the intubator. Generally, this technique should only be considered in a patient who is frankly comatose and unresponsive.

The Tactile Digital Intubation Technique

1. The right-handed operator stands on the patient's right side. Have an assistant use a gauze sponge to gently but firmly retract the tongue.
2. Insert a stylet in the ETT and bend the ETT/stylet at a 90° angle just proximal to the cuff, and place the ETT/stylet into the mouth. Alternatively, an endotracheal introducer (EI or bougie) may be used rather than the ETT/stylet combination and the ETT threaded into the airway over the EI following confirmation of EI placement in the trachea (see Chapter 12).
3. Slide the index and long fingers of the nondominant hand palm down along the tongue positioning the ETT/stylet on the palmar surface of the hand.
4. Identify the tip of the epiglottis with the tip of the long finger and direct it anteriorly.
5. Use the index finger to gently direct the ETT/stylet into the glottic opening.

Success Rates and Complications

Perhaps the most substantial limitation in performing this technique successfully is the length of the intubator's fingers relative to the patient's oropharyngeal dimensions. Biting injuries or unintentional dental injuries to the hand with the risk of infectious disease transmission may occur. The technique has only infrequently been used in the ED and most authors agree that some degree of experience is needed to perform this skill in an efficient and effective manner.

The two major tips for performing this technique are to have an assistant retract the tongue, thereby allowing the intubator the best access to the epiglottis and to ensure that the patient is sufficiently obtunded to tolerate airway manipulation.

EVIDENCE

- **Although historically recommended as the primary method for difficult airway management, NTI is an infrequently performed procedure for patients requiring emergency airway management and is now less commonly selected as a rescue method.** Because RSI has become the method of choice for intubation of emergency patients, fewer physicians routinely perform NTI. In a 1998 review of 610 intubations performed in a large ED with a level I trauma center, Sakles et al.[1] reported only eight (1.3%) NTIs. Of these patients, two attempts were unsuccessful. A review of ED intubations from 30 hospitals as part of the National Emergency Airway Registry databank project, identified 207/7,712 (2.7%) patients who required the use of rescue techniques and/or additional personnel. Rescue RSI was performed after failure of an alternative technique in 102/207 (49%) patients, whereas NTI was used as a rescue in 36/207 (17%) of patients. Although there were a greater number of rescue intubations with NTI than flexible endoscopic devices, 10/207 (4.8%), Bair et al.[2] emphasized the rapid growth in the use of the flexible endoscopic technique over other methods for both primary and rescue airway management. Although useful as a backup airway skill to maintain, NTI has a diminishing role in emergency airway management.
- **When no other alternatives are available, NTI may be performed safely in facial trauma, but clinicians should be aware of rare, yet devastating, possible complications.** Historically, facial trauma was believed to be an absolute contraindication for NTI because of the perceived associated risk of intracranial placement in the presence of cribriform plate disruption. There have been two reported cases of intracranial placement of a nasotracheal tube after facial trauma.[3,4] These case reports have been criticized for demonstrating the outcome of poor technique rather than the presence of facial trauma as the cause of these injuries.[5] At least one study has been published evaluating the risk of NTI in the presence of facial trauma. This retrospective review of 311 patients with intubation in the presence of facial fractures found that 82 patients underwent NTI.[6] The authors found no episodes of intracranial placement, significant epistaxis requiring nasal packing, esophageal intubation, or osteomyelitis. Although there is no evidence that facial trauma is not a contraindication for NTI, in the modern era of RSI and the availability of multiple alternative airway devices, the indications for NTI in the ED setting are limited.
- **Cuff inflation, neutral head position, and use of ETTs with directional tip control provide added benefit to increase success rates for NTI in both normal and difficult airways.** A number of improvements to the technique for passage of the nasotracheal tube through oropharynx and into the glottis have been suggested over the years. The most studied and successful aid to NTI appears to be the addition of cuff inflation during passage of the tube through the oropharynx until the outlet abuts the glottic opening. A prospective randomized trial evaluating successful NTI with the cuff inflated versus deflated technique demonstrated the inflated cuff technique to be superior. The results showed that 19/20 (95%) patients were intubated with the cuff inflated. In contrast, only 9/20 (45%) patients were intubated with the cuff deflated.[7] A separate study compared success rates for NTI and flexible bronchoscope in patients with an immobilized cervical spine with American Society of Anesthesiologists Class I (ASA I) and ASA II status airways while undergoing elective surgery. The authors reported that there was no significant difference in success rates between the groups. The study concluded that ETT cuff inflation could be used as an alternative to flexible bronchoscopy in patients with an immobilized cervical spine,[8] but this conclusion is not warranted by this small study, and both techniques are highly operator dependent. Other studies have demonstrated increased success with NTI using a neutral head position[9] and ETTs with directional tip control.[10] However, in the immobilized trauma patient without other identified difficult airway attributes (see Chapter 31), RSI is still considered the primary method of

airway management. In the context of specific difficult airway attributes that argue against administering a paralytic agent, either flexible endoscopic intubation or NTI, performed with the patient spontaneously breathing, may be appropriate (see Chapters 2, 3, and 15).

REFERENCES

1. Sakles JC, Laurin EG, Rantapaa AA, et al. Airway management in the emergency department: a one-year study of 610 tracheal intubations. *Ann Emerg Med.* 1998;31(3):325–332.

2. Bair AE, Filbin MR, Kulkarni RG, et al. The failed intubation attempt in the emergency department: analysis of prevalence, rescue techniques, and personnel. *J Emerg Med.* 2002;23(2):131–140.

3. Horellou MF, Mathe D, Feiss P. A hazard of naso-tracheal intubation. *Anaesthesia.* 1978;33:78.

4. Marlow TJ, Goltra DD Jr, Schabel SI. Intracranial placement of a nasotracheal tube after facial fracture: a rare complication. *J Emerg Med.* 1997;15:187–191.

5. Walls RM. Blind nasotracheal intubation in the presence of facial trauma—is it safe? *J Emerg Med.* 1997;15:243–244.

6. Rosen CL, Wolfe RE, Chew SE, et al. Blind nasotracheal intubation in the presence of facial trauma. *J Emerg Med.* 1997;15:141–145.

7. Van Elstraete AC, Pennant JH, Gajraj NM, et al. Tracheal tube cuff inflation as an aid to blind nasotracheal intubation. *Br J Anaesth.* 1993;70:691–693.

8. Van Elstraete AC, Mamie JC, Mehdaoui H. Nasotracheal intubation in patients with immobilized cervical spine: a comparison of tracheal tube cuff inflation and fiberoptic bronchoscopy. *Anesth Analg.* 1998;87(2):400–402.

9. Chung Y, Sun M, Wu H. Blind nasotracheal intubation is facilitated by neutral head position and endotracheal tube cuff inflation in spontaneously breathing patients. *Can J Anaesth.* 2003;50(5):511–513.

10. O'Connor RE, Megargel RE, Schnyder ME, et al. Paramedic success rate for blind nasotracheal intubation is improved with the use of an endotracheal tube with directional tip control. *Ann Emerg Med.* 2000;36:328–332.

18

Surgical Airway Management

Robert J. Vissers • Aaron E. Bair

INTRODUCTION

Surgical airway management is defined as the creation of an opening to the trachea by invasive, surgical means, to provide ventilation and oxygenation. There is some confusion engendered by use of the term *surgical airway management*. In some discussions, surgical airway management includes both cricothyrotomy and needle cricothyrotomy with percutaneous transtracheal ventilation (PTV). Other discussions limit surgical airway management to cricothyrotomy, and consider PTV to be simply another airway management technique. For the purposes of discussion in this chapter, surgical airway management is deemed to include cricothyrotomy (both open and wire-guided techniques), PTV, and placement of a surgical airway using a cricothyrotome, which is a device intended to place a surgical airway percutaneously, usually in one or two steps, without performance of formal cricothyrotomy.

PTV through a catheter is rarely, if ever, done in adults. It does not protect the airway and is grossly inferior to cricothyrotomy in terms of both airway protection and gas exchange. In adults, cricothyrotomy by open or Seldinger technique is preferred. PTV should be reserved for children younger than 10 years, whose anatomy is not conducive to cricothyrotomy. The faculty of The Difficult Airway Course: Emergency advised on the design of a kit that offers the instruments and equipment to perform either the Seldinger percutaneous cricothyrotomy or an open cricothyrotomy, using a cuffed tube for both methods (Melker Universal Emergency Cricothyrotomy Catheter Set, Cook Critical Care, Bloomington, IN; Fig. 18-1). Each main surgical airway technique is described in detail in the sections that follow.

Description

Cricothyrotomy is the establishment of a surgical opening in the airway through the cricothyroid membrane and placement of a cuffed tracheostomy tube or endotracheal tube (ETT).

A cricothyrotome is a kit or device that is intended to establish a surgical airway without resorting to formal cricothyrotomy. These kits use two basic approaches. One approach relies on the Seldinger technique, in which the airway is accessed through a small needle through which a flexible guide wire is passed. The airway device, with a dilator, is then passed over this guide wire and into the airway in a manner analogous with that of central line placement by the Seldinger technique. The other technique relies on the direct percutaneous placement of an airway device without the use of a Seldinger technique. There have been no clinical studies to date demonstrating the superiority of one approach over another or of any of these devices over formal surgical cricothyrotomy. However, certain attributes of the devices make them intuitively more, or less, hazardous for insertion (see the "Evidence" section).

Indications and Contraindications

The primary indication for cricothyrotomy is when a failed airway has occurred (see Chapters 2, 3) and the patient cannot be adequately ventilated or oxygenated with a bag and mask, or the patient is adequately oxygenated, but there is not another available device (e.g., fiberoptic scope, lighted stylet, intubating laryngeal mask airway [LMA]) that is believed likely to successfully secure the airway. A second indication is a method of primary airway management in patients for whom intubation is contraindicated or believed to be impossible. Thus, cricothyrotomy should be thought of as a rescue technique in most circumstances, and only infrequently will it be used as the primary method of airway management. An example of a circumstance in which cricothyrotomy is the primary method of airway management is the patient with severe lower facial trauma in whom access through the mouth or nose would be too time consuming or impossible. This patient requires immediate airway management because of the risk of aspiration of blood and secretions, and cricothyrotomy is indicated.

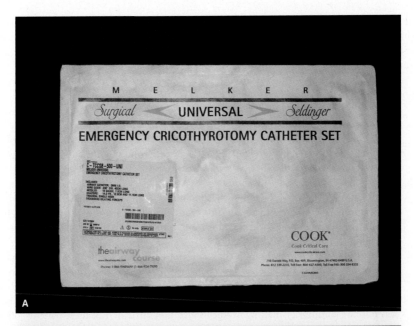

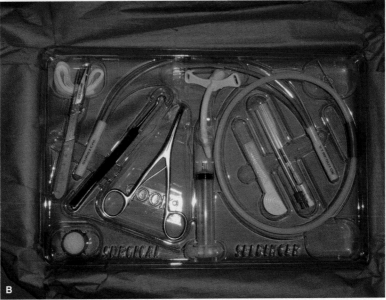

Figure 18-1 ● **A:** Melker Universal Emergency Cricothyrotomy Catheter Set (Cook Critical Care, Bloomington, IN). **B:** Opened set containing cuffed tracheostomy tube, as well as equipment for both open surgical and Seldinger techniques.

The primary hurdle to performing cricothyrotomy is simply recognizing when it is necessary to proceed with surgical airway management, and abandoning further attempts at laryngoscopy, or the use of an alternative device. Rapid sequence intubation (RSI), augmented by a variety of noninvasive airway management methods, is so successful that cricothyrotomy is often viewed as a method of last resort, to be undertaken only after multiple noninvasive attempts or techniques have failed. However, the relentless, unsuccessful pursuit of a noninvasive airway delays the initiation of a surgical airway, greatly increasing the likelihood of hypoxic injury to the patient. This fact is particularly true in the *"can't* intubate, *can't* oxygenate" (CICO) circumstance, when surgical airway management is immediately indicated and must not be delayed for attempts using other devices.

Once the decision to initiate surgical airway management has been made, there are a few fundamental considerations:

1. Will accessing the cricothyroid membrane be *effective?* In other words, will an incision at the level of the cricothyroid membrane bypass the obstruction and solve the problem? If the obstructing lesion is significantly distal to the cricothyroid membrane, performing a cricothyrotomy is a critical waste of time (see Chapter 40).

2. Will the patient's anatomy or pathologic process make cricothyrotomy *difficult* to perform? Placement of the initial skin incision is based on palpating the pertinent anatomy. If adiposity, burns, trauma, or infection make this procedure difficult, then the strategy should be adjusted accordingly. A mnemonic for difficult cricothyrotomy (SMART) is shown in Box 18-1 and is discussed in Chapter 2.

3. Which *type* of invasive technique is best in the particular circumstances (i.e., open surgical or percutaneous)? This consideration takes into account provider preference based on previous experience, equipment availability, and patient characteristics. Needle cricothyrotomy is preferred in children < 10 years of age (see Chapter 25). In obese patients, subcutaneous tissue may obscure landmarks, making needle localization difficult. For these patients, often an open surgical cricothyrotomy is a better choice.

   Contraindications to surgical airway management are few and, with one exception, are relative. That one exception is young age. Children have a small, pliable, mobile larynx and cricoid cartilage, making cricothyrotomy extremely difficult. For children younger than 10 years, unless they are teenage or adult size, needle cricothyrotomy is the surgical airway technique of choice (see Chapter 25). Relative contraindications include pre-existing laryngeal or tracheal pathology such as tumor, infections, or abscess in the area in which the procedure will be performed; hematoma or other anatomical destruction of the landmarks that would render the procedure difficult or impossible; coagulopathy; and lack of operator expertise. Cricothyrotomy has been performed successfully after systemic thrombolytic therapy. Cricothyrotomy has a high success rate when performed in the emergency department (ED) setting. The presence of an anatomical barrier, in particular, should prompt consideration of alternative techniques that might result in a successful airway. However, in cases in which no alternative method of airway management is likely to be successful or timely enough, cricothyrotomy should be performed without hesitation. The same principles apply for both the cricothyrotome and for PTV.

   The cricothyrotomes have not been demonstrated to improve success rates or time to completion, or to decrease complication rates when compared with surgical cricothyrotomy. As with formal cricothyrotomy, experience, skill, knowledge of anatomy, and adherence to proper technique are essential for success when a cricothyrotome is used.

Box 18-1. SMART Mnemonic for Difficult Cricothyrotomy

Surgery
Mass
Access/Anatomy
Radiation
Trauma

TECHNIQUE

Anatomy and Landmarks

The cricothyroid membrane is the anatomical site of access in the emergent surgical airway, regardless of the technique used. It has several advantages over the trachea in the emergent setting. The cricothyroid membrane is more anterior than the lower trachea, and there is less soft tissue between the membrane and the skin. There is less vascularity and therefore less chance of significant bleeding.

The cricothyroid membrane is identified by first locating the laryngeal prominence (notch) of the thyroid cartilage. Approximately one fingerbreadth below the laryngeal prominence, the membrane may be palpated in the midline of the anterior neck, as a soft depression between the inferior aspect of the thyroid cartilage above and the hard cricoid ring below. The relevant anatomy may be easier to appreciate in males because of the more prominent thyroid notch. The thyrohyoid space, which lies high in the neck between the laryngeal prominence and the hyoid bone, should also be identified. This will prevent the misidentification of the thyrohyoid membrane as the cricothyroid membrane, which would lead to misplacement of the tracheostomy tube above the vocal cords. In children, the cricothyroid membrane is disproportionately smaller because of a greater overlap of the thyroid cartilage over the cricoid cartilage. For this reason, cricothyrotomy is not recommended in children of age 10 years or younger.

Unfortunately, the same anatomical or physiologic abnormalities (i.e., trauma, morbid obesity, and congenital anomalies) that necessitated the surgical airway may also hinder easy palpation of landmarks. One way of estimating the location of the cricothyroid membrane is by placing four fingers on the neck, oriented longitudinally, with the small finger in the sternal notch. The membrane is approximately located under the index finger and can serve as a point at which the initial longitudinal incision is made. Except as described later in the technique for the rapid four-step cricothyrotomy, a vertical skin incision is preferred, and particularly so if anatomical landmarks are not readily apparent. Palpation through this vertical incision can then confirm the location of the cricothyroid membrane. Alternatively, identification may be facilitated by using a locator needle, attached to a syringe containing saline or lidocaine. Aspiration of air bubbles suggests entry into the airway, but it will not distinguish between the cricothyroid membrane and a lower tracheal placement.

The No-Drop Technique

The cricothyrotomy instrument set should be simple, consisting of only the equipment necessary to complete the procedure. A sample listing of recommended contents of a cricothyrotomy tray is shown in Box 18-2. Commercial kits are now available that also contain the instruments required for a cricothyrotomy (Fig. 18-1).

Box 18-2. Recommended Contents of Cricothyrotomy Tray

Trousseau dilator
Tracheal hook
Scalpel with no. 11 blade
Cuffed, nonfenestrated, no. 4 tracheostomy tube
Optional equipment: several 4 × 4 gauze sponges, two small hemostats, and surgical drapes

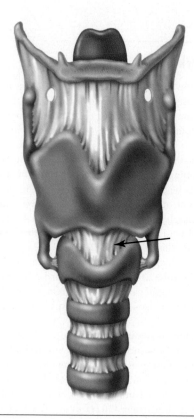

Figure 18-2 ● Anatomy of the Larynx.   The cricothyroid membrane (*arrow*) is bordered above by the thyroid cartilage and below by the cricoid cartilage.

1. *Identify the landmarks.* The cricothyroid membrane is identified using the landmarks described previously (Fig. 18-2).
2. *Prepare the neck.* If time permits, apply appropriate antiseptic solution. Local anesthesia is desirable if the patient is conscious. Infiltration of the skin and subcutaneous tissue of the anterior neck with 1% lidocaine solution will provide adequate anesthesia. If time permits and the patient is conscious and responsive, anesthetize the airway by injecting lidocaine by transcricothyroid membrane puncture (see Chapter 23). The patient will cough briefly, but the airway will be reasonably anesthetized and further cough reflexes suppressed.
3. *Immobilize the larynx.* Throughout the procedure, the larynx must be immobilized (Fig. 18-3). This is best done by placing the thumb and long finger of the nondominant hand on opposite sides of the superior laryngeal horns, the posterior superior aspect of the laryngeal cartilage. With the thumb and long finger thus placed, the index finger is ideally positioned anteriorly to relocate and reidentify the cricothyroid membrane at any time during the procedure.
4. *Incise the skin.* Using the dominant hand, a 2-cm vertical midline skin incision is performed (Fig. 18-4). Care should be taken to avoid cutting the deeper structures of the neck. The cricothyroid membrane is separated from the outside world only by skin, subcutaneous tissue, and anterior cervical fascia. An overly vigorous incision risks damage to the larynx, cricoid cartilage, and the trachea.
5. *Reidentify the membrane.* With the thumb and long finger maintaining immobilization of the larynx, the index finger can now palpate the anterior larynx, the cricothyroid membrane, and the cricoid cartilage without any interposed skin or subcutaneous tissue (Fig. 18-5). With the landmarks thus confirmed, the index finger can be left in the wound by placing it on the

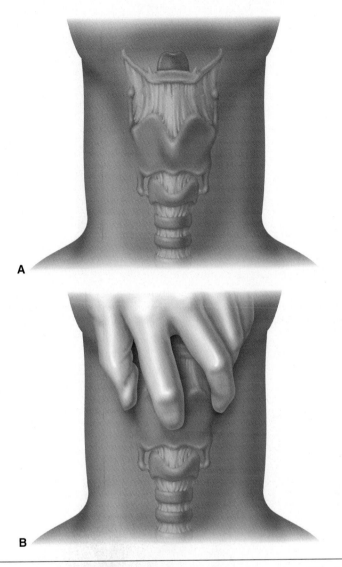

Figure 18-3 ● **A:** Surface anatomy of the airway. **B:** The thumb and long finger immobilize the superior cornua of the larynx; the index finger is used to palpate the cricothyroid membrane.

inferior aspect of the anterior larynx, thus providing a clear indicator of the superior extent of the cricothyroid membrane.

6. *Incise the membrane.* The cricothyroid membrane should be incised in a horizontal direction, with an incision at least 1 cm long (Fig. 18-6A). It is recommended to try to incise the lower half of the membrane rather than the upper half because of the relatively cephalad location of the superior cricothyroid artery and vein; however, this may be unrealistic in the emergent setting (Fig. 18-6B).

7. *Insert the tracheal hook.* The tracheal hook is rotated so that it is oriented in the transverse plane, passed through the incision, and then rotated again so the hook is oriented in a cephalad direction. The hook is then applied to the inferior aspect of the thyroid cartilage, and gentle upward and cephalad traction is applied to bring the airway immediately out to the skin incision (Fig. 18-7). If an assistant is available, this hook may be passed to the assistant to maintain immobilization of the larynx.

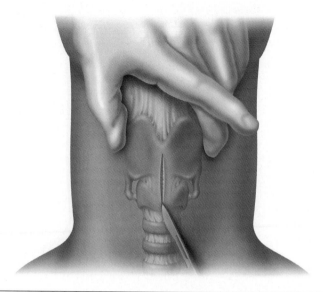

Figure 18-4 ● With the index finger moved to the side but continued firm immobilization of the larynx, a vertical midline skin incision is made, down to the depth of the laryngeal structures.

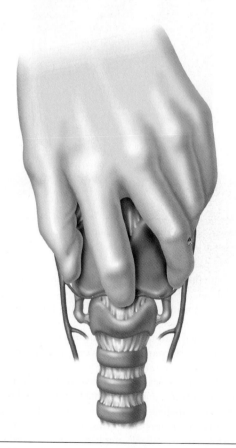

Figure 18-5 ● With the skin incised, the index finger can now directly palpate the cricothyroid membrane.

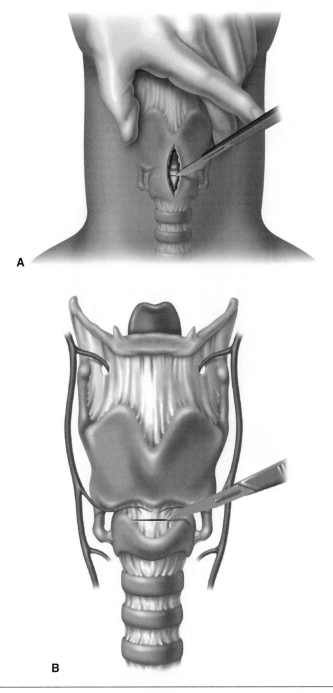

Figure 18-6 ● **A:** A horizontal membrane incision is made near the inferior edge of the cricothyroid membrane. The index finger may be swung aside or may remain in the wound, palpating the inferior edge of the thyroid cartilage, to guide the scalpel to the membrane. **B:** A low cricothyroid incision avoids the superior cricothyroid vessels, which run transversely near the top of the membrane.

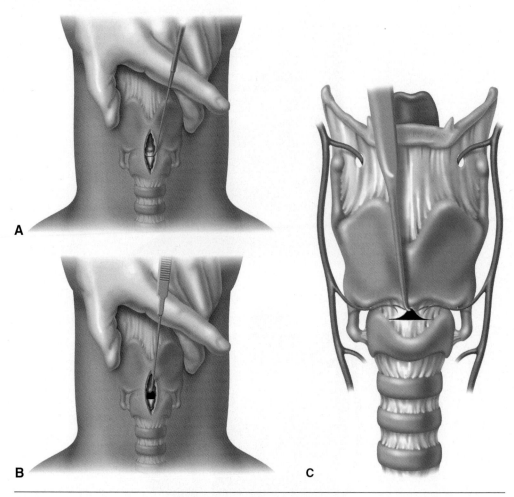

A

B

C

Figure 18-7 ● **A:** The tracheal hook is oriented transversely during insertion. **B** and **C:** After insertion, cephalad traction is applied to the inferior margin of the thyroid cartilage.

8. *Insert the Trousseau dilator.* The Trousseau dilator may be inserted in one of two ways. One method is to insert the dilator well in through the incision, directing the blades of the dilator longitudinally down the airway. The second method, which is preferred, is to insert the dilator minimally into the anterior wound with the blades oriented superiorly and inferiorly, allowing the dilator to open and enlarge the vertical extent of the cricothyroid membrane incision, which is often the anatomically limiting dimension (Fig. 18-8). When this technique is used, care must be taken not to insert the dilator too deeply into the airway because it will impede subsequent passage of the tracheostomy tube.

9. *Insert the tracheostomy tube.* The tracheostomy tube, with its inner cannula in situ, is gently inserted through the incision between the blades of the Trousseau dilator. As the tube is advanced gently following its natural curve, the Trousseau dilator is rotated to allow the blades to orient longitudinally in the airway (Fig. 18-9). The tracheostomy tube is advanced until it is firmly seated against the anterior neck. The Trousseau dilator is then carefully removed.

10. *Inflate the cuff, and confirm tube position.* With the cuff inflated, the tracheostomy tube position can be confirmed by the same methods as the ETT position. Carbon dioxide (CO_2) detection will reliably indicate correct placement of the tube and is mandatory, as for endotracheal intubation. Immediate subcutaneous emphysema with bagging suggests probable paratracheal

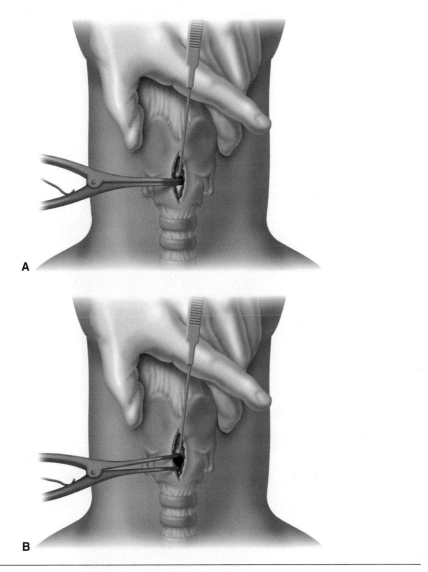

Figure 18-8 ● **A:** The Trousseau dilator is inserted a short distance into the incision. **B:** In this orientation, the dilator enlarges the opening vertically, the crucial dimension.

placement. If doubt remains, rapid insertion of a nasogastric tube through the tracheostomy tube will result in easy passage if the tube is in the trachea and obstruction if the tube has been placed through a false passage into the tissues of the neck. Auscultation of both lungs and the epigastric area is also recommended, although esophageal placement of the tracheostomy tube is exceedingly unlikely. Chest radiography should be performed to assist in the assessment of tube placement and to evaluate for the presence of barotrauma. Pneumothorax is also possible, but far less likely than the placement of the tube paratracheally.

The Rapid Four-Step Technique

This abbreviated cricothyrotomy method has been developed and adopted for training purposes at some centers. As with all techniques, the patient should be maximally oxygenated and, if given

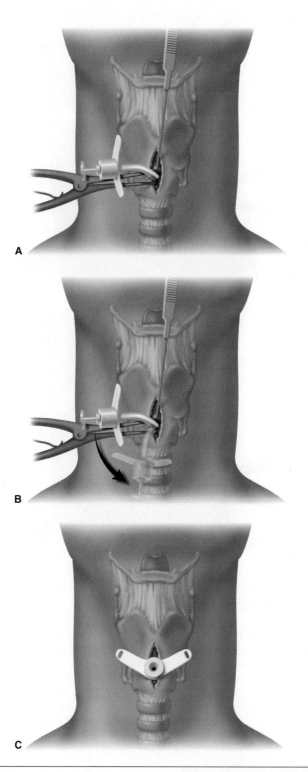

Figure 18-9 ● **A:** Insertion of the tracheostomy tube. **B:** Rotation of the Trousseau dilator to orient the blades longitudinally in the airway facilitates passage of the tracheostomy tube. **C:** Tracheostomy tube fully inserted; instruments removed.

sufficient time, the anterior neck may be prepared and locally anesthetized as for the no-drop method. From a *position at the head of the bed*, the rapid four-step technique (RFST) for cricothyrotomy proceeds sequentially as follows:

1. *Palpate and identify landmarks.* The cricothyroid membrane should be identified as described previously (Fig. 18-10). If the key landmarks are unable to be identified by palpation through the soft tissue, then a vertical skin incision is required to permit accurate identification.

2. *Make skin incision.* Once the pertinent palpable anatomy is identified, the cricothyroid membrane is incised. If the anatomy is fully appreciated through the intact skin, and there is no uncertainty about landmarks or location, then incise the skin and cricothyroid membrane simultaneously with a single horizontal incision of approximately 1.5 cm in length (Fig. 18-11A). For this type of incision, a no. 20 scalpel yields an incision that requires little widening, once used to puncture the skin and cricothyroid membrane. If the anatomy is not readily and unambiguously identified through the skin, then an initial vertical incision should be created to allow more precise palpation of the anatomy and identification of the cricothyroid membrane. In either situation, the cricothyroid membrane is incised with the no. 20 blade that is maintained in the airway, while a tracheal hook (preferably a blunt hook) is placed parallel to the scalpel on the caudad side of the blade (Fig. 18-11B). The hook is then rotated to orient it in a caudad direction to put gentle traction on the cricoid ring. The scalpel is then removed from the airway. At no time during this procedure is the incision left without instrument control of the airway. This detail is particularly important in a scenario where the patient still has the ability to respond or swallow. The newly created stoma could be irretrievably lost if the airway is uncontrolled and moves relative to the skin incision. In addition, as is the case for the no-drop method, this is a technique that relies exclusively on palpation of key structures. Bleeding will inevitably obscure visualization of the anatomy. No time should be wasted using suction or gauze or manipulating the overhead lighting.

3. *Apply traction.* The tracheal hook that has been rotated caudally and is controlling the cricoid ring is now used to lift the airway toward the skin incision. This action provides modest stoma dilation. The direction of hook pull is reminiscent of the up and away direction used with laryngoscopy (Fig. 18-12). The amount of traction force required for easy intubation (18 N or 4 lb force) is significantly lower than the force that is associated with breakage of the cricoid ring (54 N or 12 lb force). Use of the hook in this direction generally provides sufficient widening of the incision, and a Trousseau dilator is usually not required. The technique of pulling the airway upward in this way also minimizes the possibility of intubating the pretracheal potential space.

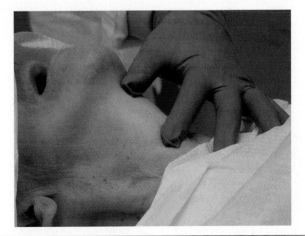

Figure 18-10 ● Palpation.   The operator's thumb is on the hyoid bone, while the cricothyroid membrane is identified using the index finger.

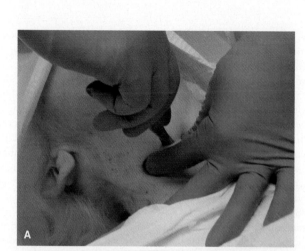

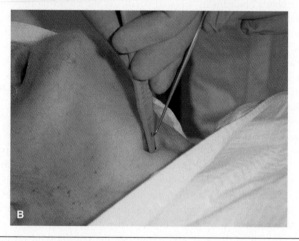

Figure 18-11 ● **Incision.**   **A:** A horizontal incision is initiated while stabilizing the larynx. **B:** Before removing the scalpel from the airway, a hook is placed on the caudal side of the scalpel, parallel to the blade.

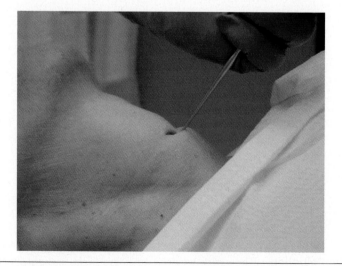

Figure 18-12 ● **Traction.**   The hook is applied to the cricoid ring and lifted.

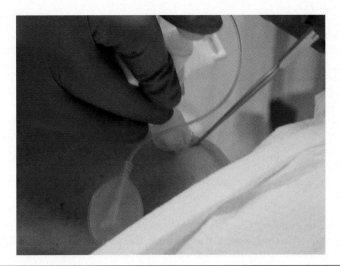

Figure 18-13 ● Intubation.   The tracheostomy tube is passed into the incision as the hook stabilizes the cricoid ring.

4. *Intubate.* With adequate control of the airway using the hook placed on the cricoid ring, tracheostomy tube is readily placed into the airway and secured (Fig. 18-13). Confirmation techniques proceed as described in the no-drop technique.

Complications

Because of the high success rate of RSI, cricothyrotomy is infrequently performed in EDs, so reports of complications are difficult to evaluate. In the National Emergency Airway Registry (NEAR II) study, only 0.8% of 8,937 ED intubations were managed by cricothyrotomy, although the incidence was higher in trauma patients (1.7%).

The most important complication for the patient in the context of surgical airway management is when delayed decision making after initial intubation failure leads to prolonged, ineffective intubation attempts that result in hypoxic injury. Failure to rapidly place the tracheotomy tube into the trachea or misplacement of the tube into the soft tissues of the neck is more a failure of technique than a complication and must be recognized immediately, as is the case with any misplaced ETT. Complications such as pneumothorax, significant hemorrhage requiring operative intervention, laryngeal or tracheal injury, infection, and long-term complications, such as subglottic stenosis or permanent voice change, are relatively infrequent. In general, the incidence of all complications, immediate and delayed, and major or minor, is approximately 20%, although published reports range from 0% to 54%. Emergency cricothyrotomy has higher complication rate than elective cricothyrotomy. However, most of these complications are minor, particularly when compared with the consequences of a persistently failed airway.

There is insufficient evidence to determine whether the overall complication rate is lower when the traditional no-drop technique of cricothyrotomy is used versus the RFST. Box 18-3 lists complications of surgical airway management.

Alternatives to Open Surgical Techniques

Seldinger technique

When an alternative to open cricothyrotomy is desired, we recommend using a Seldinger technique. The Melker Universal Emergency Cricothyrotomy Catheter Set uses a modified Seldinger technique to assist in the placement of a tracheal airway (Fig. 18-14). This method is

Box 18-3. Complications of Surgical Airway Management
Hemorrhage Pneumomediastinum Laryngeal/tracheal injury Cricoid ring laceration Barotrauma (especially when jet ventilation is used) Infection Voice change Subglottic stenosis

similar to the one commonly used in the placement of central venous catheters and offers some familiarity to the operator uncomfortable with or inexperienced in the surgical cricothyrotomy techniques described previously. Devices that incorporate an inflatable cuff are recommended (Fig. 18-14B).

1. *Identify landmarks.* The cricothyroid membrane is identified by the method described earlier. The nondominant hand is used to control the larynx and maintain identification of the landmarks.
2. *Prepare neck.* Antiseptic solution is applied to the anterior neck, and if time permits, infiltration of the site with 1% lidocaine with epinephrine is recommended.
3. *Insert locator needle.* The locator needle is then inserted into the cricothyroid membrane in a slightly caudal direction (Fig. 18-14C). The needle is attached to a syringe and advanced with the dominant hand, while negative pressure is maintained on the syringe. The sudden aspiration of air indicates placement of the needle into the tracheal lumen.
4. *Insert guide wire.* The syringe is then removed from the needle. A soft-tipped guide wire is inserted through the needle into the trachea in a caudal direction (Fig. 18-14D). The needle is then removed, leaving the wire in place. Control of the wire must be maintained at all times.
5. *Incise skin.* A small skin incision is then made adjacent to the wire. This facilitates passage of the airway device through the skin (Fig. 18-14E). Alternatively, the skin incision may be made vertically over the membrane before insertion of the needle and guide wire.
6. *Insert the airway and dilator.* The airway catheter (3 to 6 mm internal diameter [ID]) with an internal dilator in place is inserted over the wire into the trachea (Fig. 18-14F). If resistance is met, the skin incision should be deepened and a gentle twisting motion applied to the airway device (Fig. 18-14G). When the airway device is firmly seated in the trachea, the wire and dilator are removed together (Fig. 18-14H).
7. *Confirm tube location.* If the device has a cuff, inflate it at this time. Tube location is confirmed in the usual manner, including mandatory end-tidal CO_2 detection. The airway must then be secured properly. The devices are radiopaque on radiographs.

Direct airway placement devices

Numerous commercial cricothyrotome devices are available. These purport to place an airway simply and rapidly, but none of these has an adequate safety and performance record to warrant a recommendation for emergency use, and the incidence of injury to the airway is higher than when a Seldinger technique is used. These devices, such as Nu-Trake and Pertrach, generally involve multiple steps in the insertion, using a large device that functions as both introducer and airway. The details of the operation of these devices may be obtained from the manufacturer and are provided as inserts with the kits. These devices offer no clear advantage in technique, are rarely (if ever) as easily placed as is claimed, and are more likely to

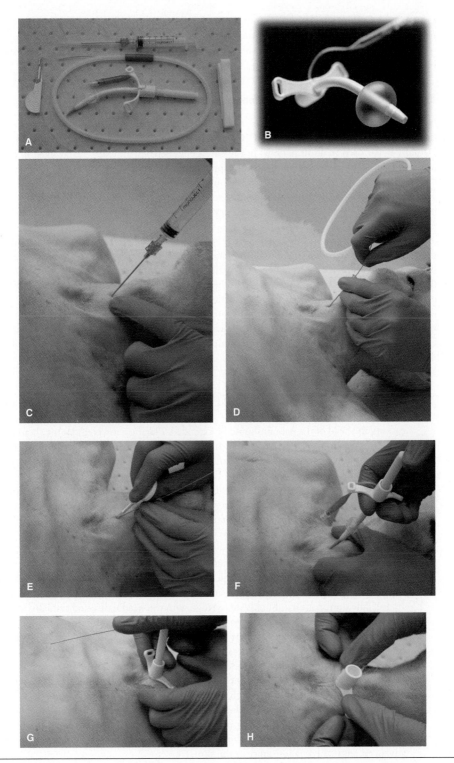

Figure 18-14 ● **A:** Kit contents. **B:** Cuffed tube. **C:** Needle insertion. **D:** Wire placement through needle. **E:** Small incision. **F:** Airway with dilator inserted with wire guidance. **G:** Airway inserted to the hub using a gentle twisting motion. **H:** Wire and dilator removed as one (Melker Universal Cricothyrotomy Kit, Cook Critical Care, Bloomington, IN).

cause traumatic complications during their insertion than those that use a Seldinger technique, primarily because of the cutting characteristics of the airway device. In particular, cricothyrotomes recommended for children should be approached with extreme caution and are not recommended.

Percutaneous transtracheal ventilation technique

Needle cricothyrotomy with percutaneous transtracheal ventilation (PTV) is a surgical airway that may be used to temporize in the CICO situation, particularly in children. Although PTV is virtually never used in adult patients in the emergency setting, and very rarely even in children, it is a simple, relatively effective means of supporting oxygenation. Advantages of this technique over cricothyrotomy may include speed, a simpler technique, and less bleeding. PTV can also provide an alternative for operators unable to perform a cricothyrotomy. Age is not a contraindication to PTV, which is the surgical airway of choice for children younger than 10 years (see Chapter 25).

Several other aspects of this technique that differ from cricothyrotomy are important to consider. To provide ventilation, supraglottic patency must be maintained to allow for exhalation. In the case of complete upper-airway obstruction, air stacking from PTV will cause barotrauma; therefore, cricothyrotomy is preferable. Another significant difference is that the catheter in PTV does not provide airway protection. Also, suctioning cannot adequately be performed through the percutaneous catheter. PTV has been associated with a significant incidence of barotrauma and is rarely used as a rescue device, particularly with the widespread use of other devices such as the LMA. PTV is therefore best considered a temporizing means of rescue oxygenation until a more definitive airway can be obtained.

1. **Procedure**
   a. *Identify the landmarks.* The anatomy and landmarks used in needle cricothyrotomy are identical to those described previously for a surgical cricothyrotomy. If there are no contraindications, the head of the patient should be extended. Placing a towel under the shoulders may facilitate cervical hyperextension. The area overlying the cricothyroid membrane should be prepared with an antiseptic solution and, if time permits, anesthetized with 1% lidocaine and epinephrine.
   b. *Immobilize the larynx.* Use the thumb and the middle fingers of the nondominant hand to stabilize the larynx and cricoid cartilage while using the index finger to palpate the cricothyroid membrane. It is essential to maintain control of the larynx throughout the procedure.
   c. *Insert transtracheal needle.* A large-bore intravenous (IV) catheter (12G to 16G) is attached to a 20-ml syringe, which may be empty or partially filled with a clear liquid. A 15° angle can be created by bending the needle/catheter combination 2.5 cm from the distal end of the IV catheter, or a commercially available catheter can be used (Fig. 18-15A). A commercial catheter may be preferred because it is reinforced with wire coils to prevent kinking (Fig. 18-16). The dominant hand holds the syringe with the needle directed caudally in the long axis of the trachea at a 30° angle to the skin (Fig. 18-15B). While maintaining negative pressure on the syringe, the needle is inserted through the cricothyroid membrane into the trachea. As soon as the needle enters the trachea, the syringe will easily fill with air. If a liquid is used, bubbles will appear. Any resistance implies that the catheter remains in the tissue. In the awake patient, lidocaine may be used in the syringe and then injected into the tracheal lumen to suppress the cough reflex.
   d. *Advance catheter.* Once entry into the trachea is confirmed, the catheter can be advanced. The needle may be partially or completely withdrawn before advancement; however, the needle should not be advanced with the catheter. A small incision can assist with catheter advancement if there is resistance at the skin.
   e. *Confirm location.* The catheter should be advanced to the hub and controlled by hand at all times. Air should be reaspirated to confirm once again the location of the catheter within the trachea.

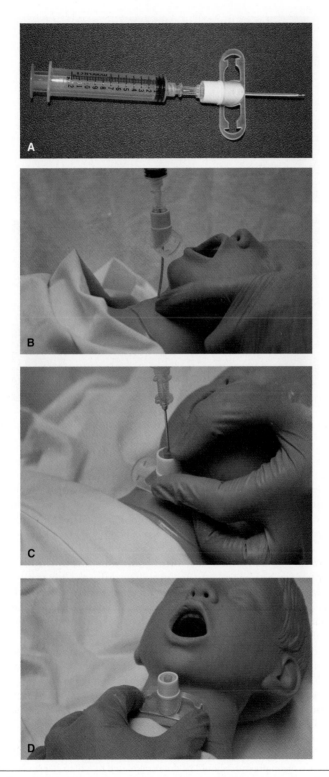

Figure 18-15 ● **A:** Nonkinking catheter for jet ventilation. **B:** Needle insertion. **C:** Removal of needle. **D:** Tracheotomy catheter placed.

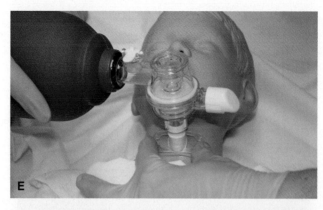

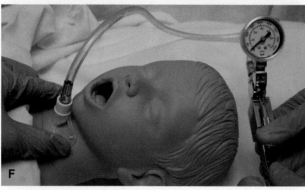

Figure 18-15 ● **(continued)** E: Oxygenation with bag. F: Oxygenation with jet ventilator (Acutronic, Germany).

f. *Connect to bag or jet ventilation.* The catheter may be connected to a bag ventilator using a preexisting adapter, or if there is only a Luer lock present, the adapter from a 3-0 pediatric ETT will fit the Luer lock (Fig. 18-15E). For jet ventilation, the catheter is connected to the female end of the tubing of the jet ventilation system by a Luer lock. The hub should not be secured in place by anything other than a human hand until a definitive airway is established (Fig. 18-15F). Firm, constant pressure must be applied by hand to ensure that proper positioning is maintained and to create a seal at the skin to minimize air leak.

g. *Perform jet ventilation.* In the adult, the jet ventilation system should be connected to an oxygen source of 50 psi with a continuously adjustable regulator to allow the pressure to be titrated so the lowest effective pressure (often about 30 psi) required to safely deliver a tidal volume is used. In general, inspiration is <1 second followed by 3 seconds of expiration. Because the gas flow through a 14G needle at 50 psi is 1,600 ml per second, <1 second of inspiratory time is required for an adequate tidal volume in a normally compliant lung. Recent research demonstrates that effective oxygenation may occur with considerably <30 psi pressure, and the lowest pressure that results in effective oxygenation should be used. Exhalation depends on the elastic recoil of the lung, which is a relatively low-driving pressure. Therefore, the recommended inspiratory-to-expiratory ratio (I:E) is 1:3. It is important to maintain upper-airway patency to allow for exhalation and avoid air trapping and barotrauma. All patients should have an oral and nasal airway placed. For small adults and children, oxygen pressure should be downregulated to <20 to 30 psi, if possible. For children younger than 5 years, a bag should be used for ventilation, connected to the catheter using the ETT adapter from a 3.0-mm-ID ETT (see Chapter 25).

2. **Equipment**
   a. Transtracheal catheters. A large-bore IV catheter is acceptable. The proper placement is made easier by placing a small angle 2.5 cm from the tip. Commercially available devices include precurved (Acutronic, Germany) and nonkinkable wire-coiled (Cook Critical Care, Bloomington, IN) catheters (Figs. 18-15A and 18-16). The wire-coiled catheter will not kink when bent; therefore, it provides a more secure airway.
   b. *PTV systems.* The PTV system consists of a high-pressure oxygen source (usually central wall oxygen pressure of 50 psi), high-pressure oxygen tubing, a regulator to control the driving pressure, an on–off valve to control inspiratory time, high-pressure tubing, and a Luer lock to connect to the catheter (Fig. 18-17).

   A regulator to control the driving pressure is optional but recommended. This device is particularly useful where barotrauma is a concern and in pediatrics, where the inspiratory pressures should be reduced to <20 to 30 psi, if possible. Although a system can be assembled

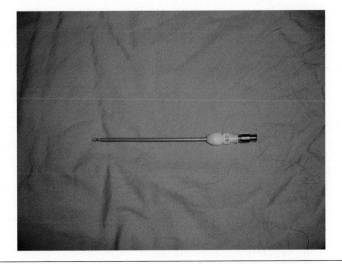

Figure 18-16 ● Nonkinkable wire-coiled TTJV catheter (Cook Critical Care, Bloomington, IN).

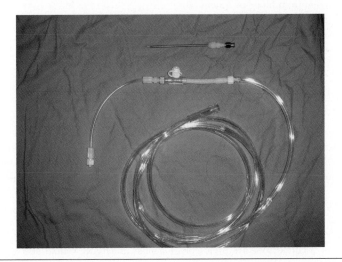

Figure 18-17 ● Disposable jet ventilator system with high-pressure oxygen tubing, on–off valve, and PVC tubing with Luer lock. Note that this device does not include a pressure regulator (Cook Critical Care, Bloomington, IN).

inexpensively from readily available materials, a commercially made, preassembled system is recommended. The reliability and control inherent in the commercial devices are well worth the marginal increase in cost.

A PTV system can also be connected to a low-flow portable oxygen tank when circumstances require mobility. When the flow is set at the maximal 15 L per minute and no flow is allowed, the pressure temporarily increases to 120 psi. Once flow is released, high flow occurs momentarily and then rapidly decreases to the steady state of 5 to 10 psi. Adequate tidal volumes may be achieved through a 14G catheter in the first 0.5 second. A shorter I:E ratio of 1:1 is recommended.

Another setup using manual ventilation with a self-inflating reservoir bag has been described, using standard equipment found in any ED. Bag ventilation may be connected directly to the percutaneous transtracheal catheter in two ways. The male end of a 15-mm ETT adapter from a 3-mm-ID ETT will fit directly into the catheter. Alternatively, the male end of a plungerless 3-ml syringe will fit into the catheter, and the male end of an 8-mm-ID ETT adapter will then insert into the female end of the empty syringe. Ventilation is temporary at best, and partial arterial CO_2 pressure will increase at a rate 2 to 4 mm Hg per minute. Even the simple assembly of this system is more time consuming to be done during the event, so it must be preassembled. This arrangement may have particular utility in the pediatric patient younger than 5 years when excessive pressures may be delivered through a PTV device, even when a regulator to control inspiratory pressures is available. In general, children younger than 5 years should receive PTV through a ventilation bag; children of age 5 to 12 years receive ventilation by bag or using PTV at <30 mm Hg; and those older than 12 years to adult receive at a pressure range from 30 to 50 mm Hg. A catheter of <3 mm ID will be insufficient to adequately oxygenate the adult patient using a bag, and 50 psi pressurized oxygen is required.

3. **Complications specific to PTV**

There is insufficient experience with PTV to properly identify, quantify, or classify complications. Insufflation of gases at high pressure has significant likelihood of inflicting injury to the airway mucosa or deeper tissues and must be undertaken with extreme caution. Known complications of PTV include the following:

a. Subcutaneous emphysema
b. Barotrauma
c. Reflex cough with each ventilation (may be aborted with lidocaine)
d. Catheter kinking
e. Obstruction from blood or mucus
f. Esophageal puncture
g. Mucosal damage if nonhumidified gas is used

TIPS AND PEARLS

Surgical airway management is rarely the method of first choice for patients requiring emergency airway management. However, there is a population of patients for whom surgical airway management will literally make the difference between life and death. Therefore, providers for patients requiring emergency airway management must be proficient with surgical airway management.

Although appealing on the surface, there may be little advantage to using a Seldinger-based method rather than a formal, surgical cricothyrotomy set. Time of performance of the procedure, complication rates, degree of difficulty, and success rates are all comparable. Seldinger technique devices that use a cuffed tube are preferable. Personal preference should also guide selection. A commercial kit is available which offers all instruments and equipment to perform both the Seldinger-based insertion and a formal, open, cricothyrotomy by either the standard "no-drop" or Rapid

Four-Step Technique (Melker Universal Emergency Cricothyrotomy Catheter Set; Fig. 18-1). There is no evidence that any cricothyrotome can be placed with acceptable success and safety in a child younger than 10 to 12 years, regardless of the design of the device or the claims of the manufacturer.

PTV is virtually never indicated in the adult patient and establishment of a more functional surgical airway using a percutaneous technique or by formal cricothyroidotomy is vastly preferable. In children younger than 10 years, the opposite is true. In this age group, PTV is the primary surgical airway management method of choice. Despite the rarity of use of PTV in the ED, centers providing emergency care to children should have a PTV set readily available and providers should be familiar with how to connect and use it. The wire-coiled catheter designed for the PTV cannula resists kinking and so is preferable to a standard IV catheter.

Of the methods described in this chapter, only a formal surgical cricothyrotomy and variations of the recently modified Melker set result in the placement of a cuffed tube within the trachea. The other techniques described here must be considered temporary at best. Placement of a tracheostomy tube or ETT through a formal surgical cricothyrotomy incision results in a definitive airway for the patient.

The No.4 cuffed tracheostomy tube, which has an inside diameter of 5 mm, can be used for virtually all cases of adult cricothyrotomy in the ED. The tube is of adequate size to provide ventilation in virtually all circumstances, and its outside dimensions are such that it will almost always be easily inserted. For large adult men, a No.6 can be used.

EVIDENCE

- **Which technique is best?** There is limited literature that effectively compares different techniques of invasive surgical airway management. The relatively rare performance of an emergency surgical airway, compounded with the urgency of the circumstance, may explain the absence of any controlled clinical trials comparing techniques in the emergency setting. Comorbid injuries or illnesses often preclude long-term assessment of sequelae, and the few studies performed do not compare or identify specific invasive techniques.[1] As such, the current level of evidence for or against a particular technique exists as expert consensus based on collective experience, limited descriptive series, or studies in cadaveric and animal models.[2-10]

    Several studies have directly compared the percutaneous, wire-guided technique to the traditional open, or no-drop, technique in cadavers.[11,12,14-16] Eisenburger et al.,[11] studying the performance of intensive care trainees, and Chan et al.,[12] in a similar study of emergency residents and attendings, compared the two techniques in randomized, crossover studies and found no difference in times to completion among groups. Immediate complications were also similar. Interestingly, despite evidence of superiority by any objective measure, the majority of participants in Chan et al.'s[12] study stated a preference for the percutaneous, wire-guided technique. Other cadaveric studies have had conflicting results regarding which approach is more rapid.[15,16] Complication rates between the traditional open technique and Seldinger technique appear to be similar.[12,13] Therefore, the operator should choose the technique he or she is most comfortable with and expert at, and which is readily available in the department.

- **Rapid four-step or no-drop technique for open cricothyrotomy?** Each approach has its proponents. The no-drop technique has been in use for decades and has withstood the test of time. The RFST is proposed to be an improvement over the no-drop technique based on the following:

    ○ The RFST requires only one person to perform the procedure. Ideally, the no-drop technique requires *two* people (i.e., one operator and one assistant). The assistant is responsible for not dropping the tracheal hook as it stabilizes the trachea. Without an assistant, the operator must maintain the no-drop approach with the Trousseau dilator while inserting the tube, which is not a desirable circumstance.

○ The RFST can be readily performed from the head of the bed without having to move to the patient's side, where the operator is best positioned for the no-drop technique.

○ The RFST requires only a simple hook and a scalpel, which may be available even in the absence of a formal cricothyrotomy kit. This is a minimal advantage because the standard cricothyrotomy kit is also simple containing only three basic instruments (scalpel, hook, and dilator).

There are no controlled human trials comparing these approaches; however, case series suggest RFST is an acceptable approach in the emergency setting.[10,15,17,18] In a randomized, crossover, cadaveric study comparing the two techniques, Holmes et al.[19] found the RFST to be significantly faster (43 vs. 134 seconds, $p < .001$), without a significant difference in immediate complications. In a similar study, Davis et al.[20] also found the RFST to be faster. One study comparing complications of the RFST and the standard technique found the overall rate of complications (38%) to be similar, but the incidence of major complications (e.g., complete transection of the cricoid cartilage, posterior tracheal, or esophageal perforation) 6% higher for the RFST.[15]

Potential disadvantages of the RFST:

○ The RFST relies on a single, relatively small incision to hasten the placement of the ETT. Although literature exists that supports the routine use of this technique, the location of the initial incision is of critical importance.[10,17,18] Most of the reported complications related to the RFST in patients have been related to the initial incision being made too small and then requiring time-consuming revision of the incision.[10] If the initial incision is misplaced or initially made too small and subsequently requires revision, then any proposed time-saving advantage is lost. When the anatomy precludes the ability to confidently landmark the cricothyroid space, it may be prudent to proceed with the traditional vertical incision, which allows digital palpation of the landmark structures within the neck, or localization of the airway by needle aspiration.

○ Concerns over a possible higher incidence of cricoid ring damage and esophageal perforation have been raised, but larger studies are needed to determine whether this possibility is real.[19,20] The use of a double hook may significantly reduce the potential for cricoid ring injury.[20,21]

Overall, the evidence does not support the use of one technique over the other. The choice of the RFST against the no-drop method will be made by the operator on the basis of training, experience, and judgment, and either approach is acceptable, each having some advantages and disadvantages and neither being clearly superior.

● **Can a procedure done so rarely be taught, retained, and used successfully?** Ultimately, any discussion of the technical merits of a procedure will be irrelevant if hesitancy on the part of the provider results in significant delay in establishing a definitive airway. Fortunately, this potential hesitancy is readily overcome by technical proficiency. Anyone responsible for emergency airway management should choose an invasive method, learn it, and practice it at regular intervals to maintain proficiency.

The success of RSI and the proliferation of alternative airway devices has led to a concern over gaining and maintaining competency in invasive airway management.[22–24] Retrospective studies suggest a current cricothyrotomy rate of approximately 1% of all emergency airways. The reasons for this low incidence have been attributed to emergency medicine training, the success of RSI, and reduced transport rate for blunt traumatic arrests.[22,24] Regardless of the cause, this incidence is believed to be too low to ensure adequate training, yet highlights the probability that all emergency physicians will be called on to perform an invasive airway at some point in their career.

To address this issue, some authors have advocated the performance of invasive airway techniques on the newly dead.[25] Many physicians have received cricothyrotomy and endotracheal intubation training on the recently deceased without consent from the family. This practice, however, has raised ethical concerns and is no longer considered an acceptable practice at many institutions. Olsen et al.[26] studied the feasibility of obtaining family consent for teaching cricothyrotomy on the newly dead in the ED. Consent was obtained for postmortem cricothyrotomy in 20 of 51 deaths (39%) in a large teaching hospital over a 7-month period. It is unclear how feasible this approach would be in other settings, but it does represent a potential opportunity to practice in a way that most closely approximates the true anatomy.

To ensure familiarity with the equipment and technique, it is likely that practice must occur outside the clinical setting. Koppel and Reed[27] reported that although 80% of anesthesiology programs instruct their residents on cricothyrotomies, 60% use lectures only, a poor teaching technique for developing proficiency in manual skills. One study attempted to determine the minimum training required to perform cricothyrotomy in 40 seconds or less on a manikin. One hundred and two physicians performed 10 procedures, and by the fifth attempt, 96% plateaued in their success.[28]

There are no studies that have identified the optimal interval between training episodes for retention, although one small report suggested increased retention when repeated monthly versus every 3 months.[29] Studies in cadavers performed primarily to compare different techniques have also identified a similarly rapid learning curve; however, the time to procedure completion was greater (73 to 102 seconds).[11,14]

There are no studies examining the clinical correlation of these training techniques; however, the high success rates of emergency cricothyrotomies suggest that retention and application have occurred. Based on the limited available literature, we make the following recommendations regarding the learning and retention of invasive airway techniques:

o Identify a preferred method of invasive airway management to learn; select one that is immediately available to you.
o Practice the technique one to two times per year on live animal models, animal tracheas, patient simulators, or manikins, depending on availability.
o Practice the procedure five times at each training session.
o When appropriate, consider requesting consent for cricothyrotomy on the newly dead.

Tracheas may be ordered from a slaughterhouse at relatively low cost, and the technique may be attempted multiple times on each specimen. Simulators represent a significant purchase cost; however, they are useful for training multiple critical skills and are increasingly commonly available at teaching institutions because prices have become much lower. Models specifically for cricothyrotomy training are also available. Live animal models and cadavers are generally used only in formal residency training sessions and specialized procedural courses because of significant expense and limited access.

• **When is a surgical airway indicated?** The failed airway algorithm (see Chapter 3) suggests that cricothyrotomy should be a considered, even in a "*can't* intubate, *can* oxygenate" situation, when it is clear that alternative approaches have failed or are judged likely to fail. However, it helps to recognize that a given provider attempting laryngoscopy may have a certain "emotional inertia" when it comes to changing strategies. First, one must acknowledge that a laryngoscopist may not want to recognize that his or her laryngoscopy has failed. In addition, the hesitancy to perform an infrequently used technique may conspire to tempt the provider to have just "one more look." Such perseveration on a single method of intubation can have disastrous results. Although some rescue devices may serve as a bridge in some circumstances, anatomy and urgency often preclude their use, and insistence on attempting to try alternative devices, in a desaturating CICV patient, can be disastrous. In all likelihood, the main complication associated with cricothyrotomy, or other invasive airways, is not doing it soon enough.

• **Is there a role for surgical airways in the prehospital setting?** Although its use is rare, cricothyrotomy has been widely taught and employed in the prehospital environment. The data are limited but suggest that the technique can be used in this setting; however, there appears to be higher incidence of complications and poor outcomes compared to the hospital setting.[32,33] There are less data on the use of percutaneous cricothyrotomes. Cadaveric studies suggest that this technique may be associated with fewer complications than open cricothyrotomy when used by prehospital providers.[34] Field studies for percutaneous cricothyrotomes and needle

PTV are very limited and inconclusive. A recent position paper on the use of alternate airways in the out-of-hospital setting, from the National Association of EMS Physicians,[35] also concluded that there is insufficient evidence to either support or refute the need for all agencies to have a surgical airway technique available. If cricothyrotomy is to be used in an emergency medical services system, training, skill retention, individual case review, and systemwide quality management are essential. A field cricothyrotomy might be viewed as analogous to a police officer discharging a firearm. Each event is significant and worthy of thoughtful review.

REFERENCES

1. McGill J, Clinton JE, Ruiz E. Cricothyrotomy in the emergency department. *Ann Emerg Med*. 1982;11:361–364.

2. Esses BA, Jafek BW. Cricothyroidotomy: a decade of experience in Denver. *Ann Otol Rhinol Laryngol*. 1987;96:519–524.

3. Walls RM. Cricothyroidotomy. In: Campbell WH, ed. *Emergency Medicine Clinics of North America*. Philadelphia, PA: WB Saunders; 1988:725–736.

4. Erlandson MJ, Clinton JE, Ruiz E, et al. Cricothyrotomy in the emergency department revisited. *J Emerg Med*. 1989;7:115–118.

5. DeLaurier GA, Hawkins ML, Treat RC, et al. Acute airway management: role of cricothyroidotomy. *Am Surg*. 1990;56:12–15.

6. Salvino CK, Dries D, Gamelli R, et al. Emergency cricothyroidotomy in trauma victims. *J Trauma*. 1993;34:503–505.

7. Hawkins ML, Shapiro MB, Cue JI, et al. Emergency cricothyrotomy: a reassessment. *Am Surg*. 1995;61:52–55.

8. Bair AE, Filbin MR, Kulkarni RG, et al. The failed intubation attempt in the emergency department: analysis of prevalence, rescue techniques, and personnel. *J Emerg Med*. 2002;23:131–140.

9. Bair AE, Panacek EA, Wisner DH, et al. Cricothyrotomy: a 5-year experience at one institution. *J Emerg Med*. 2003;24:151–156.

10. Isaacs JH Jr. Emergency cricothyrotomy: long-term results. *Am Surg*. 2001;67:346–349.

11. Eisenburger P, Laczika K, List M, et al. Comparison of conventional surgical versus Seldinger technique emergency cricothyrotomy performed by inexperienced clinicians. *Anesthesiology*. 2000;92:687–690.

12. Chan TC, Vilke GM, Bramwell KJ, et al. Comparison of wire-guided cricothyrotomy versus standard surgical cricothyrotomy technique. *J Emerg Med*. 1999;17:957–962.

13. Benkhadra M, Lenfant F, Nemetz W, et al. A comparison of two emergency cricothyroidotomy kits in human cadavers. *Anesth Analg*. 2008;106:182.

14. Johnson DR, Dunlap A, McFeely P, et al. Cricothyrotomy performed by prehospital personnel: a comparison of two techniques in a human cadaver model. *Am J Emerg Med*. 1993;11:207–209.

15. Schaumann N, Lorenz V, Schellongowski P, et al. Evaluation of Seldinger technique emergency cricothyroidotomy versus standard surgical cricothyroidotomy in 200 cadavers. *Anesthesiology*. 2005;102:7.

16. Schober P, Hegemann MC, Schwarte LA, et al. Emergency cricothyrotomy-a comparative study of different techniques in human cadavers. *Resuscitation*. 2009;80:204.

17. Brofeldt BT, Panacek EA, Richards JR. An easy cricothyrotomy approach: the rapid four-step technique. *Acad Emerg Med*. 1996;3:1060–1063.

18. Brofeldt BT, Osborn ML, Sakles JC, et al. Evaluation of the rapid four-step cricothyrotomy technique: an interim report. *Air Med J*. 1998;17:127–130.

19. Holmes JF, Panacek EA, Sakles JC, et al. Comparison of 2 cricothyrotomy techniques: standard method versus rapid 4-step technique. *Ann Emerg Med*. 1998;32:442–447.

20. Davis DP, Bramwell KJ, Hamilton RS, et al. Safety and efficacy of the rapid four-step technique for cricothyrotomy using a Bair Claw. *J Emerg Med*. 2000;19:125–129.

21. Bair AE, Laurin EG, Karchin A, et al. Cricoid ring integrity: implications for emergent cricothyrotomy. *Ann Emerg Med*. 2003;41:333–337.

22. Chang RS, Hamilton RJ, Carter WA. Influence of an emergency medicine residency on the role of cricothyrotomy. *Acad Emerg Med*. 1996;3:534.

23. Knopp RK, Waeckerle JF, Callaham ML. Rapid sequence intubation revisited. *Ann Emerg Med*. 1998;31:398–400.

24. Chang RS, Hamilton RJ, Carter WA. Declining rate of cricothyrotomy in trauma patients with an emergency medicine residency: implications for skills training. *Acad Emerg Med*. 1998;5:247–251.

25. Knopp RK. Practicing cricothyrotomy on the newly dead. *Ann Emerg Med*. 1995;25:694–695.

26. Olsen J, Spilger S, Windisch T. Feasibility of obtaining family consent for teaching cricothyrotomy on the newly dead in the emergency department. *Ann Emerg Med*. 1995;25:660–665.

27. Koppel J, Reed A. Formal instruction in difficult airway management. *Anesthesiology*. 1995;83: 1343–1346.

28. Wong DT, Prabhu AJ, Coloma M, et al. What is the minimum training required for successful cricothyroidotomy? *Anesthesiology*. 2003;98:349–353.

29. Prabhu AJ, Correa R, Wong DT, et al. What is the optimal training interval for a cricothyrotomy? *Can J Anaesth*. 2001;48:A59.

30. Sagarin MJ, Barton ED, Chng YM, et al. Airway management by US and Canadian emergency medicine residents: a multicenter analysis of more than 6,000 endotracheal intubation attempts. *Ann Emerg Med*. 2005;46(4):328–336.

31. Sakles JC, Laurin EG, Rantapaa AA, et al. Airway management in the emergency department: a one-year study of 610 tracheal intubations. *Ann Emerg Med*. 1998;31(3):325–332.

32. Bulger EM, Copass MK, Maier RV, et al. An analysis of advanced prehospital airway management. *J Emerg Med*. 2002;23(2):183–189.

33. Fortune JB, Judkins DG, Scanzaroli D, et al. Efficacy of prehospital surgical cricothyrotomy in trauma patients. *J Trauma*. 1997;42(5):832–836.

34. Keane MF, Brinsfield KH, Dyer KS, et al. A laboratory comparison of emergency percutaneous and surgical cricothyrotomy by prehospital personnel. *Prehosp Emerg Care*. 2004;8(4):424–426.

35. O'Connor RE. Alternate airways in the out-of-hospital setting: position statement of the National Association of EMS Physicians. *Prehosp Emerg Care*. 2007;11(1):54–55.

19

Rapid Sequence Intubation

Ron M. Walls

INTRODUCTION

Definition

Rapid sequence intubation (RSI) is the administration, after preoxygenation, of a potent induction agent followed immediately by a rapidly acting neuromuscular blocking agent (NMBA) to induce unconsciousness and motor paralysis for tracheal intubation. The technique is predicated on the fact that the patient has not fasted before intubation and, therefore, is at risk for aspiration of gastric contents. The preoxygenation phase begins before drug administration and permits a period of apnea to occur safely between the administration of the drugs and intubation of the trachea, without the need for positive-pressure ventilation. In other words, the purpose of RSI is to render the patient unconscious and paralyzed and then to intubate the trachea without the use of bag-mask ventilation, which may cause gastric distention and increase the risk of aspiration. Sellick maneuver (posterior pressure on the cricoid cartilage to occlude the esophagus and prevent passive regurgitation) formerly was recommended, but it has been shown to impair glottic visualization in some cases, and the evidence supporting its use is dubious, at best. We no longer recommend routine use of this maneuver during emergency intubation.

Indications and Contraindications

RSI is the cornerstone of emergency airway management and is the technique of choice when emergency intubation is indicated, and the patient does not have difficult airway features felt to contraindicate the use of an NMBA (see Chapters 2 and 3). When a contraindication to succinylcholine is present, rocuronium is recommended as the NMBA (see Chapter 22). Some practitioners eschew the use of succinylcholine and routinely use rocuronium for all intubations; this is a matter of preference, for there are both pros and cons to this approach.

TECHNIQUE

RSI can be thought of as a series of discrete steps, referred to as the seven Ps. These are shown in Box 19-1.

1. *Preparation*
   Before initiating the sequence, the patient is thoroughly assessed for difficulty of intubation (see Chapter 2). Fallback plans in the event of failed intubation are established, and the necessary equipment is located. The patient is in an area of the emergency department that is organized and equipped for resuscitation. Cardiac monitoring, BP monitoring, and pulse oximetry should be used in all cases. Continuous capnography provides additional valuable monitoring information, particularly after intubation. The patient has at least one, and preferably two, secure, well-functioning intravenous (IV) lines. Pharmacologic agents are drawn up in properly

---

Box 19-1. The Seven Ps of RSI

1. **P**reparation
2. **P**reoxygenation
3. **P**retreatment
4. **P**aralysis with induction
5. **P**ositioning
6. **P**lacement with proof
7. **P**ostintubation management

labeled syringes. Vital equipment is tested. If a video or fiberoptic laryngoscope is to be used, it is turned on and image quality is verified. If a direct laryngoscope is to be used, the blade of choice is affixed to the laryngoscope handle and clicked into the "on" position to ensure that the light functions and is bright. The endotracheal tube (ETT) of the desired size is prepared, and the cuff tested for leaks. If difficult intubation is anticipated, a tube 0.5 mm less in internal diameter (ID) should also be prepared. Selection and preparation of the tube, as well as the use of the intubating stylet and bougie, are discussed in Chapter 12. Throughout this preparatory phase, the patient is receiving preoxygenation as described in the next section.

2. *Preoxygenation*

Preoxygenation is essential to the "no bagging" principle of RSI. Preoxygenation is the establishment of an oxygen reservoir within the lungs, blood, and body tissue to permit several minutes of apnea to occur without arterial oxygen desaturation. The principle reservoir is the functional residual capacity in the lungs, which is approximately 30 ml per kg. Administration of 100% oxygen for 3 minutes replaces this predominantly nitrogenous mixture of room air with oxygen, allowing several minutes of apnea time before hemoglobin saturation decreases to <90% (Fig. 19-1). Similar preoxygenation can be achieved much more rapidly by having the patient take eight vital capacity breaths (the greatest volume breaths the patient can take) while receiving 100% oxygen.

Obese patients are best preoxygenated when placed approximately 25° to 30° upright, and oxyhemoglobin desaturation is significantly delayed if oxygen is continuously administered at 5 L per minute by nasal cannula throughout the intubation sequence. In nonobese patients, desaturation also is delayed and reduced by continuous administration of oxygen at 5 L per minute during apnea.

The time to desaturation for an individual patient varies, depending on particular patient attributes, with children, morbidly obese patients, chronically ill (especially cardiopulmonary) patients, and late-term pregnant women desaturating significantly more rapidly than an average healthy adult does.

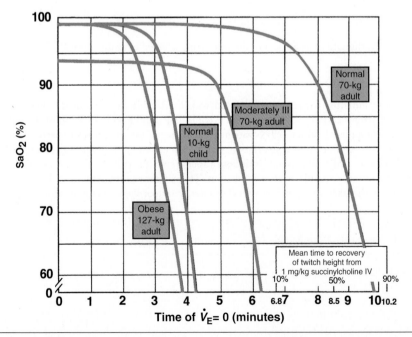

Figure 19-1 ● Time to Desaturation for Various Patient Circumstances. (From Benumof J, Dagg R, Benumof R. Critical hemoglobin desaturation will occur before return to an unparalyzed state following 1 mg/kg IV succinylcholine. *Anesthesiology.* 1997;87:979.)

Note the bars indicating recovery from succinylcholine paralysis on the bottom right of Figure 19-1. This demonstrates the fallacy of the oft-cited belief that a patient will quite likely recover sufficiently from succinylcholine-induced paralysis to breathe on his or her own before sustaining injury from hypoxemia, even if intubation and mechanical ventilation are both impossible. Although many patients will recover adequate neuromuscular function to breathe on their own before catastrophic desaturation, many others, including almost all children, will not, and even those who do are dependent on optimal preoxygenation before paralysis.

A healthy, fully preoxygenated 70-kg adult will maintain oxygen saturation at >90% for 8 minutes, whereas an obese adult will desaturate to 90% in <3 minutes. A 10-kg child will desaturate to 90% in <4 minutes. The time for desaturation from 90% to 0% is even more important and is much shorter. The healthy 70-kg adult desaturates from 90% to 0% in <120 seconds, and the small child does so in 45 seconds. A late-term pregnant woman is a high oxygen user, has a reduced functional residual capacity, and has an increased body mass, so she desaturates quickly in a manner analogous to that of the obese patient. Particular caution is required in this circumstance because both the obese patient and the pregnant woman may also be difficult to intubate and to bag-mask ventilate.

Most emergency departments do not use systems that are capable of delivering 100% oxygen. Typically, emergency department patients are preoxygenated using the "100% non-rebreather mask," which delivers approximately 65% to 70% oxygen (see Chapter 5). In physiologically well patients in whom difficult intubation is not anticipated, this percentage is often sufficient and adequate preoxygenation is achieved. However, higher inspired fractions of oxygen are often desirable and can be delivered by active breathing through the demand valve of bag-mask systems equipped with a one-way exhalation valve, or by specially designed high-concentration oxygen delivery devices. Oxygen delivery is discussed in detail in Chapter 5. The use of pulse oximetry throughout intubation enables the physician to monitor the level of oxygen saturation eliminating guesswork.

3. *Pretreatment*

Pretreatment is the administration of drugs to mitigate adverse effects associated with the intubation or the patient's underlying comorbidities. These adverse effects include bronchospastic reactivity of the airways to the ETT in patients with reactive airways disease, the intracranial pressure (ICP) response to airway manipulation in patients with elevated ICP, and systemic release of sympathetic adrenergic amines (the reflex sympathetic response to laryngoscopy [RSRL]). The pretreatment drugs are shown in Box 19-2 and discussed in detail in Chapter 20. Because there are three classes of patients for whom pretreatment is indicated, the mnemonic "ABC" can be used: **A**sthma (representing reactive airways disease), **B**rain (representing elevated ICP), and **C**ardiovascular (representing those at risk from RSRL; i.e., patients with ischemic heart disease, vascular disease [especially cerebrovascular disease], hypertension, and vascular events, such as aortic dissection, intracranial hemorrhage, etc.). The two drugs, fentanyl and lidocaine, and their relationship to the ABC conditions can be represented in a Venn diagram (Fig. 19-2). The pretreatment agents, when indicated, are administered 3 minutes before the induction and neuromuscular blocking agents.

4. *Paralysis with induction*

In this phase, a rapidly acting induction agent is given in a dose adequate to produce prompt loss of consciousness (see Chapter 21). Administration of the induction agent is immediately followed by the NMBA, usually succinylcholine (see Chapter 22). If succinylcholine is

---

Box 19-2. Pretreatment Drugs for RSI

Fentanyl	When sympathetic responses should be blunted (e.g. increased ICP, aortic dissection, intracranial hemorrhage, and ischemic heart disease)
Lidocaine	For reactive airways disease or increased ICP

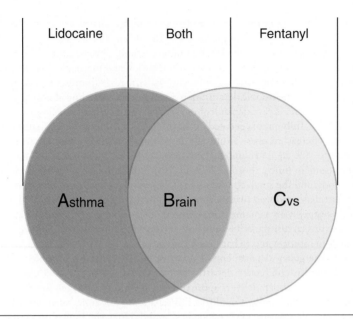

Figure 19-2 ● **Pretreatment Agents for RSI—the ABC Approach.** CVS, cardiovascular system.

contraindicated, rocuronium is used. Both the induction agent and the NMBA are given by IV push. RSI involves neither the slow administration of the induction agent nor a titration-to-end point approach. The sedative agent and dose are selected with the intention of rapid IV administration of the drugs. Although rapid administration of the induction agent can increase the likelihood and severity of side effects, especially hypotension, the entire technique is predicated on rapid loss of consciousness, rapid neuromuscular blockade, and a brief period of apnea without interposed assisted ventilation before intubation. Therefore, the induction agent is given as a rapid push followed immediately by a rapid push of the NMBA. Within a few seconds of the administration of the induction agent and NMBA, the patient will begin to lose consciousness, and respiration will decline, and then cease.

5. *Positioning*

   After 20 to 30 seconds, the patient is apneic and becoming flaccid. If succinylcholine has been used as the NMBA, fasciculations will be observed during this time. The oxygen mask used for preoxygenation remains in place to prevent the patient from acquiring even a partial breath of room air. At this point, the patient is positioned optimally for intubation, with consideration for cervical spine immobilization in trauma. Some patients, as discussed in Section VIII of this manual, will be sufficiently compromised that they require assisted ventilation almost continuously throughout the sequence to maintain oxygen saturations over 90%. Such patients, especially those with profound hypoxemia, are ventilated with bag and mask at all times except when laryngoscopy is occurring. Morbidly obese patients will maintain high oxygen saturations longer if they receive oxygen at 5 L per minute through nasal cannula throughout laryngoscopy. It is likely that this benefit pertains also to other patients. When bag-mask ventilation is performed on an unresponsive patient, the application of Sellick maneuver may minimize the volume of gases passed down the esophagus to the stomach, possibly decreasing the likelihood of regurgitation.

6. *Placement with proof*

   At 45 seconds after the administration of the succinylcholine, or 60 seconds if rocuronium is used, test the patient's jaw for flaccidity and intubate. Because preoxygenation endows most patients with several *minutes* of safe apnea time, the intubation can be performed gently and carefully and multiple attempts, if needed, often are possible without any need to provide additional oxygenation by bag and mask. Tube placement is confirmed as described in Chapter 12. End-tidal carbon dioxide ($ETCO_2$) detection is mandatory. A capnometer, such as a colorimetric $ETCO_2$ detector, is sufficient for this purpose. Continuous capnography provides additional and ongoing information.

7. *Postintubation management*

   After placement is confirmed, the ETT is secured in place. Mechanical ventilation should be initiated as described in Chapter 7. A chest radiograph should be obtained to assess pulmonary status and ensure that mainstem intubation has not occurred. Hypotension is common in the postintubation period and is often caused by diminished venous blood return as a result of the increased intrathoracic pressure that attends mechanical ventilation, exacerbated by the hemodynamic effects of the induction agent. Although this form of hypotension often is self-limited and responds to IV fluids, more ominous causes should be sought. BP should be measured, and if significant hypotension is present, the management steps in Table 19-1 should be considered.

   Long-term sedation almost always is indicated. Long-term paralysis, however, generally is avoided, except when necessary. Use of a sedation scale, such as the Richmond Agitation Sedation Scale, to optimize patient comfort helps guide decision making regarding the necessity of neuromuscular blockade (Box 19-3). Sedation and analgesia are administered to reach the desired level, and neuromuscular blockade is used only if the patient then requires it for management. Use of a sedation scale prevents the use of neuromuscular blockade for patient control when the cause of the patient's agitation is inadequate sedation. A sample sedation protocol is shown in Figure 19-3. Maintenance of intubation and mechanical ventilation requires both sedation and analgesia, and these can be titrated to patient response. A reasonable sedation starting point is lorazepam 0.05 mg per kg or midazolam 0.1-0.2 mg per kg, combined with an analgesic such as fentanyl 2 μg per kg, morphine 0.2 mg per kg, or hydromorphone (Dilaudid) 0.03 mg per kg. Fentanyl may be preferable because of its superior hemodynamic stability. When an NMBA is required, a full paralytic dose should be used (e.g., vecuronium 0.1 mg per kg). Sedation and analgesia are difficult to titrate when the patient is paralyzed, and "topping up" doses should be administered regularly, before physiologic stress (hypertension and tachycardia) is evident. For patients requiring serial examination, particularly patients with neurologic conditions, propofol by infusion is preferable because it can be discontinued or

TABLE 19-1
Hypotension in the Postintubation Period

Cause	Detection	Action
Pneumothorax	Increased PIP, difficulty bagging, decreased breath sounds, and decreasing oxygen saturation	Immediate thoracostomy
Decreased venous return	Worst in patients with high PIPs secondary to high intrathoracic pressure or those with marginal hemodynamic status before intubation	Fluid bolus and treatment of airway resistance (bronchodilators); increase the inspiratory flow rate to allow increased expiratory time; try $\downarrow V_T$, respiratory rate, or both if SpO_2 is adequate, and decrease the dose of sedation agent(s)
Induction agents	Other causes excluded	Fluid bolus and decrease the dose of sedation agent(s)
Cardiogenic	Usually in compromised patient; ECG; exclude other causes	Fluid bolus (caution), pressors, and decrease the dose of sedation agent(s)

Box 19-3. Richmond Agitation Sedation Scale

Score	Term	Description	
+4	Combative	Overtly combative, violent, and immediate danger to staff	
+3	Very agitated	Pulls or removes tube(s) or catheter(s) and is aggressive	
+2	Agitated	Frequent nonpurposeful movement and fights ventilator	
+1	Restless	Anxious but movements not aggressive and vigorous	
0	Alert and calm		
−1	Drowsy	Not fully alert, but has sustained awakening (eye opening/eye contact) to *voice* (>10 s)	Verbal stimulation
−2	Light sedation	Briefly awakens with eye contact to *voice* (<10 s)	
−3	Moderate sedation	Movement or eye opening to *voice* (but no eye contact)	
−4	Deep sedation	No response to voice, but movement or eye opening to *physical* stimulation	Physical stimulation
−5	Unarousable	No response to *voice* or *physical* stimulation	

Procedure for Richmond Agitation Sedation Scale Assessment
1. Observe patient.
   a. Patient is alert, restless, or agitated. **(score 0 to +4)**
2. If not alert, state patient's name and *say* to open eyes and look at speaker.
   b. Patient awakens with sustained eye opening and eye contact. **(score −1)**
   c. Patient awakens with eye opening and eye contact, but not sustained. **(score −2)**
   d. Patient has any movement in response to voice but no eye contact. **(score −3)**
3. When no response to verbal stimulation, physically stimulate patient by shaking shoulder and/or rubbing sternum.
   e. Patient has any movement to physical stimulation. **(score −4)**
   f. Patient has no response to any stimulation. **(score −5)**

Adapted from Sessler CN, Gosnell M, Grap MJ, et al. The Richmond Agitation-Sedation Scale: validity and reliability in adult intensive care patients. *Am J Respir Crit Care Med*. 2002;166:1338–1344; and Ely EW, Truman B, Shintani A, et al. Monitoring sedation status over time in ICU patients: the reliability and validity of the Richmond Agitation Sedation Scale (RASS). *JAMA*. 2003;289:2983–2991.

decreased with rapid recovery of consciousness. Propofol infusion can be started at 25 to 50 μg/kg/minute and titrated. An initial bolus of 0.5 to 1 mg per kg may be given if rapid sedation is desired. Analgesia is required, as above, because propofol is not an analgesic.

Timing the Steps of RSI

Successful RSI requires a detailed knowledge of the sequence of steps to be taken and also of the time required for each step to achieve its purpose. Preoxygenation requires at least 3 minutes for maximal effect. If necessary, eight vital capacity breaths (if possible) can accomplish equivalent

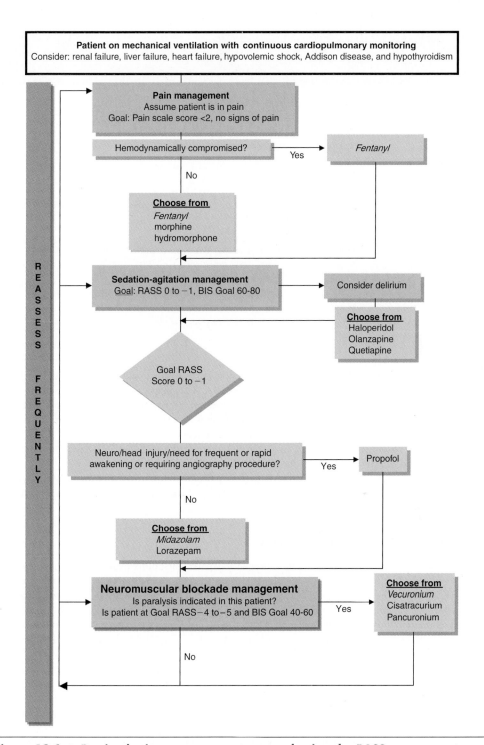

Figure 19-3 ● Postintubation management protocol using the RASS score.   See also Box 19-3 for description of the Sedation Scale (RASS). BIS: Bispectral Index. (The protocol, reproduced with permission, was developed for use at Brigham and Women's Hospital, Boston, MA.)

TABLE 19-2 Rapid Sequence Intubation	
Time	**Action (seven Ps)**
Zero minus 10 min	**P**reparation: *Assemble all necessary equipment, drugs, etc.*
Zero minus 5 min	**P**reoxygenation
Zero minus 3 min	**P**retreatment
Zero	**P**aralysis with induction: *Administer induction agent by IV push, followed immediately by paralytic agent by IV push*
Zero plus 20–30 s	**P**ositioning: *Position patient for optimal laryngoscopy; continue oxygen supplementation at 5 L/min by nasal after apnea ensues*
Zero plus 45 s	**P**lacement with proof: *Assess mandible for flaccidity; perform intubation; confirm placement*
Zero plus 1 min	**P**ostintubation management: *Long-term sedation with paralysis only if indicated*

preoxygenation in <30 seconds. It is recommended that pretreatment drugs be given 3 minutes before the administration of the sedative and NMBA. The pharmacokinetics of the sedatives and neuromuscular blockers would suggest that a 45-second interval between administration of these agents and initiation of endotracheal intubation is optimal, extending to 60 seconds if rocuronium is used. Thus, the entire sequence of RSI can be described as a series of timed steps. For the purposes of discussion, *time zero* is the time at which the sedative agent and NMBA are pushed. The recommended sequence is shown in Table 19-2.

An example of RSI performed for a generally healthy 40-year-old, 80-kg patient is shown in Table 19-3. Other examples of RSI for particular patient conditions are in the corresponding sections throughout this manual.

Success Rates and Adverse Events

RSI has a very high success rate in the emergency department, approximately 99% in most modern series. The National Emergency Airway Registry (NEAR), an international multicenter study of >8,500 emergency department intubations, reported >99% success for RSI when used on patients with medical emergencies and >97% for trauma patients. RSI success rates are higher than those for other emergency airway management methods, and RSI is the main rescue technique when other methods, such as blind nasotracheal intubation, fail. The NEAR investigators classify events related to intubation as follows:

- Immediate complications such as witnessed aspiration, broken teeth, airway trauma, and undetected esophageal intubation
- Technical problems such as mainstem intubation, cuff leak, and recognized esophageal intubation
- Physiologic alterations such as pneumothorax, pneumomediastinum, cardiac arrest, and dysrhythmia

This system allows witnessed complications to be identified and all adverse events to be captured, but avoids the incorrect attribution of various technical problems (e.g., recognized esophageal intubation or tube cuff failure) or physiologic alterations (e.g., cardiac arrest in a

---

TABLE 19-3
RSI for Healthy 80-kg Patient

Time	Action (seven Ps)
Zero minus 10 min	**P**reparation
Zero minus 5 min	**P**reoxygenation
Zero minus 3 min	**P**retreatment: *None indicated*
Zero	**P**aralysis with induction: *Etomidate 24 mg IV push; succinylcholine 120 mg IV push*
Zero plus 20–30 s	**P**ositioning: *Position patient for optimal laryngoscopy; continue oxygen supplementation at 5 L/min*
Zero plus 45 s	**P**lacement with proof: *Confirm with ETCO$_2$, physical examination*
Zero plus 1 min	**P**ostintubation management: *Long-term sedation/paralysis as indicated*

---

patient who was *in extremis* before intubation was undertaken and which may or may not be attributable to the intubation) as complications. Overall, event rates are low in the NEAR studies; immediate complications are seen in approximately 3% of RSI patients. Hypotension and alterations in heart rate can result from the pharmacologic agents used or from stimulation of the larynx with resultant reflexes. Other studies have reported consistent results. The most catastrophic complication of RSI is unrecognized esophageal intubation, which is rare in the emergency department, but occurs with alarming frequency in some prehospital studies. This situation underscores the importance of confirming tube placement described in Chapter 12. It is incumbent on the person who performs RSI to be able to establish an airway and maintain mechanical ventilation. This process may require a surgical airway as the final rescue from a failed oral intubation attempt (see Chapter 3). Aspiration of gastric contents can occur but is uncommon. Overall, the true complication rate of RSI in the emergency department is low and the success rate is exceedingly high, especially when one considers the serious nature of the illnesses for which patients are intubated, as well as the limited time and information available to the clinician performing the intubation.

"Accelerated" and "Immediate" RSI and "Delayed Sequence Intubation"

When rapid intubation is required, the RSI sequence can be compressed so the steps are conducted much more rapidly than the standard RSI outlined previously.

1. Accelerated RSI
   - Shorten preoxygenation to 30 seconds by using eight vital capacity breaths
   - Shorten the pretreatment interval to 1 or 2 minutes from 3 minutes
2. Immediate RSI
   - Preoxygenate with eight vital capacity breaths
   - Eliminate pretreatment
      An alternative to RSI, so-called delayed sequence intubation has been advocated for use in emergency intubations when the patient is significantly hypoxemic, or at risk for precipitous oxyhemoglobin desaturation. The technique involves administration of the induction agent, followed

by several minutes of oxygenation using pressure support mask ventilation (such as bi-level positive airway pressure or continuous positive airway pressure). When oxygenation is felt to be optimal, the operator pushes the NMBA and intubates as for RSI. Although the technique has gained some attention, it is without support of an evidence base, and its safety is not established. Other than for highly selected cases and in the presence of a truly expert and experienced clinician, we cannot recommend its use.

EVIDENCE

- **What is the optimal method for preoxygenation?** Standard preoxygenation has traditionally been achieved by 3 minutes of normal tidal volume breathing of 100% oxygen. Pandit et al.[1] showed that eight vital capacity breaths achieves similar preoxygenation to that of 3 minutes of normal tidal volume breathing and that both of these methods are superior to four vital capacity breaths. The time to desaturation of oxyhemoglobin to 95% is 5.2 minutes after eight vital capacity breaths versus 3.7 minutes after 3 minutes of tidal volume breathing and 2.8 minutes after four vital capacity breaths.[2,3] Preoxygenation of normal healthy patients can produce an average of 8 minutes of apnea time before desaturation to 90% occurs, but the times are much less (as little as 3 minutes) in patients with cardiovascular disease, obese patients, and small children.[4]

  Sufficient recovery from succinylcholine paralysis cannot be relied on before desaturation occurs, even in properly preoxygenated healthy patients.[4,5] Term pregnant women also desaturate more rapidly than nonpregnant women do and desaturate to 95% in <3 minutes, compared with 4 minutes for nonpregnant controls. Preoxygenating in the upright position prolongs desaturation time in nonpregnant women to 5.5 minutes, but does not favorably affect term pregnant patients.[2,6]

- **How should obese patients be preoxygenated?** Obese patients desaturate more rapidly than nonobese patients.[4] Two techniques have emerged that maximize the time to desaturation for obese patients. First, preoxygenation of the morbidly obese (body mass index > 40 kg per m^2) in the 25° head up position achieves higher arterial oxygenation saturations and significantly prolongs desaturation time to 92%, to about 3½ minutes versus 2½ minutes over those patients preoxygenated in the supine position.[7] Second, providing continuous oxygen by nasal cannula during the apneic phase is known to prolong maintenance of high oxyhemoglobin saturation in normal patients. In one study, despite preoxygenation using only four vital capacity breaths, 15 patients receiving 5 L per minute of oxygen through a nasopharyngeal catheter did not desaturate at all, maintaining oxyhemoglobin saturations of 100% for 6 minutes, versus their "no oxygen" comparison group, which desaturated to 95% in an average of a little >3½ minutes.[8] In obese patients, the effect may be even more important because of the rapid desaturation these patients otherwise exhibit. When obese patients receive continuous oxygen at 5 L per minute during the apneic phase of intubation, desaturation is delayed to about 5¼ versus 3¾ minutes for a nonoxygenated comparison group and 8/15 oxygenated patients versus 1/15 nonoxygenated patients maintained oxyhemoglobin saturation of 95% or higher for 6 minutes.[9] Surprisingly, although the use of noninvasive positive-pressure ventilation for preoxygenation of obese patients shortened the time required for preoxygenation, it did not prolong the time to desaturation to 95%.[10] On balance, we recommend the use of noninvasive positive-pressure ventilation for the preoxygenation of obese patients, and for those in whom ambient pressure oxygenation at 100% FiO_2 fails to achieve acceptable oxygen saturation. For all obese patients, we recommend the use of continuous apneic oxygenation with nasal cannula at 5 L per minute flowrate. For nonobese patients, continuous oxygenation also makes sense, particularly if the airway is anticipated to be difficult.

- **Pretreatment drugs, induction agents, and NMBAs:** Evidence regarding the use of pretreatment drugs, induction agents, and NMBAs are discussed in the "Evidence" sections of the relevant chapters.

- **Sellick maneuver:** Two meta-analyses of the studies of Sellick maneuver, one in 1997, the other in 2007, are in agreement that there is no solid evidence supporting its routine use during RSI.[11,12] Similarly, a 2010 study of 402 trauma patients suggests that, at the least, the maneuver has as much potential for harm as for good.[13] Sellick maneuver may be applied improperly or not at all during a significant proportion of emergency department RSIs.[14] Even when applied by experienced practitioners, Sellick maneuver can increase peak inspiratory pressure (PIP) and decrease tidal volume or even cause complete obstruction during bag-mask ventilation.[15] The practice, though, is so embedded in emergency medicine and anesthesia cultures, that practitioners have been slow to abandon it.
- **Is RSI superior to intubation with sedation alone?** This is also discussed in the evidence sections for Chapter 22. The most powerful evidence supporting the use of an NMBA in addition to an induction agent comes from dosing studies of NMBAs, of which there are many. The results uniformly are the same. Intubation is more successful because of better intubating conditions when an NMBA is used, when compared to the use of an induction agent alone. These results are even more compelling when one realizes that the depth of anesthesia in these studies is invariably deeper than that obtained with use of a single dose of an induction agent for emergency intubation. In a study of 180 general anesthesia patients, 0% of patients who received no succinylcholine had excellent intubating conditions versus 80% of patients receiving 1.5 mg per kg of succinylcholine.[16] Seventy percent of the "no NMBA" group had intubating conditions characterized as "poor." In a different study by the same investigators, "acceptable" intubating conditions were achieved in 32% of patients with general anesthesia but no NMBA versus over 90% of patients receiving any effective dose of succinylcholine.[17] In a rocuronium dosing study, 13/20 saline placebo patients had unacceptable intubating conditions versus 1/20 patients who received rocuronium 1.2 mg per kg.[18] Bozeman et al.[19] compared the use of etomidate alone to etomidate plus succinylcholine in a prehospital flight paramedic program and found that RSI outperformed etomidate-alone intubations by all measures of ease of intubation. Li et al.[20] found significant improvement in intubation success rates when RSI was introduced in the emergency department. Bair et al.[21] analyzed 207 (2.7%) failed intubations among 7,712 intubations in the NEAR registry and found that the greatest proportion of rescue procedures (49%) involved the use of RSI to achieve intubation after failure of oral or nasotracheal intubation by non-RSI methods.
- **What about RSI for children?** A multicenter report by the NEAR investigators identified 156 pediatric intubations from among 1,288 total intubations. Eighty-one percent of the pediatric intubations were performed using RSI.[22] A study of 105 children younger than 10 years (average age, 3 years) who underwent RSI with etomidate as the induction agent showed stable hemodynamics and high success and safety profiles.[23]

REFERENCES

1. Pandit JJ, Duncan T, Robbins PA. Total oxygen uptake with two maximal breathing techniques and the tidal volume breathing technique: a physiologic study of preoxygenation. *Anesthesiology.* 2003;99:841–846.

2. Baraka AS, Taha SK, Aouad MT, et al. Preoxygenation: comparison of maximal breathing and tidal volume breathing techniques. *Anesthesiology.* 1999;91:612–616.

3. Ramez Salem M, Joseph NJ, Crystal GJ, et al. Preoxygenation: comparison of maximal breathing and tidal volume techniques. *Anesthesiology.* 2000;92:1845–1847.

4. Benumof JL, Dagg R, Benumof R. Critical hemoglobin desaturation will occur before return to an unparalyzed state following 1 mg/kg intravenous succinylcholine. *Anesthesiology.* 1997;87(4):979–982.

5. Heier T, Feiner JR, Lin J, et al. Hemoglobin desaturation after succinylcholine-induced apnea: a study of the recovery of spontaneous ventilation in healthy volunteers. *Anesthesiology.* 2001;94:754–759.

6. Hayes AH, Breslin DS, Mirakhur RK, et al. Frequency of haemoglobin desaturation with the use of succinylcholine during rapid sequence induction of anaesthesia. *Acta Anaesthesiol Scand*. 2001;45:746–749.

7. Dixon BJ, Dixon JB, Carden JR, et al. Preoxygenation is more effective in the 25 degrees head-up position than in the supine position in severely obese patients: a randomized controlled study. *Anesthesiology*. 2005;102(6):1110–1115.

8. Taha SK, Siddik-Sayyid SM, El-Khatib MF, et al. Nasopharyngeal oxygen insufflation following pre-oxygenation using the four deep breath technique. *Anaesthesia*. 2006;61(5):427–430.

9. Ramachandran SK, Cosnowski A, Shanks A, et al. Apneic oxygenation during prolonged laryngoscopy in obese patients: a randomized, controlled trial of nasal oxygen administration. *J Clin Anesth*. 2010;22(3):164–168.

10. Delay JM, Sebbane M, Jung B, et al. The effectiveness of noninvasive positive pressure ventilation to enhance preoxygenation in morbidly obese patients: a randomized controlled study. *Anesth Analg*. 2008;107(5):1707–1713.

11. Brimacombe JR, Berry AM. Cricoid pressure. *Can J Anaesth*. 1997;44:414–425.

12. Ellis DY, Harris T, Zideman D. Cricoid pressure in emergency department rapid sequence tracheal intubations: a risk-benefit analysis. *Ann Emerg Med*. 2007;50:653–665.

13. Harris T, Ellis DY, Foster L, et al. Cricoid pressure and laryngeal manipulation in 402 pre-hospital emergency anaesthetics: essential safety measure or a hindrance to rapid safe intubation? *Resuscitation*. 2010;81:810–816.

14. Olsen JC, Gurr DE, Hughes M. Video analysis of emergency medicine residents performing rapid-sequence intubations. *J Emerg Med*. 2000;18(4):469–472.

15. Allman KG. The effect of cricoid pressure application on airway patency. *J Clin Anesth*. 1995;7(3):197–199.

16. Naguib M, Samarkandi AH, El-Din ME, et al. The dose of succinylcholine required for excellent endotracheal intubating conditions. *Anesth Analg*. 2006;102(1):151–155.

17. Naguib M, Samarkandi A, Riad W, et al. Optimal dose of succinylcholine revisited. *Anesthesiology*. 2003;99(5):1045–1049.

18. Kirkegaard-Nielsen H, Caldwell JE, Berry PD. Rapid tracheal intubation with rocuronium: a probability approach to determining dose. *Anesthesiology*. 1999;91(1):131–136.

19. Bozeman WP, Kleiner DM, Huggett V. A comparison of rapid-sequence intubation and etomidate-only intubation in the prehospital air medical setting. *Prehosp Emerg Care*. 2006;10(1):8–13.

20. Li J, Murphy-Lavoie H, Bugas C, et al. Complications of emergency intubation with and without paralysis. *Am J Emerg Med*. 1999;17(2):141–143.

21. Bair AE, Filbin MR, Kulkarni RG, et al. The failed intubation attempt in the emergency department: analysis of prevalence, rescue techniques, and personnel. *J Emerg Med*. 2002;23(2):131–140.

22. Sagarin MJ, Chiang V, Sakles JC, et al. Rapid sequence intubation for pediatric emergency airway management. *Pediatr Emerg Care*. 2002;18(6):417–423.

23. Guldner G, Schultz J, Sexton P, et al. Etomidate for rapid-sequence intubation in young children: hemodynamic effects and adverse events. *Acad Emerg Med*. 2003;10:134–139.

20

Pretreatment Agents

David A. Caro • Stephen Bush

INTRODUCTION

Pretreatment refers to the administration of drugs 3 minutes before the paralysis step of rapid sequence intubation (RSI) in an attempt to attenuate the adverse effects of laryngoscopy and intubation, mainly intracranial pressure (ICP) rise, blood pressure changes, and increases in airways resistance. The timing of pretreatment agents and a brief overview of their use are provided in Chapter 19.

The acts of intubation, laryngoscopy, and tracheal intubation are exceedingly stimulating, leading to as much as a doubling of heart rate and systolic blood pressure. Increases in left ventricular (LV) ejection velocity leads to an increase in arterial wall shear forces. Bradycardia, particularly in children younger than 1 year, may also occur. Laryngoscopy and endotracheal intubation may cause a rise in ICP, and the stimulation of the upper airway reflexes may incite coughing, laryngospasm, or bronchospasm.

The mechanisms behind these responses are believed to include the 9th and 10th cranial nerves. Sympathetic activation releases norepinephrine from adrenergic nerve terminals and epinephrine from the adrenal glands. The subsequent elevation in blood pressure may be exacerbated by the activation of the renin–angiotensin system. Parasympathetic activation can result in bronchoconstriction and coughing. The clinical relevance of these responses is not clear, but there is some evidence that these responses to laryngoscopy and intubation can contribute to adverse outcomes.

A wide variety of pharmacologic agents have been studied in an attempt to identify agents that can blunt these reflexes in both elective and emergency airway management. Practically, lidocaine ultra–short–acting opioids, such as fentanyl (Sublimaze) and its derivatives, and atropine are the most appropriate for emergency intubations. Of these, lidocaine and the ultra–short–acting opioids have undergone the most evaluation. Although these drugs may be helpful when given before intubation in both elective and emergency airway management situations, few formal studies have examined the ability of the drugs to mitigate responses and improve outcome in the context of emergency RSI.

Table 20-1 lists the recommendations for the use of lidocaine and fentanyl in emergency RSI. Lidocaine blunts reflexive rises in ICP during intubation, and mitigates reactive increases in small- and medium-size airways resistance in patients with reactive airways disease who are undergoing intubation. Fentanyl and other ultra–short–acting opioids have been reported to blunt the reflex sympathetic response to laryngoscopy (RSRL) in a dose-related fashion. Control of this sympathetic response attenuates the magnitude of the rise in ICP by mitigating blood pressure increases during laryngoscopy and intubation. Similarly, patients at risk from the adverse effects of a sudden rise in blood pressure, myocardial oxygen demand, or LV ejection velocity may benefit from attenuating sympathetic activation. For example, patients with coronary artery disease, neurovascular events such as intracranial hemorrhage, or major vascular disorders such as aortic dissection should ideally not be exposed to the effects of a sudden and significant release of catecholamines.

Atropine is used to treat bradycardia when it occurs (after excluding hypoxia as a possible cause). The empiric administration of atropine to children younger than 1 year who will be receiving succinylcholine is considered a reasonable (optional) practice (see Chapter 4).

LIDOCAINE

Lidocaine functions by blocking fast sodium channels in neurons. It is an amide local anesthetic agent that is metabolized in the liver and excreted in the urine. A single intravenous (IV) dose need not be adjusted in renal failure patients. IV lidocaine is absolutely contraindicated in patients allergic to amide local anesthetic agents (exceedingly rare) and in patients with high-grade heart

TABLE 20-1
Pretreatment Agent Summary

Drug	Dose	Time to onset	Duration of action	Elimination	Special considerations
Lidocaine	1.5 mg/kg IV	45–90 s	10–20 min	Metabolism: hepatic (90%) Excretion: renal	Category B in pregnancy. Readily crosses the blood–brain barrier and the placenta
Fentanyl	3 mcg/kg IV	2–3 min	30–60 min	Metabolism: hepatic (90%) and small intestine Excretion: renal	Certain cytochrome P-450 (CYP) isoenzyme 3A4 inhibitors will prolong action (e.g., macrolides, azoles, protease inhibitors)

block or bradycardia unless a pacemaker has been placed. Lidocaine can aggravate hypovolemic and cardiogenic shock, and is relatively contraindicated in Wolff–Parkinson–White syndrome. Box 20-1 shows the drugs for which severe drug interactions have been reported with lidocaine.

Adverse effects are rare, but include central nervous system (CNS) toxicity (seizures and coma) and cardiac conduction abnormalities (severe bradycardia and dysrhythmias), and cardiogenic shock when used at high doses. The available evidence supports the use of lidocaine at a dose of 1.5 mg per kg to suppress the cough reflex and to mitigate the ICP response to upper airway manipulation, laryngoscopy, and intubation. The recommendation regarding ICP is based predominantly on the results of older studies of patients with elevated ICP undergoing various airway procedures, including tracheal suctioning and laryngoscopy, although there is some conflict in the literature. No studies have directly addressed its use in emergency RSI, and none has used patient outcome as a primary end point. However, we recommend the use of lidocaine for patients with elevated ICP. This is based on the cough suppression effect, the potential to reduce the ICP response during laryngoscopy and intubation, and the fact that the drug at the recommended dose is safe and commonly used, and therefore unlikely to cause patient harm or lead to medication error. Lidocaine also appears to diminish the reflex bronchospasm that may occur with the intubation of patients with reactive airways disease. We believe that the evidence is sufficient recommend the use of lidocaine as a pretreatment agent in patients with reactive airways disease who are undergoing intubation. The recommendations for the use of lidocaine as a pretreatment agent for emergency RSI are shown in Box 20-2.

Box 20-1. Severe Drug-Drug Interactions for Lidocaine

Dofetilide (class III antiarrhythmic)—can cause dysrhythmias
Monoamine oxidase inhibitors—can cause hypotension
Amiodarone—can cause bradycardia (other antiarrhythmics may also cause additive effects)

Box 20-2. Recommendations for Lidocaine as a Pretreatment Agent for RSI

- Patients with reactive airways disease
- Patients with elevated ICP

FENTANYL AND OTHER ULTRA–SHORT-ACTING OPIOIDS

Given in sufficiently high doses, most sedative/hypnotic agents will attenuate the RSRL. However, the drug dose required to produce this degree of CNS depression will usually produce significant hypotension.

Fentanyl (Sublimaze) is an opioid receptor agonist that selectively activates the μ-receptor. It is metabolized in the liver and has first-phase redistribution within 5 minutes, and an elimination half-life of 7 hours. Fentanyl has a time to onset of 2 to 3 minutes and duration of action of approximately 30 to 60 minutes. It is a class C drug in pregnancy. Major side effects include dose-related respiratory depression and hypotension in patients who are dependent on sympathetic tone.

Fentanyl attenuates the sympathetic response to laryngoscopy with minimal side effects other than dose-related respiratory depression, which is rarely an issue in the doses used for RSI pretreatment. Fentanyl does not release histamine and has no direct effect on the pulmonary response to laryngoscopy. Fentanyl has been shown to have a partial attenuating effect on the RSRL at doses as low as 2 mcg per kg IV.

For emergency intubation, we recommend fentanyl in a dose of 3 mcg per kg IV 3 minutes before the induction and paralytic agents for patients who might be adversely affected by a systemic release of catecholamines. Patients with increased ICP frequently lose the ability to autoregulate, and consequently, increases in blood pressure may exacerbate the ICP elevation. Patients with intracranial hemorrhage, ischemic heart disease, known or suspected cerebral or aortic aneurysm, or dissection or rupture of a great vessel are similarly at risk from an acute hypertensive response.

Fentanyl should be given as the last of the pretreatment drugs, over a period of 30 to 60 seconds, to minimize the likelihood of significant respiratory depression. Whenever fentanyl is given, watch the patient for signs of hypoventilation before administration of the sedative and paralytic agents. Because fentanyl is given to reduce sympathetic tone, extreme caution must be used in the hemodynamically compromised patient who is dependent on sympathetic tone to maintain hemodynamic stability (e.g., compensated or decompensated shock). Fentanyl is not recommended in pediatric RSI because the administration would further complicate the resuscitation, and the benefit for children has not been demonstrated.

Muscle wall rigidity is a unique and idiosyncratic response to opioids and is probably related to the dose and speed of opioid administration, the concomitant use of nitrous oxide, and the absence of muscle relaxants. It is not reversible with naloxone (Narcan). It is usually seen with fentanyl doses well in excess of 500 mcg (0.5 mg) and primarily affects the chest and abdominal wall musculature. The rigidity tends to occur very quickly after the patient begins to lose consciousness, and it is abolished by the administration of paralyzing doses of succinylcholine, once the abnormality is recognized. Rigidity has not been reported with the use of fentanyl in the emergency department. Because fentanyl is used in relatively low doses for emergency RSI, it is exceedingly unlikely that any muscle rigidity will occur.

Recommendations for the use of fentanyl as a pretreatment agent for emergency RSI are given in Box 20-3. Three important caveats apply to the use of fentanyl as a pretreatment agent during RSI:

1. Avoid fentanyl pretreatment if the patient is in compensated or decompensated shock, or minimally hemodynamically stable and dependent on sympathetic drive.

Box 20-3. Recommendations for Fentanyl as a Pretreatment Agent for RSI

- Patients with elevated ICP (at risk from increasing blood pressure)
- Patients with cardiovascular disease at risk from increased blood pressure and cardiac force of contraction (ischemic coronary disease, aneurysmal disease, great vessel rupture or dissection, and intracranial hemorrhage)

---

2. Be prepared for dose-related respiratory depression.
3. Give fentanyl as the final pretreatment agent and administer over 30 to 60 seconds.

OTHER POTENTIAL PRETREATMENT AGENTS

The β-2 agonist, albuterol, can mitigate the bronchospastic response to airway manipulation, and is used for this purpose for elective anesthesia in the operating room, and for elective bronchoscopy. We do not classify it as a pretreatment agent for emergency RSI because it is universally given to patients with severe asthma, regardless of whether the patient is ultimately intubated.

Atropine should be immediately available as a rescue agent when intubation is undertaken. Bradycardia has also been reported in adults receiving a second dose of succinylcholine, and is believed to result from stimulation of cardiac muscarinic receptors. Whether this uncommonly observed bradycardia is caused directly by succinylcholine, by manipulation of the airway, or by the patient's underlying condition or comorbidity is unknown. Profound bradycardia and cardiac arrest can occur during intubation of critically ill patients.

β-Blockers (e.g., esmolol [Brevibloc]) have been shown to be beneficial in attenuating the sympathetic response to laryngoscopy. They are not effective in attenuating any rise in ICP, except that caused by elevations in blood pressure. β-Blockers may increase airways resistance, especially in patients with reactive airways disease, and they are negative inotropes, and so are contraindicated in clinical situations in which maximum cardiac output is mandatory. Thus, although these agents are capable of blunting the sympathetic response to laryngoscopy, we do not recommend them for use as routine pretreatment agents for emergency RSI. On balance, fentanyl is a more appropriate agent for this purpose.

Neuromuscular blocking agents are used in some instances to "defasciculate" a patient undergoing RSI with succinylcholine. The benefits of this practice are unclear, as are the magnitude of the side effects of succinylcholine that defasciculation are intended to blunt. We do not recommend defasciculation of patients receiving succinylcholine as the neuromuscular blocking agent for RSI.

SUMMARY AND RECOMMENDATIONS

1. Pretreatment agents are used to attenuate the adverse physiologic responses to laryngoscopy and intubation.
2. As is discussed in Chapter 19, there are three classes of patients for who pretreatment is indicated. Use the mnemonic ABC: *A*sthma (representing reactive airways disease), *B*rain (representing elevated ICP), and *C*ardiovascular (representing those at risk from reflex sympathetic responses to laryngoscopy [i.e., patients with ischemic heart disease, vascular disease (especially cerebrovascular disease), hypertension, and vascular events, such as rupture or dissection of a

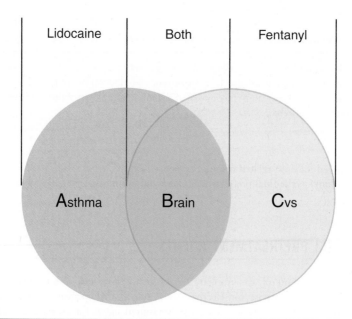

Figure 20-1 ● **The ABC Approach to Pretreatment.**

great vessel]). The two drugs, lidocaine and fentanyl, and their relationship to the ABC conditions, are shown in Figure 20-1.

3. Ideally, any pretreatment agent should be administered 3 minutes before the sedative agent to match peak drug effect with airway manipulation. Even if time is short, there may be some benefit to giving lidocaine pretreatment. Fentanyl, if indicated, can be given after intubation, if there was not sufficient time to give it as a pretreatment agent.

EVIDENCE

- **Does lidocaine mitigate cough and bronchospasm in susceptible patients?** Lidocaine appears to diminish the reflex bronchospasm that may occur with intubation in patients with reactive airways disease. There are high quality studies that show that IV lidocaine at a dose of 1.5 mg per kg IV can effectively suppress the cough reflex in humans.[1,2]
- **Does lidocaine attenuate the rise in ICP seen with airway manipulation?** Data on the effect of lidocaine on the increase in ICP with intubation is conflicting. Three best evidence reviews of the use of lidocaine in head injury patients undergoing RSI found that high-quality evidence is lacking.[2–4] Conflicting data exist in the literature. On balance, there is suggestive evidence that lidocaine may mitigate the ICP response to airway manipulation, and the drug is commonly used and safe in the doses recommended. We continue to recommend lidocaine for use in patients with elevated ICP pending evidence to the contrary.
- **What evidence is there that an opioid may cause other unwanted effects when used as a pretreatment drug?** High-dose fentanyl (100 mcg per kg, or approximately 30 times the dose used in emergency RSI) caused 8% of patients undergoing cardiac surgery to develop extreme thoracic and abdominal rigidity.[5] There is a single case report of rigidity in a patient who received fentanyl (approximately 2 mcg per kg) while taking venlafaxine.[6] Fentanyl has been widely used for procedural sedation in doses similar to those used for RSI, and reports of muscle rigidity are absent, even from large series.[7,8]

- **What is the evidence for the use of atropine to prevent bradycardia in pediatric patients undergoing RSI?** No relevant, systematic reviews are currently published. Multiple, small studies were identified.[9–15] The five highest-quality studies have patient populations of 20 to 90. Three studies showed drops in heart rate even with atropine.[10–12] A good-quality retrospective review of 143 pediatric intubations with RSI demonstrated six episodes of bradycardia, three of whom had received atropine pretreatment.[16] The data continue to be difficult to interpret. Although there exists a potential for bradycardia during intubation of pediatric patients, either with or without succinylcholine, atropine has not been shown to prevent this, and there are no grounds to support the routine use of atropine for pediatric intubation with succinylcholine. Many practitioners continue to use atropine for children under age 1 year, though."

REFERENCES

1. Butler J, Jackson R. Best evidence topic report. Lignocaine as a pretreatment to rapid sequence intubation in patients with status asthmaticus. *Emerg Med J*. 2005;22:732.

2. Butler J, Jackson R. Towards evidence based emergency medicine: best BETs from Manchester Royal Infirmary. Lignocaine premedication before rapid sequence induction in head injuries. *Emerg Med J*. 2002;19:554.

3. Robinson N, Clancy M. In patients with head injury undergoing rapid sequence intubation, does pretreatment with intravenous lignocaine/lidocaine lead to an improved neurological outcome? A review of the literature. *Emerg Med J*. 2001;18:453–457.

4. Brooks D, Anderson CM, Carter MA, et al. Clinical practice guidelines for suctioning the airway of the intubated and nonintubated patient. *Can Respir J*. 2001;8:163–181.

5. Caspi J, Klausner JM, Safadi T, et al. Delayed respiratory depression following fentanyl anesthesia for cardiac surgery. *Crit Care Med*. 1988;16:238–240.

6. Roy S, Fortier LP. Fentanyl-induced rigidity during emergence from general anesthesia potentiated by venlafexine. *Can J Anaesth*. 2003;50:32–35.

7. Roback MG, Wathen JE, Bajaj L, et al. Adverse events associated with procedural sedation and analgesia in a pediatric emergency department: a comparison of common parenteral drugs. *Acad Emerg Med*. 2005;12:508–513.

8. Sacchetti A, Senula G, Strickland J, et al. Procedural sedation in the community emergency department: initial results of the ProSCED registry. *Acad Emerg Med*. 2007;14:41–46.

9. Barrington KJ, Finer NN, Etches PC. Succinylcholine and atropine for premedication of the newborn infant before nasotracheal intubation: a randomized, controlled trial. *Crit Care Med*. 1989;17:1293–1296.

10. Kelly MA, Finer NN. Nasotracheal intubation in the neonate: physiologic responses and effects of atropine and pancuronium. *J Pediatr*. 1984;105:303–309.

11. Oei J, Hari R, Butha T, et al. Facilitation of neonatal nasotracheal intubation with premedication: a randomized controlled trial. *J Paediatr Child Health*. 2002;38:146–150.

12. Roberts KD, Leone TA, Edwards WH, et al. Premedication for nonemergent neonatal intubations: a randomized, controlled trial comparing atropine and fentanyl to atropine, fentanyl, and mivacurium. *Pediatrics*. 2006;118:1583–1591.

13. Desalu I, Kushimo OT, Bode CO. A comparative study of the haemodynamic effects of atropine and glycopyrrolate at induction of anaesthesia in children. *West Afr J Med*. 2005;24:115–119.

14. Shorten GD, Bissonnette B, Hartley E, et al. It is not necessary to administer more than 10 micrograms.kg-1 of atropine to older children before succinylcholine. *Can J Anaesth*. 1995;42:8–11.

15. McAuliffe G, Bissonnette B, Boutin C. Should the routine use of atropine before succinylcholine in children be reconsidered? *Can J Anaesth*. 1995;42:724–729.

16. Fastle RK, Roback MG. Pediatric rapid sequence intubation: incidence of reflex bradycardia and effects of pretreatment with atropine. *Pediatr Emerg Care*. 2004;20:651–655.

21

Sedative Induction Agents

David A. Caro • Katren R. Tyler

INTRODUCTION

Agents used to sedate, or "induce," patients for intubation during rapid sequence intubation (RSI) are properly called sedative induction agents because induction of general anesthesia is at the extreme of the spectrum of their sedative actions. In this chapter, we refer to this family of drugs as "induction agents." The ideal induction agent would smoothly and quickly render the patient unconscious, unresponsive, and amnestic in one arm/heart/brain circulation time. Such an agent would also provide analgesia, maintain stable cerebral perfusion pressure and cardiovascular hemodynamics, be immediately reversible, and have few, if any, adverse side effects. Unfortunately, such an induction agent does not exist. Most induction agents meet the first criterion because they are highly lipophilic and, therefore, have a rapid onset within 15 to 30 seconds of intravenous (IV) administration. Their clinical effect is likewise terminated quickly as the drug rapidly redistributes to less well-perfused tissues. All induction agents have the potential to cause myocardial depression and subsequent hypotension. These effects depend on the particular drug; the patient's underlying physiologic condition; and the dose, concentration, and speed of injection of the drug. The faster the drug is administered (IV push), the larger the concentration of drug that saturates those organs with the greatest blood flow (i.e., brain and heart), and the more pronounced the effect. Because RSI requires rapid administration of a preselected dose of the induction agent, the choice of drug and the dose must be individualized to capitalize on desired effects, while minimizing those that might adversely affect the patient. Some patients are so unstable that the primary goal is to produce amnesia rather than anesthesia because to produce the latter might lead to severe hypotension and organ hypoperfusion.

The induction agents include ultra–short-acting barbiturates: thiopental (Pentothal) and methohexital (Brevital); benzodiazepines: principally midazolam (Versed); and miscellaneous agents: etomidate (Amidate), ketamine (Ketalar), and propofol (Diprivan). Thiopental (Pentothal) is no longer available for clinical use in the United States, Canada, or the rest of the developed world. Other agents, such as the opioid analgesic fentanyl (Sublimaze), can function as anesthetic induction agents when used in large doses (e.g., for fentanyl 30 μg [0.03 mg] per kg); however, they are rarely, if ever, used for that purpose during emergency intubation, and so are not discussed here.

General anesthetic agents act through two principal mechanisms: (1) an increase in inhibition through γ-aminobutyric acid. A receptors (e.g., benzodiazepines, barbiturates, propofol, etomidate, isoflurane, enflurane, and halothane), and (2) a decreased excitation through N-methyl-D-aspartate (NMDA) receptors (e.g., ketamine, nitrous oxide, and xenon). Dexmedetomidine is a relatively selective α_2-adrenergic agonist (like clonidine) with sedative properties, and is used in the operating room and ICU settings for procedural sedation (e.g., awake intubation), as a component of balanced anesthesia, and for the sedation of intubated patients. Dexmedetomidine is not an induction agent and its role in emergency medicine for procedural sedation is yet to be determined.

The IV induction agents discussed in this chapter share important pharmacokinetic characteristics. Induction agents are highly lipophilic and because the brain is a highly perfused, lipid dense organ, a standard induction dose of each agent in a euvolemic, normotensive patient will produce induction within 30 seconds. The blood–brain barrier is freely permeable to medications used to induce anesthesia. The observed clinical duration of each drug is measured in minutes because of the drugs' distribution half-life ($t_{1/2}\alpha$), characterized by distribution of the drug from the central circulation to well-perfused tissues, such as brain. The redistribution of the drug from brain to fat and muscle terminates its CNS effects. The elimination half-life ($t_{1/2}\beta$, usually measured in hours) is characterized by each drug's reentry from fat and lean muscle into plasma down a concentration gradient leading to hepatic metabolism and renal excretion. Generally, it requires four to five elimination half-lives to completely clear the drug from the body.

The dosing of induction agents in nonobese adults should be based on ideal body weight (IBW) in kilograms. In clinical practice, the actual body weight is a reasonable enough approximation to IBW for the purposes of dosing these agents.

For obese patients, the situation is more complicated. The high lipophilicity of the induction agents combined with the increased volume of distribution (V_d) of these drugs in obesity argues for actual body weight dosing (see Chapter 39). Opposing this, however, is the significant cardiovascular depression that would occur if such a large quantity of drug is injected as a single bolus. Balancing these two considerations, and given the paucity of actual pharmacokinetic studies in obese patients, the best approach is to use Lean Body Weight (LBW) for dosing of most induction agents, decreasing to IBW if the patient is hemodynamically compromised, or for drugs with significant hemodynamic depression, such as propofol. LBW is obtained by adding 0.3 of the patient's excess weight (actual body weight minus IBW) to the IBW, and using the sum as the dosing weight. This is in contrast to succinylcholine, which is dosed at total body weight. Drug dosing for obese patients is discussed in Chapter 39.

Aging affects the pharmacokinetics of induction agents. In elderly patients, lean body mass and total body water decrease while total body fat increases, resulting in an increased volume of distribution, an increase in $t_{1/2}\beta$, and an increased duration of drug effect. In addition, the elderly are more sensitive to the hemodynamic and respiratory depressant effects of these agents, and the induction doses should be reduced to approximately one-half to three-fourths of the dose used in their healthy, younger counterparts.

ETOMIDATE

Etomidate (Amidate)				
Usual emergency induction dose (mg/kg)	Onset (s)	$t_{1/2}\alpha$ (min)	Duration (min)	$t_{1/2}\beta$ (h)
0.3	15–45	2–4	3–12	2–5

Clinical Pharmacology

Etomidate is an imidazole derivative that is primarily a hypnotic and has no analgesic activity. With the exception of ketamine, etomidate is the most hemodynamically stable of the currently available induction agents. It exerts its effect by enhancing GABA activity at the GABA–receptor complex, inhibiting excitatory stimuli. Etomidate attenuates underlying elevated intracranial pressure (ICP) by decreasing cerebral blood flow (CBF) and cerebral metabolic oxygen demand ($CMRO_2$). Its hemodynamic stability preserves cerebral perfusion pressure. Etomidate may not be the most cerebroprotective of the various available induction agents (that attribute probably resides with the barbiturates), but its hemodynamic stability and favorable CNS effects make it an excellent choice for patients with elevated ICP.

Etomidate does not release histamine and is safe for use in patients with reactive airways disease. However, it lacks the direct bronchodilatory properties of ketamine, which may be a preferable agent in these patients.

Indications and Contraindications

Etomidate has become the induction agent of choice for most emergent RSIs because of its rapid onset, its hemodynamic stability, its positive effect on $CMRO_2$ and cerebral perfusion pressure, and its rapid recovery. As with any induction agent, dosage should be adjusted in hemodynamically compromised patients. Etomidate is a U.S. Food and Drug Administration (FDA) pregnancy category C drug.

Etomidate is not FDA approved for use in children, but many series report safe and effective use in pediatric patients.

Dosage and Clinical Use

In euvolemic and hemodynamically stable patients, the normal induction dose of etomidate is 0.3 mg per kg IV push. In compromised patients, the dose should be reduced commensurate with the patient's clinical status; reduction to 0.2 mg per kg is usually sufficient. In morbidly obese patients, the induction dose should be based on lean body weight, by using IBW and adding a correction of 30% of the weight.

Adverse Effects

Pain on injection is common because of the diluent (propylene glycol) and can be somewhat mitigated by having a fast-flowing IV solution running in a large vein. Myoclonic movement during induction is common and has been confused with seizure activity. It is of no clinical consequence and generally terminates promptly as the neuromuscular blocking agent takes effect.

The most significant and controversial side effect of etomidate is its reversible blockade of 11-β-hydroxylase, which decreases both serum cortisol and aldosterone levels. This side effect has been more common with continuous infusions of etomidate in the ICU setting than with a single-dose injection used for emergency RSI. The risks and benefits of the use of etomidate in patients with sepsis are discussed in detail in the "Evidence" section at the end of the chapter.

KETAMINE

Ketamine (Ketalar)				
Usual emergency induction dose (mg/kg)	Onset (s)	$t_{1/2}\alpha$ (min)	Duration (min)	$t_{1/2}\beta$ (h)
1.5	45–60	11–17	10–20	2–3

Clinical Pharmacology

Ketamine is a phencyclidine derivative that provides significant analgesia, anesthesia, and amnesia, with minimal effect on respiratory drive. The amnestic effect is not as pronounced as that seen with the benzodiazepines. Ketamine is believed to interact with the NMDA receptors at the GABA–receptor complex, promoting neuroinhibition and subsequent anesthesia. Action on opioid receptors accounts for its profound analgesic effect. Ketamine releases catecholamines, stimulates the sympathetic nervous system, and therefore augments heart rate and BP in those patients who are not catecholamine-depleted secondary to the demands of their underlying disease. Furthermore, increases in mean arterial pressure may offset any rise in ICP, resulting in a relatively stable cerebral perfusion pressure. This is discussed in detail in the "Evidence" section. In addition to its catecholamine-releasing effect, ketamine directly relaxes bronchial smooth muscle, producing bronchodilation. Ketamine is primarily metabolized in the liver, producing one active metabolite, norketamine, which is metabolized and excreted in the urine.

Indications and Contraindications

Ketamine is the induction agent of choice for patients with reactive airways disease who require tracheal intubation. Ketamine is an excellent induction agent for patients who are hypovolemic, hypotensive, or hemodynamically unstable, including those with sepsis. In normotensive or hypertensive patients with ischemic heart disease, catecholamine release may adversely increase myocardial oxygen demand, but it is unlikely that this effect is detrimental in patients with significant hypotension, in whom additional catecholamine release may support the blood pressure. Ketamine's preservation of upper airway reflexes makes it appealing for awake laryngoscopy and intubation in the difficult airway patient where the dose is titrated to effect. The effects of ketamine on ICP will be discussed in the "Evidence" section. The pregnancy category of ketamine has not been established by the FDA so it is not currently recommended for use in pregnant women.

Dosage and Clinical Use

The induction dose of ketamine for RSI is 1 to 2 mg per kg IV. In patients who are catecholamine depleted, doses >1.5 mg per kg IV may cause myocardial depression and exacerbate hypotension. For sedation, ketamine is titrated to effect beginning with 0.2 mg per kg IV. Because of its generalized stimulating effects, ketamine enhances laryngeal reflexes and increases pharyngeal and bronchial secretions. These secretions may uncommonly precipitate laryngospasm, and may interfere with upper airway examination during awake intubation, but are not an issue during RSI. Atropine 0.01 mg per kg IV or glycopyrrolate (Robinul) 0.01 mg per kg IV may be administered 15 to 20 minutes before ketamine to promote a drying effect for awake intubation, when feasible. Ketamine is available in three separate concentrations: 10, 50, and 100 mg per ml. Care should be taken to ensure that only one concentration is stored in the emergency department.

Adverse Effects

Hallucinations may occur on emergence from ketamine and are more common in the adult than in the child. They may be attenuated by the concomitant or subsequent administration of a benzodiazepine, if desired. Such emergence reactions occur infrequently in the emergency department as most patients are subsequently sedated with either a benzodiazepine, or with propofol, after the airway has been secured.

PROPOFOL

Propofol (Diprivan)				
Usual emergency induction dose (mg/kg)	Onset (s)	$t_{1/2}\alpha$ (min)	Duration (min)	$t_{1/2}\beta$ (h)
1.5	15–45	1–3	5–10	1–3

Clinical Pharmacology

Propofol is an alkylphenol derivative (i.e., an alcohol) with hypnotic properties. It is highly lipid soluble. Propofol enhances GABA activity at the GABA–receptor complex. It decreases $CMRO_2$ and ICP. Propofol does not cause histamine release. Propofol causes a reduction in BP through vasodilation and direct myocardial depression. The ensuing hypotension, or the resultant decrease in cerebral perfusion pressure, may be detrimental in a compromised patient. The manufacturer recommends that rapid bolus dosing (either single or repeated) be avoided in patients who are elderly, debilitated, or ASA Class III or IV in order to minimize undesirable cardiovascular depression, including hypotension. It must be used cautiously for emergency RSI in hemodynamically unstable patients.

Indications and Contraindications

Propofol is an excellent induction agent in a stable patient. Its adverse potential for hypotension and reduction in cerebral perfusion pressure limits its role as an induction agent in emergent RSI. Propofol has been used successfully as an induction agent during tracheal intubation for reactive airways disease. There are no absolute contraindications to the use of propofol. Propofol is delivered as an emulsion in soybean oil and lecithin. Patients who are allergic to eggs generally react to the ovalbumin and not to lecithin, so propofol is not contraindicated in patients with egg allergy. Propofol is a pregnancy category B drug, and has become the induction agent of choice in pregnant patients.

Dosage and Clinical Use

The induction dose of propofol is 1.5 mg per kg IV in a euvolemic, normotensive patient. Because of its predictable tendency to reduce mean arterial BP, doses are reduced by 1/3 to 1/2 when propofol is given as an induction agent for emergency RSI in compromised or elderly patients.

Adverse Effects

Propofol causes pain on injection, which can be attenuated by injecting the medication through a rapidly running IV in a large vein (e.g., antecubital). Premedication of the vein with lidocaine (2 to 3 ml of 1% lidocaine) will also minimize the pain of injection. Propofol and lidocaine are compatible in the same syringe and can be mixed in a 10:1 ratio (10 ml of propofol to 1 ml of 1% lidocaine). Propofol can cause mild clonus to a greater degree than thiopental, but less than etomidate or methohexital. Venous thrombophlebitis at the injection site may occasionally occur.

METHOHEXITAL

Ultra–Short-Acting Barbiturates					
	Usual emergency induction dose (mg/kg)	Onset (s)	$t_{1/2}\alpha$ (min)	Duration (min)	$t_{1/2}\beta$ (h)
Methohexital (Brevital)	1.5	<30	5–6	5–10	2–5

Clinical Pharmacology

Thiopental was once the prototypical barbiturate used for anesthetic induction. In January 2011, however, thiopental was removed from clinical use in the United States, Canada, the United Kingdom, Australia, and New Zealand, citing concerns from the manufacturer that clinical supplies could be used in lethal injection. Methohexital is a close relative of thiopental and remains in clinical use. Both are ultra–short-acting CNS depressants that induce hypnosis (sleep) but not analgesia. Recovery after a small dose is rapid with some somnolence and retrograde amnesia. Repeated IV doses lead to prolonged anesthesia because fatty tissues act as a reservoir. Methohexital is two to three times more potent than thiopental, 1.5 mg of methohexital being equal to 4 mg of thiopental. The $t_{1/2}\beta$ for methohexital is shorter than that for thiopental.

At low doses, ultra–short-acting barbiturates decrease GABA dissociation from its receptor, which enhances GABA's neuroinhibitory activity. At higher doses, they can directly stimulate the GABA receptor itself. Barbiturates are cerebroprotective, causing a dose-dependent decrease in cerebral metabolic oxygen consumption and a parallel decrease in CBF and ICP, provided cerebral perfusion pressure is maintained.

Thiopental and methohexital are largely degraded in the liver. Neither have active metabolites.

Indications and Contraindications

Thiopental was widely used as an induction agent in the past, but it has largely been supplanted by etomidate and propofol. It is currently unavailable for clinical use. Methohexital is primarily used for procedural sedation and is rarely used for induction.

Dosage and Clinical Use

The dosing of ultra–short-acting barbiturates depends on the hemodynamic status of the patient and the concomitant use of other agents in RSI. The recommended induction dose of methohexital in the euvolemic, normotensive patient is 1.5 mg per kg IV. For procedural sedation or an assisted laryngoscopy, half this dose should be used.

The ultra–short-acting barbiturates should be avoided entirely in frankly hypotensive patients for whom other drugs, such as etomidate or ketamine, may preserve greater hemodynamic stability. With the widespread adoption of etomidate, which has significant cardiovascular stability, the ultra–short-acting barbiturates are rarely used as induction agents for emergent RSI.

Adverse Effects

The principal side effects of barbiturates include central respiratory depression, venodilation, and myocardial depression. Barbiturates cause a dose-related release of histamine that rarely is clinically significant, but may cause or exacerbate bronchospasm in patients with reactive airways disease. Ketamine is the preferred induction agent for patients with reactive airways disease. Methohexital causes more excitatory phenomena (twitching and hiccups) than thiopental.

Inadvertent intra-arterial injection or subcutaneous extravasation of ultra–short-acting barbiturates can result in chemical endarteritis and distal thrombosis, ischemia, and tissue necrosis because they have a highly alkaline pH (>10). If extravasation occurs, 40 to 80 mg of papaverine (Cerespan) in 20 ml normal saline or 10 ml of 1% lidocaine (Xylocaine) should be injected intra-arterially proximal to the site to inhibit smooth muscle spasm. Consider local infiltration of an α-adrenergic blocking agent, such as phentolamine, into the vasospastic area.

BENZODIAZEPINES

Short-Acting Benzodiazepines					
	Usual emergency induction dose (mg/kg)	**Onset (s)**	$t_{1/2}\alpha$ **(min)**	**Duration (min)**	$t_{1/2}\beta$ **(h)**
Midazolam Versed	0.2–0.3	60–90	7–15	15–30	2–6

Clinical Pharmacology

Although chemically distinct from the barbiturates, the benzodiazepines also exert their effects through the GABA–receptor complex. Benzodiazepines specifically stimulate the benzodiazepine receptor, which in turn modulates GABA, the primary neuroinhibitory transmitter. The benzodiazepines provide amnesia, anxiolysis, central muscle relaxation, sedation, anticonvulsant effects, and hypnosis. Although the benzodiazepines generally have similar pharmacologic profiles, they differ in selectivity, which makes their clinical usefulness variable. The benzodiazepines have potent, dose-related amnestic properties, perhaps their greatest asset for emergency indications. The three benzodiazepines of interest for emergency applications are midazolam (Versed), diazepam (Valium), and lorazepam (Ativan). Of the three, midazolam is the most lipid soluble and is the only benzodiazepine suitable for use as an induction agent for emergent RSI. Midazolam rarely is used as an induction agent for emergent RSI, however, because its time to clinical effectiveness is much longer than is the case for any of the other commonly used induction agents. When IV midazolam is given as an anesthetic induction agent, induction of anesthesia occurs in approximately 1.5 minutes when narcotic premedication has been used, and in 2 to 2.5 minutes without narcotic premedication. This slow onset of action is mitigated by the profound amnestic effects of midazolam. Its pharmacokinetic attributes, however, make it a poor induction agent, and it cannot be recommended for this purpose. Midazolam has one significant active metabolite, 1-hydroxy-midazolam, which may contribute to the net pharmacologic activity of midazolam. Clearance of midazolam is reduced in association with old age, congestive heart failure, and liver disease. The elimination half-life of midazolam $(t_{1/2}\beta)$ may be prolonged in renal impairment. The benzodiazepines do not release histamine, and allergic reactions are very rare.

Indications and Contraindications

The primary indications for benzodiazepines are to promote amnesia and sedation. In this regard, the benzodiazepines are unparalleled. Midazolam's primary use in the emergency department and elsewhere in the hospital is for procedural sedation. Lorazepam is used primarily for treatment of seizures and alcohol withdrawal, and both agents are used for sedation and anxiolysis in a variety of settings, including postintubation.

Because of their dose-related reduction in systemic vascular resistance and direct myocardial depression, dosage must be adjusted in volume-depleted or hemodynamically compromised patients. Studies have shown that the correct induction dose of midazolam, 0.3 mg per kg, is rarely used. Even at this dose, midazolam is a poor induction agent for emergent RSI because of delay in onset of action and adverse hemodynamic effects.

All benzodiazepines are FDA pregnancy category D.

Dosage and Clinical Use

Although midazolam is occasionally used as an induction agent in the operating room, we do not recommend its use for emergent RSI. Even in the correct induction dose for hemodynamically stable patients of 0.2 to 0.3 mg per kg IV push, the onset is slow, and so the drug is not suited to emergency applications. Midazolam should be reserved for sedative applications, and its use in emergency RSI is not advised because superior agents are readily available. Similarly, diazepam and lorazepam are not recommended for emergent RSI because of their slow onset of action.

Adverse Effects

With the exception of midazolam, the benzodiazepines are insoluble in water and are usually in solution in propylene glycol. Unless injected into a large vein, pain and venous irritation on injection can be significant.

EVIDENCE

- **Is etomidate safe to use in septic patients?** Etomidate has become the preferred agent for emergent RSI in North America and in much of the rest of the world because of its simple dosing strategies, reliable onset of action, and cardiovascular stability.[1,2] The debate about the safety of etomidate in patients with sepsis has been raging for much of the last decade. The debate regarding the safety of etomidate in patients with sepsis has occurred within the larger discussion of critical illness relative corticosteroid insufficiency (CIRCI) and the role of corticosteroids in the management of critically ill patients.[3] CIRCI, however, is more complicated than a simple reduction in circulating cortisol levels, and likely stems from a dysfunction at the level of the hypothalamic pituitary axis. Many of the features of CIRCI are still being identified, but likely include decreased production of corticotropin-releasing hormone, adrenocorticotropic hormone (ACTH), cortisol, and perhaps critically, dysfunction of the glucocorticoid receptors.[3]

  Confounding this is the inability to precisely characterize the nature and role of adrenal insufficiency in critical illness and how this may or may not relate to total cortisol levels or response to ACTH.[2,3] The current consensus recommendations are to base decisions related to glucocorticoid administration on clinical evaluation and not on laboratory testing.[3]

  A single dose of etomidate causes a reversible inhibition of adrenal hormone synthesis by blocking 11-β-hydroxylase. It was for this reason that etomidate infusions ceased to be used for ICU sedation in the early 1980s.[4] Following a single dose of etomidate, there is an immediate inhibition of adrenal hormone synthesis that lasts 12 to 24 hours, and may extend as long as 72 hours in some patients.[1] What remains unclear is whether there are any significant clinical sequelae from the transient inhibition of adrenal hormonal synthesis.

  For the most part, there is broad agreement that in patients without sepsis or sepsis-like syndromes, the advantages of etomidate significantly outweigh concerns about possible inhibition of adrenal hormone synthesis.

  For patients with sepsis or with sepsis-like syndromes, there remains much debate as to the potential risks of etomidate. The literature is significantly divided. Much of the data has emerged from observational studies[2,5–9] and post hoc analyses.[10,11] There have been many review articles[12–14] and several meta-analyses.[13] However, very few patients have been enrolled in randomized controlled trials, and several studies used cortisol levels as the primary outcomes[1,2] and did not address mortality or length of stay. In 2009, Jabre et al.[15] published an RCT comparing 234 patients in the etomidate group and 235 in a ketamine group. Although the percentage of patients with adrenal insufficiency was significantly higher in the etomidate group, they found no serious adverse events with either study drug.[15] The number of patients with sepsis as the final diagnosis was 41 in the etomidate group and 35 in the ketamine group. In August 2010, a comprehensive metanalysis concluded that although etomidate suppresses adrenal function transiently, there is no significant mortality effect based on the current data.[1]

  In November 2010, Tekwani et al.[16] published an RCT comparing etomidate ($n = 61$) and midazolam ($n = 59$) as induction agents in patients with a primary infectious cause for their illness, with primary outcome measure of hospital length of stay and secondary outcomes of ICU length of stay, ventilator days, and mortality. They found no significant differences in their primary or secondary outcomes. To date, no study has been adequately powered to detect a small difference in mortality or in hospital, ICU, or ventilator length of stay.[1]

  The debate over the safety of etomidate in sepsis patients has expanded in recent years. There is recognition that some degree of adrenal insufficiency occurs in many patients with critical illness, and that measurement of total cortisol levels is likely oversimplifying the problem.

  For the emergency physician who relies upon etomidate for the simple dosing regimen, rapid onset of action, and lack of cardiovascular compromise, even in patients who are hemodynamically unstable, there are three main choices in the patient with presumptive sepsis:

- *Avoid etomidate use entirely in patients who are presumed to be septic.* Some advocates of this approach emerged early in the debate,[10,11,17,18] but as further data have emerged, the possible risk of etomidate use in septic patients appears to have been overstated and a clinical equipoise has developed.[1,2,15] The risk of using etomidate must be balanced against the risk of an alternative agent. Only ketamine provides hemodynamic stability comparable with etomidate,[5,15] and ketamine is not available in many settings where emergent intubation is performed.

- *Routinely administer glucocorticoids to patients with septic shock who have received etomidate.* The emerging recognition of the relationship between critical illness and adrenal insufficiency (CIRCI) has made this question both simpler and more complex. Studies of supplemental corticosteroids in patients with sepsis have had equivocal results.[19,20] Although it has been posited that glucocorticoids should be given immediately after the administration of etomidate when the adrenal suppression is likely to be greatest[10], there is no evidence that this approach improves patient outcome.[5,18] The current international consensus is that supplemental "glucocorticoids should be considered in the management of septic patients when they have responded poorly to fluid resuscitation and vasopressor agents."[3]

- *Communicating clearly to critical care staff that the patient was given a dose of etomidate for induction.* It is almost impossible to argue against this common sense approach.

- **Which induction agents are the most hemodynamically stable when used for RSI?** In RSI, a predetermined dose of an induction agent is given at the same time as a muscle relaxant. The physician makes his or her best estimation of the dose of induction agent required and the dose is not titrated. The physician aims to give a large enough dose of induction agent to prevent awareness, while minimizing the risk of hemodynamic collapse. Although virtually all induction agents *could be used* for RSI, not all are appropriate. We want to avoid both patient awareness and hemodynamic compromise. The ideal induction agent in RSI will have rapid and reliable onset and few adverse (particularly hemodynamic) effects.[21]

    Etomidate results in the least variation in BP and heart rate when compared with the other agents used for rapid induction of anesthesia.[22] This cardiovascular stability is seen in both children and adults, including the elderly.[23–25] The drug is delivered to the CNS in a timely and dependable manner. It is for these reasons that etomidate remains the standard choice for RSI.[21]

    Propofol is a very popular induction agent for elective procedures, when the induction dose is titrated against the patient response. It is a poor choice of induction agent for RSI in hemodynamically compromised patients, who run the risk of further hemodynamic deterioration coupled with awareness during intubation.[21]

    Thiopental, for many years the staple induction agent for RSI, is no longer available for clinical use in North America, the United Kingdom, Europe, or Australasia (P. Liston, Thiopental not available UK or Australia 2011, *personal communication*) following manufacturers concerns about thiopental use in lethal injection.

    Benzodiazepines are generally not suitable as induction agents in RSI. Midazolam is 95% protein bound. Both midazolam and lorazepam require closure of an imidazole ring to have enough lipid solubility to cross the blood–brain barrier, which take as long as 10 minutes. Some authors have referred to benzodiazepines as being "almost useless" for RSI.[21]

    Ketamine offers several advantages as an induction agent in hemodynamically compromised patients. Ketamine is a sympathomimetic agent, increasing heart rate, arterial pressure, and cardiac output in animal models. Data on the use of ketamine as an induction agent in RSI are sparse. Conversely, there is significant clinical experience using ketamine for RSI, although much of it is in the resource-poor developing world or in warfare, neither of which lend themselves to clinical trials.[21] In 2009, Jabre et al.[15] published the largest clinical trial to date involving ketamine 2 mg per kg for RSI in adults, and comparing it to etomidate 0.3 mg per kg, both with succinylcholine as the neuromuscular blocking (NMB) agent. There were no significant hemodynamic differences between the two groups. The study concluded that ketamine is a safe alternative to etomidate for endotracheal intubation in critically ill patients, and should be considered in those with sepsis.

In the hemodynamically unstable patient, ketamine or etomidate offer the most reliable method of rapidly achieving unconsciousness while limiting further hemodynamic compromise.

- **What is the risk of ketamine in the brain-injured patient?** For many years, the use of ketamine was thought to be contraindicated in brain-injured patients because of the risk of increasing intracranial pressure through increased CBF. Subsequent animal models and later clinical data have refuted this earlier hypothesis.[21,26–28]

In uninjured brains, CPP = MAP – ICP where CPP is the cerebral perfusion pressure; MAP is the mean arterial pressure; and ICP is the intracranial pressure. Following brain injury, there is a loss of cerebral autoregulation and CBF is largely dependent on cerebral perfusion pressure, which in turn is largely dependent on mean arterial pressure. Consequently, agents such as etomidate and ketamine that maintain MAP will maintain CBF. This is particularly true in patients with polytrauma where traumatic brain injury and shock may coexist.[21] The dangers of hypotension on the injured brain are well known, and any mechanism by which hypotension can be avoided in traumatic brain injury should be encouraged.[29,30] In ventilated patients with controlled ventilation, ketamine does not increase ICP.[27,28] In addition to the neuroprotective effects of maintaining CBF through cerebral perfusion pressure, ketamine has also been found to have other neuroprotective properties. A comprehensive review of the available experimental and clinical evidence for the neuroprotective properties of ketamine was recently published.[28] Animal models show that ketamine inhibits the NMDA-receptor activation, reduces neuronal apoptosis, and reduces the systemic inflammatory response to tissue injury.[28,31] In the last few years, increasing clinical evidence of the safety of ketamine in brain-injured patients has emerged. It is becoming increasingly clear that ketamine is likely not dangerous in brain-injured patients, and instead may confer advantages over other agents. Most clinical data come from neurosurgical units with invasive intracranial pressure using ketamine as a sedative agent.[26–28]

Very little of these data have been generated using ketamine as an induction agent in the emergency department setting. There are not yet sufficient data to support using ketamine induction for RSI in all brain-injured patients. If the brain-injured patient is also hypotensive, then ketamine is an excellent choice.

- **What is the best induction agent for patients with severe bronchospasm?** Most of the data on the use of induction agents in asthma comes from the anesthesia literature in elective surgical cases, from animal models, and from experience using ketamine as a sedating agent in intubated asthmatic patients.[32–35] Although ketamine is widely accepted and recommended as the induction agent of choice for severe asthma, the data on ketamine use for induction in RSI in asthmatic patients in the emergency department are sparse. Etomidate caused a mild increase in airway resistance in a very small study of nonasthmatic intubated patients.[35] Midazolam data are lacking. Ketamine and propofol both cause bronchodilation in asthmatic patients.[32,34,36] In the emergency department, severe bronchospasm raises concerns of significantly decreased venous return and cardiovascular collapse, especially following intubation. While propofol may have some bronchodilatory properties, this possible benefit is outweighed in the unstable asthmatic patient by risks of hemodynamic instability, making ketamine the best choice for induction agent in severe bronchospasm. Etomidate also is a good choice as an induction agent in severe bronchospasm because of its excellent hemodynamic stability. Following intubation, either propofol or ketamine are excellent choices for sedation in the patient with severe bronchospasm.

REFERENCES

1. Hohl CM, Kelly-Smith CH, Yeung TC, et al. The effect of a bolus dose of etomidate on cortisol levels, mortality, and health services utilization: a systematic review. *Ann Emerg Med.* 2010;56:105–113.e5.

2. Dmello D, Taylor S, O'Brien J, et al. Outcomes of etomidate in severe sepsis and septic shock. *Chest.* 2010;138:1327–1332.

3. Marik PE, Pastores SM, Annane D, et al. Recommendations for the diagnosis and management of corticosteroid insufficiency in critically ill adult patients: consensus statements from an international task force by the American College of Critical Care Medicine. *Crit Care Med.* 2008;36:1937–1949.

4. Ledingham IM, Watt I. Influence of sedation on mortality in critically ill multiple trauma patients. *Lancet.* 1983;1:1270.

5. Ray DC, McKeown DW. Effect of induction agent on vasopressor and steroid use, and outcome in patients with septic shock. *Crit Care.* 2007;11:R56.

6. Ehrman R, Wira C, Lomax A, et al. Etomidate use in severe sepsis and septic shock patients does not contribute to mortality. *Intern Emerg Med.* 2011;6:253–257.

7. Tekwani KL, Watts HF, Chan CW, et al. The effect of single-bolus etomidate on septic patient mortality: a retrospective review. *West J Emerg Med.* 2008;9:195–200.

8. Tekwani KL, Watts HF, Rzechula KH, et al. A prospective observational study of the effect of etomidate on septic patient mortality and length of stay. *Acad Emerg Med.* 2009;16:11–14.

9. Baird CRW, Hay AW, McKeown DW, et al. Rapid sequence induction in the emergency department: induction drug and outcome of patients admitted to the intensive care unit. *Emerg Med J.* 2009;26:576–579.

10. Annane D. ICU physicians should abandon the use of etomidate! *Intensive Care Med.* 2005;31:325–326.

11. Cuthbertson BH, Sprung CL, Annane D, et al. The effects of etomidate on adrenal responsiveness and mortality in patients with septic shock. *Intensive Care Med.* 2009;35:1868–1876.

12. Edwin SB, Walker PL. Controversies surrounding the use of etomidate for rapid sequence intubation in patients with suspected sepsis. *Ann Pharmacother.* 2010;44:1307–1313.

13. Albert SG, Ariyan S, Rather A. The effect of etomidate on adrenal function in critical illness: a systematic review. *Intensive Care Med.* 2011;37:901–910.

14. Kulstad EB, Kalimullah EA, Tekwani KL, et al. Etomidate as an induction agent in septic patients: red flags or false alarms? *West J Emerg Med.* 2010;11:161–172.

15. Jabre P, Combes X, Lapostolle F, et al. Etomidate versus ketamine for rapid sequence intubation in acutely ill patients: a multicentre randomised controlled trial. *Lancet.* 2009;374:293–300.

16. Tekwani KL, Watts HF, Sweis RT, et al. A comparison of the effects of etomidate and midazolam on hospital length of stay in patients with suspected sepsis: a prospective, randomized study. *Ann Emerg Med.* 2010;56:481–489.

17. Jackson WL Jr. Should we use etomidate as an induction agent for endotracheal intubation in patients with septic shock?: a critical appraisal. *Chest.* 2005;127:1031–1038.

18. Mohammad Z, Afessa B, Finkielman JD. The incidence of relative adrenal insufficiency in patients with septic shock after the administration of etomidate. *Crit Care.* 2006;10:R105.

19. Sprung CL, Annane D, Keh D, et al. Hydrocortisone therapy for patients with septic shock. *N Engl J Med.* 2008;358:111–124.

20. Annane D, Sebille V, Charpentier C, et al. Effect of treatment with low doses of hydrocortisone and fludrocortisone on mortality in patients with septic shock. *JAMA.* 2002;288:862–871.

21. Morris C, Perris A, Klein J, et al. Anaesthesia in haemodynamically compromised emergency patients: does ketamine represent the best choice of induction agent? *Anaesthesia.* 2009;64:532–539.

22. Jellish WS, Riche H, Salord F, et al. Etomidate and thiopental-based anesthetic induction: comparisons between different titrated levels of electrophysiologic cortical depression and response to laryngoscopy. *J Clin Anesth*. 1997;9:36–41.

23. Sokolove PE, Price DD, Okada P. The safety of etomidate for emergency rapid sequence intubation of pediatric patients. *Pediatr Emerg Care*. 2000;16:18–21.

24. Guldner G, Schultz J, Sexton P, et al. Etomidate for rapid-sequence intubation in young children: hemodynamic effects and adverse events. *Acad Emerg Med*. 2003;10:134–139.

25. Benson M, Junger A, Fuchs C, et al. Use of an anesthesia information management system (AIMS) to evaluate the physiologic effects of hypnotic agents used to induce anesthesia. *J Clin Monit Comput*. 2000;16:183–190.

26. Bar-Joseph G, Guilburd Y, Tamir A, et al. Effectiveness of ketamine in decreasing intracranial pressure in children with intracranial hypertension. *J Neurosurg Pediatr*. 2009;4:40–46.

27. Himmelseher S, Durieux ME. Revising a dogma: ketamine for patients with neurological injury? *Anesth Analg*. 2005;101:524–534.

28. Hudetz JA, Pagel PS. Neuroprotection by ketamine: a review of the experimental and clinical evidence. *J Cardiothorac Vasc Anesth*. 2010;24:131–142.

29. Schreiber MA, Aoki N, Scott BG, et al. Determinants of mortality in patients with severe blunt head injury. *Arch Surg*. 2002;137:285–290.

30. Zafar SN, Millham FH, Chang Y, et al. Presenting blood pressure in traumatic brain injury: a bimodal distribution of death. *J Trauma*. 2011; 71:1179–1184.

31. Harbeck-Seu A, Brunk I, Platz T, et al. A speedy recovery: amphetamines and other therapeutics that might impact the recovery from brain injury. *Curr Opin Anaesthesiol*. 2011;24:144–153.

32. Burburan SM, Xisto DG, Rocco PR. Anaesthetic management in asthma. *Minerva Anestesiol*. 2007;73:357–365.

33. Hemmingsen C, Nielsen PK, Odorico J. Ketamine in the treatment of bronchospasm during mechanical ventilation. *Am J Emerg Med*. 1994;12:417–420.

34. Stather DR, Stewart TE. Clinical review: mechanical ventilation in severe asthma. *Crit Care*. 2005;9:581–587.

35. Eames WO, Rooke GA, Wu RS, et al. Comparison of the effects of etomidate, propofol, and thiopental on respiratory resistance after tracheal intubation. *Anesthesiology*. 1996;84:1307–1311.

36. Conti G, Ferretti A, Tellan G, et al. Propofol induces bronchodilation in a patient mechanically ventilated for status asthmaticus. *Intensive Care Med*. 1993;19:305.

22

Neuromuscular Blocking Agents

David A. Caro • Erik G. Laurin

INTRODUCTION

Neuromuscular blockade is the cornerstone of rapid sequence intubation (RSI) optimizing conditions for tracheal intubation while minimizing the risks of aspiration or other adverse physiologic events. NMBAs do not provide analgesia, sedation, or amnesia. As a result, they are paired with a sedative-induction agent for RSI. Similarly, appropriate sedation is essential when maintaining neuromuscular blockade postintubation.

Cholinergic nicotinic receptors on the postjunctional membrane of the motor endplate play the primary role in stimulating muscular contraction. Under normal circumstances, the presynaptic neuron synthesizes acetylcholine (ACH) and stores it in small packages (vesicles). Nerve stimulation results in these vesicles migrating to the prejunctional nerve surface, rupturing and discharging ACH into the cleft of the motor endplate. The ACH attaches to the nicotinic receptors, promoting depolarization that culminates in a muscle cell action potential and muscular contraction. As the ACH diffuses away from the receptor, the majority of the neurotransmitter is hydrolyzed by acetylcholinesterase (ACHE). The remainder undergoes re-uptake by the prejunctional neuron.

NMBAs are either agonists ("depolarizers" of the motor endplate) or antagonists (competitive agents, also known as "nondepolarizers"). Agonists work by persistent depolarization of the endplate, exhausting the ability of the receptor to respond. Antagonists, on the other hand, attach to the receptors and competitively block access of ACH to the receptor while attached. Because they are in competition with ACH for the motor endplate, antagonists can be displaced from the endplate by increasing concentrations of ACH, the end result of reversal agents (cholinesterase inhibitors such as neostigmine, edrophonium, and pyridostigmine) that inhibit ACHE and allow ACH to accumulate and reverse the block.

SUCCINYLCHOLINE

Depolarizing (Non-Competitive) NMBA: Succinylcholine					
Intubating dose (mg/kg)	Onset (s)	$t_{1/2}\alpha$ (min)	Duration (min)	$t_{1/2}\beta$ (h)	Pregnancy category
1.5	45	<1	6–10	2–5	C

The ideal muscle relaxant to facilitate tracheal intubation would have a rapid onset of action, rendering the patient paralyzed within seconds; a short duration of action, returning the patient's normal protective reflexes within 3 to 4 minutes; no significant adverse side effects; and metabolism and excretion independent of liver and kidney function. Unfortunately, such an agent does not exist. Succinylcholine (SCh) comes closest to meeting these desirable goals. Despite the historic and well-known adverse effects of SCh and the continuous advent of new competitive NMBAs, SCh remains the drug of choice for emergency RSI in both adults and children.

Clinical Pharmacology

SCh is comprised of two molecules of ACH linked by an ester bridge, and as such, is chemically similar to ACH. It stimulates all nicotinic and muscarinic cholinergic receptors of the sympathetic and parasympathetic nervous system to varying degrees, not just those at the neuromuscular junction. For example, stimulation of cardiac muscarinic receptors can cause bradycardia, especially when repeated doses are given to small children. Although SCh can be a negative inotrope, this effect is so minimal as to have no clinical relevance. SCh causes the release of trace amounts of histamine, but this effect is also not clinically significant. Initially, SCh depolarization manifests as fasciculations, but this is followed rapidly by complete motor paralysis. The onset, activity, and duration of action of SCh are independent of the activity of ACHE and instead depend on rapid hydrolysis by pseudocholinesterase (PCHE), an enzyme of the liver and plasma that is not present at the neuromuscular junction. Therefore, diffusion away from the neuromuscular junction motor endplate and back into the vascular compartment is ultimately responsible for SCh metabolism. This extremely important pharmacologic concept explains why only a fraction of the initial intravenous (IV) dose of SCh ever reaches the motor endplate to promote paralysis. As a result, larger, rather than smaller, doses of SCh are used for emergency RSI. Incomplete paralysis may jeopardize the patient by compromising respiration while failing to provide adequate relaxation to facilitate tracheal intubation. Succinylmonocholine, the initial metabolite of SCh, sensitizes the cardiac muscarinic receptors in the sinus node to repeat does of SCh, which may cause bradycardia that is responsive to atropine. At room temperature, SCh retains 90% of its activity for up to 3 months. Refrigeration mitigates this degradation. Therefore, if SCh is stored at room temperature, it should be dated and stock should be rotated regularly.

Indications and Contraindications

SCh is the NMBA of choice for emergency RSI because of its rapid onset and relatively brief duration of action. A personal or family history of malignant hyperthermia (MH) is an absolute contraindication to the use of SCh. Inherited disorders that lead to abnormal or insufficient cholinesterases prolong the duration of the block and contraindicate SCh use in elective anesthesia, but are not ordinarily an issue in emergency airway management. Certain conditions, described in "Adverse Effects" below, place patients at risk for SCh-related hyperkalemia and represent absolute contraindications to SCh. These patients should be intubated using a competitive, nondepolarizing NMBA. Relative contraindications to the use of SCh are dependent on the skill and proficiency of the intubator and the individual patient's clinical circumstance. The role of difficult airway assessment in the decision regarding whether a patient should undergo RSI is discussed in Chapters 2 and 7.

Dosage and Clinical Use

In the normal-size adult patient, the recommended dose of SCh for emergency RSI is 1.5 mg per kg IV. In a rare, life-threatening circumstance when SCh must be given intramuscularly (IM) because of inability to secure venous access, a dose of 4 mg per kg IM may be used. Absorption and delivery of drug will be dependent on the patient's circulatory status. IM administration may result in a prolonged period of vulnerability for the patient, during which respirations will be compromised, but relaxation is not sufficient to permit intubation. Active bag-mask ventilation will usually be required before laryngoscopy in this circumstance.

SCh is dosed on a total body weight basis. In the emergency department, it may be impossible to know the exact weight of a patient, and weight estimates, especially of supine patients, have been shown to be notoriously inaccurate. In those uncertain circumstances, it is better to err on the side of a higher dose of SCh to ensure adequate patient paralysis. The serum half-life of SCh is <1 minute, so doubling the dose increases the duration of block by only 60 seconds. SCh is safe up to a cumulative dose of 6 mg per kg. At doses >6 mg per kg, the typical phase 1 depolarization block of SCh becomes a phase 2 block, which changes the pharmacokinetic displacement of SCh from the motor endplate. Although the electrophysiologic features of a phase 2 block resemble that of a nondepolarizing or competitive block (train-of-four fade and posttetanic potentiation) the block remains nonreversible. This prolongs the duration of paralysis but is otherwise clinically irrelevant. The risk of an inadequately paralyzed patient who is difficult to intubate because of an inadequate dose of SCh greatly outweighs the minimal potential for adverse effects from excessive dosing.

In children younger than 10 years, length-based dosing is recommended, but if weight is used as the determinant, the recommended dose of SCh for emergency RSI is 2 mg per kg IV, and in the newborn (younger than 12 months), the appropriate dose is 3 mg per kg IV. Some practitioners routinely administer atropine to children younger than 12 months who are receiving SCh, but there is no high-quality evidence to support this practice. There is similarly no evidence that it is harmful, so it is considered. When adults or children of any age receive a second dose of SCh, bradycardia may occur, and atropine should be readily available.

Adverse Effects

The recognized side effects of SCh include fasciculations, hyperkalemia, bradycardia, prolonged neuromuscular blockade, Malignant Hyperthermia, and trismus/masseter muscle spasm. Each is discussed separately.

1. **Fasciculations**

   Fasciculations are believed to be produced by stimulation of the nicotinic ACH receptors. Fasciculations occur simultaneously with increases in intracranial pressure (ICP), intraocular pressure, and intragastric pressure, but these are not the result of concerted muscle activity. Of these, only the increase in ICP is potentially clinically important.

   The exact mechanisms by which these effects occur are not well elucidated. In the past, it was recommended that non-depolarizing agents be given in advance of SCh to mitigate ICP elevation, but there is insufficient evidence to support this practice.

   The relationship between muscle fasciculation and subsequent postoperative muscle pain is controversial. Studies have been variable with respect to prevention of fasciculations and subsequent muscle pain. Although there exists a theoretical concern regarding the extrusion of vitreous in patients with open globe injuries who are given SCh, there are no published reports of this potential complication. Anesthesiologists continue to use SCh as a muscle relaxant in cases of open globe injury, with or without an accompanying defasciculating agent. Similarly, the increase in intragastric pressure that has been measured has never been shown to be of any clinical significance, perhaps because it is offset by a corresponding increase in the lower esophageal sphincter pressure.

2. **Hyperkalemia**

   Under normal circumstances, serum potassium increases minimally (0 to 0.5 mEq per L) when SCh is administered. In certain pathologic conditions, however, a rapid and dramatic increase in serum potassium can occur in response to SCh. These pathologic hyperkalemic responses occur by two distinct mechanisms: receptor upregulation and rhabdomyolysis. In either situation, potassium increase may approach 5 to 10 mEq per L within a few minutes and result in hyperkalemic dysrhythmias or cardiac arrest.

   Two forms of postjunctional receptors exist: mature (junctional) and immature (extrajunctional). Each receptor is composed of five proteins arranged in a circular fashion around a common channel. Both types of receptors contain two α-subunits. ACH must attach to both α-subunits to open the channel and effect depolarization and muscle contraction. When receptor upregulation occurs, the mature receptors at and around the motor endplate are gradually converted over a 4- to 5-day period to immature receptors that propagate throughout the entire muscle membrane. Immature receptors are characterized by low conductance and prolonged channel opening times (four times longer than mature receptors), resulting in increasing release of potassium. Most of the entities associated with hyperkalemia during emergency use of SCh are the result of receptor upregulation. Interestingly, these same extrajunctional nicotinic receptors are relatively refractory to nondepolarizing agents, so larger doses of vecuronium, pancuronium, or rocuronium may be required to produce paralysis. This is not an issue in emergency RSI, where full intubating doses several times greater than the ED_{95} for paralysis are used.

   Hyperkalemia also may occur with rhabdomyolysis, most often that associated with myopathies, especially inherited forms of muscular dystrophy. When severe hyperkalemia occurs related to rhabdomyolysis, the mortality approaches 30%, almost three times higher than that in cases of receptor upregulation. This mortality increase may be related to coexisting cardiomyopathy. SCh is a toxin to unstable membranes in any patient with a myopathy and should be avoided.

Patients with the following conditions are at risk of SCh-induced hyperkalemia:

I. Receptor Upregulation

   a. **Burns**—In burn victims, the extrajunctional receptor sensitization becomes clinically significant 5 days postburn. It lasts an indefinite period of time, at least until there is complete healing of the burned area. If the burn becomes infected or healing is delayed, the patient remains at risk for hyperkalemia. It is prudent to avoid SCh in burned patients beyond day 5 postburn if any question exists regarding the status of their burn. The percent of body surface area burned does not correlate well with the magnitude of hyperkalemia. Significant hyperkalemia has been reported in patients with as little as 8% total body surface area burn (less than the surface of one arm), but this is rare. The majority of emergent intubations for burn patients are performed within the safe 5-day window period. Should a later intubation become necessary, however, rocuronium or vecuronium provide excellent alternatives.

   b. **Denervation**—The patient who suffers a denervation event, such as spinal cord injury or stroke, is at risk for hyperkalemia from approximately the fifth day postevent, until 6 months postevent. Patients with progressive neuromuscular disorders, such as multiple sclerosis or amyotrophic lateral sclerosis, are perpetually at risk for hyperkalemia. Likewise, patients with transient neuromuscular disorders, such as Guillain-Barre syndrome or wound botulism, can develop hyperkalemia after day 5, depending on the severity of their disease. As long as the neuromuscular disease is dynamic, there will be augmentation of the extrajunctional receptors, which increases the risk for hyperkalemia. These specific clinical situations should be considered absolute contraindications to SCh during the designated time periods.

   c. **Crush injuries**—The data regarding crush injuries are scant. The hyperkalemic response begins about 5 days postinjury, similar to denervation, and persists for several months after healing seems complete. The mechanism appears to be receptor upregulation.

   d. **Severe infections**—This entity seems to relate to established, serious infections, usually in the ICU environment. The mechanism is receptor upregulation, but the initiating event is not established. Total body muscular disuse atrophy and chemical denervation of the ACH receptors, particularly related to long-term infusions of NMBAs, appear to drive the pathologic receptor changes. Again, the at-risk time period begins 5 days after initiation of the infection and continues indefinitely as long as the disease process is dynamic. Intraabdominal sepsis has most prominently been identified as the culprit, but any serious, prolonged, debilitating infection should prompt concern.

II. Myopathy

   SCh is absolutely contraindicated in patients with inherited myopathies, such as muscular dystrophy. Myopathic hyperkalemia can be devastating because of the combined effects of receptor upregulation and rhabdomyolysis. This is a particularly difficult problem in pediatrics, when a child with occult muscular dystrophy receives SCh. SCh has a black box warning advising against its use in elective pediatric anesthesia, but it continues to be the muscle relaxant of choice for emergency intubation. Any patient suspected of a myopathy should be intubated with nondepolarizing muscle relaxants rather than SCh.

III. Pre-existing Hyperkalemia

   Hyperkalemia, per se, is not an absolute contra-indication to SCh. There is no evidence that SCh is harmful in patients with pre-existing hyperkalemia, but who are not otherwise at risk of severe SCh-induced hyperkalemia by one of the mechanisms described in the preceding secion. There is widespread concern that patients with acute hyperkalemia secondary to acute renal failure or diabetic ketoacidosis are more likely to exhibit cardiac dsysrhythmias from SCh administration than patients with chronic or recurrent hyperkalemia. There is, however, no evidence to support this claim. Patients with pre-existing hyperkalemia are subject to the same potential rise of 0 to 0.5 mEq per L of potassium as for "normal" patients. The only study that examined the use of SCh in patients with chronic renal failure (including documented hyperkalemia before intubation) failed to identify any adverse effects related to SCh.

A reasonable approach is to assume that SCh is safe to use in patients with renal failure unless the ECG (either monitor tracing or 12-lead ECG) shows evidence of acute hyperkalemia (peaked T waves or prolongation of QRS).

3. **Bradycardia**

   In both adults and children, repeated doses of SCh may produce bradycardia, and administration of atropine may become necessary.

4. **Prolonged neuromuscular blockade**

   Prolonged neuromuscular blockade may result from an acquired PCHE deficiency, a congenital absence of PCHE, or the presence of an atypical form of PCHE, any of the three of which will delay the degradation of SCh and prolong paralysis. Acquired PCHE deficiency may be a result of liver disease, chronic cocaine abuse, pregnancy, burns, oral contraceptives, metoclopramide, bambuterol, or esmolol. A 20% reduction in normal levels will increase apnea time about 3 to 9 minutes. The most severe variant (0.04% of population) will result in prolonged paralysis for 4 to 8 hours.

5. **Malignant hyperthermia**

   A personal or family history of MH is an absolute contraindication to the use of SCh. MH is a myopathy characterized by a genetic skeletal muscle membrane abnormality of the Ry^1 ryanodine receptor. It can be triggered by halogenated anesthetics, SCh, vigorous exercise, and even emotional stress. Following the initiating event, its onset can be acute and progressive, or delayed for hours. Generalized awareness of MH, earlier diagnosis, and the availability of dantrolene (Dantrium) have decreased the mortality from as high as 70% to <5%. Acute loss of intracellular calcium control results in a cascade of rapidly progressive events manifested primarily by increased metabolism, muscular rigidity, autonomic instability, hypoxia, hypotension, severe lactic acidosis, hyperkalemia, myoglobinemia, and disseminated intravascular coagulation. Temperature elevation is a late manifestation. The presence of more than one of these clinical signs is suggestive of MH.

   Masseter spasm, once claimed to be the hallmark of MH, is not pathognomonic. SCh can promote isolated masseter spasm as an exaggerated response at the neuromuscular junction, especially in children.

   The treatment for MH consists of discontinuing the known or suspected precipitant and the immediate administration of dantrolene sodium (Dantrium). Dantrolene is essential to successful resuscitation and must be given as soon as the diagnosis is seriously entertained. Dantrolene is a hydantoin derivative that acts directly on skeletal muscle to prevent calcium release from the sarcoplasmic reticulum without affecting calcium reuptake. The initial dose is 2.5 mg per kg IV, repeated every 5 minutes until muscle relaxation occurs or the maximum dose of 10 mg per kg is administered. Dantrolene is free of any serious side effects. In addition, measures to control body temperature, acid–base balance, and renal function must be used. All cases of MH require constant monitoring of pH, arterial blood gases, and serum potassium. Immediate and aggressive management of hyperkalemia with the administration of calcium gluconate, glucose, insulin, and sodium bicarbonate may be necessary. Interestingly, full paralysis with nondepolarizing NMBAs will prevent SCh-triggered MH. MH has never been reported related to the use of SCh in the emergency department. The MH emergency hotline number is 1–800-MH-HYPER 1-800-644-9737 (United States and Canada) 24 hours a day, 7 days a week. Ask for "index zero." The e-mail address for the Malignant Hyperthermia Association of the United States (MHAUS) is mhaus@norwich.net, and the Web site is www.mhaus.org.

6. **Trismus/masseter muscle spasm**

   On occasion, SCh may cause transient trismus/masseter muscle spasm, especially in children. This manifests as jaw muscle rigidity associated with limb muscle flaccidity. Pretreatment with defasciculating doses of nondepolarizing NMBAs will not prevent masseter spasm. If masseter spasm interferes with intubation, an intubating dose of a competitive nondepolarizing agent (e.g., rocuronium 1 mg per kg) should be administered and will relax the involved muscles. The patient may require bag-mask ventilation until relaxation is complete and intubation is possible. Masseter spasm should prompt serious consideration of the diagnosis of MH (see previous discussion).

COMPETITIVE NEUROMUSCULAR BLOCKING AGENTS

Nondepolarizing (Competitive) NMBAs				
	Intubating dose (mg/kg)	Time to intubation level paralysis (s)	Duration (min)	Pregnancy category
Vecuronium	0.01 to prime, then 0.15	75–90	60–75	C
Rocuronium	1	60	40–60	B

Clinical Pharmacology

The nondepolarizing, or competitive, NMBAs compete with and block the action of ACH at the motor endplate postjunctional cholinergic nicotinic receptors. The blockade is accomplished by competitively binding to one or both of the α-subunits in the receptor, preventing ACH access to both α-subunits, which is required for muscle depolarization. This competitive α blockade is characterized by the absence of fasciculations, and the reversal of paralysis by ACHE inhibitors that normally prevent the metabolism of ACH. As a result, ACH reaccumulates at the motor endplate, and is once again able to promote muscular contraction. For the most part, these drugs are eliminated by Hoffman degradation (atracurium and cisatracurium), or excreted unchanged in bile (vecuronium and rocuronium), although there is limited liver metabolism and renal excretion of both vecuronium and rocuronium.

The nondepolarizing NMBAs are divided into two groups: the benzylisoquinoline compounds (e.g., D-tubocurarine, atracurium, and mivacurium) and the aminosteroid compounds (e.g., vecuronium, pancuronium, and rocuronium). Of the two groups, the aminosteroid compounds are the only agents commonly used for emergency RSI and postintubation paralysis.

In general, the aminosteroid compounds do not release histamine and do not cause ganglionic blockade. They vary inversely regarding their potency and time to onset (more potent agents require longer time to onset), and they exhibit differences in their vagolytic effects (i.e., moderate in pancuronium, slight in rocuronium, and absent in vecuronium).

These compounds are further subdivided based on their duration of action, which is determined by their metabolism and excretion. None has the brief duration of action of SCh. Pancuronium is longer lasting than vecuronium or rocuronium. Although pancuronium is excreted primarily by the kidney, 10% to 20% is metabolized in the liver. Vecuronium is more lipophilic, hence more easily absorbed. It is eliminated primarily in bile and is very stable cardiovascularly. Rocuronium is lipophilic and excreted in bile. We recommend only rocuronium or vecuronium for emergency RSI (see Chapter 19).

The nondepolarizing NMBAs can be reversed by administering ACHE inhibitors such as neostigmine (Prostigmine) 0.06 to 0.08 mg per kg IV after significant (40%) spontaneous recovery has occurred. Atropine 0.01 mg per kg IV or glycopyrrolate (Robinul) 0.01 mg per kg IV should be given routinely to block excessive muscarinic stimulation (SLUDGE syndrome - Salivation, Lacrimation, Urination, Diarrhea, Gastrointestinal Upset, Emesis). Reversal of blockade virtually never is indicated following emergency airway management.

A new selective rocuronium reversal agent, sugammadex, is approved in Europe, but not in the USA, at the time of this writing. Its hollow, cone-shaped polysaccharide molecular structure encapsulates rocuronium thereby reversing the neuromuscular block without the muscarinic side effects of the ACHE inhibitors. Spontaneous breathing is restored in approximately 1 minute, compared to more than 5 minutes with the ACHE inhibitors. In addition, sugammadex is rapidly effective, regardless of the extent of the neuromuscular block, and it is not necessary for any spontaneous recovery to occur before reversal is initiated. Approval and adoption of sugammadex may lead to abandonment of SCh for emergency intubation. See "Evidence" section for details.

Indications and Contraindications

The competitive NMBAs serve a multipurpose role in emergency airway management. Although they have been widely used as pretreatment agents to attenuate increases in ICP that occurs in response to SCh administration, we no longer recommend them for this purpose. Rocuronium is the preferred agent for emergency RSI when SCh is contraindicated, but vecuronium also is a reasonable choice. Any of the competitive agents is appropriate for maintenance of paralysis after intubation, when this is desired. The only contraindication to a competitive NMBA is known prior anaphylaxis to that agent. Patients with myasthenia gravis are sensitive to NMBAs and may experience greater, or more prolonged, paralysis at any given dose.

Dosage and Clinical Use

Rocuronium, 1.0 mg per kg IV, is the drug of choice for RSI when SCh is contraindicated. It produces intubation-level paralysis consistently within 60 seconds, especially when an adequate dose of induction (sedative) agent is used, because the induction agent also causes substantial relaxation. If rocuronium is not available, vecuronium can be given using a priming regimen. A priming dose of 0.01 mg per kg is given, followed 3 minutes later by an intubating dose of 0.15 mg per kg. Pancuronium is not recommended for emergency RSI because of its long time of onset.

For postintubation management when continued neuromuscular blockade is desired, vecuronium 0.1 mg per kg IV or pancuronium 0.1 mg per kg IV is appropriate, in concert with adequate sedation (see Chapters 19 and 21). Table 22-1 lists the onset and duration of action for routine paralyzing doses of all commonly used NMBAs. The onset times and durations are for the specific doses listed, which are lower than the doses used for intubation.

Adverse Effects

Of the three aminosteroid compounds, pancuronium is the least expensive but may be less desirable because it tends to produce tachycardia. The competitive NMBAs are generally less desirable for intubation than SCh because of either delayed time to paralysis, prolonged duration of action, or both. Their onset can be shortened by administering the larger intubating dose (as opposed to the ED95 dose [Table 22-1] used for surgical paralysis), but this further prolongs the duration of action. Availability of rapidly effective reversal agents, such as sugammadex, may greatly expand the role of competitive NMBAs in emergency RSI.

EVIDENCE

- **What is the advantage to RSI with an NMBA versus intubation with deep sedation alone?** RSI with an NMBA is the current standard of care for emergency intubation. Multiple prospective studies confirm the high success rate of RSI with NMBAs when performed by experienced operators,[1-4] with a lower rate of complications compared to intubation using sedatives alone.[5,6]
- **Are any of the nondepolarizing NMBAs as good as SCh for emergency RSI?** Multiple studies have compared SCh with rocuronium and vecuronium for intubation. All have concluded that the two drugs are similar but not identical.[7-10] A recent Cochrane review of rocuronium versus SCh for RSI concluded that SCh produces slightly better intubating conditions and has a statistically significantly reduced number of intubation attempts when compared with intubating doses of rocuronium.[11] The Cochrane review included 26 papers, of which only two used true RSI (intubation in <60 seconds), and none of the intubations were performed by emergency physicians in the emergency department. There are few data comparing SCh and rocuronium for emergency department RSI by emergency physicians, but one study of 520 intubations found SCh produced slightly better intubating conditions than rocuronium.[8] The

TABLE 22-1
Onset and Duration of Action of Neuromuscular Blocking Drugs

Drug	Dose (mg/kg)	Time to maximal blockade (min)	Time to recovery (min) 25%	75%
Quaternary amine				
SCh	1.0	1.1	8	11 (90%)
Benzylisoquinolinium compounds				
Tubocurarine	0.5	3.4	—	130
Metocurine	0.4	4.1	107	—
Atracurium	0.4	2.4	38	52
Doxacurium	0.05	5.9	83	116
Mivacurium	0.15	1.8	16	25
Cisatracurium	0.1	7.7	46	63
Aminosteroid compounds				
Pancuronium	0.08	2.9	86	—
Vecuronium	0.1	2.4	44	56
Rocuronium	0.6	1.0	43	66

From Hunter JM. Drug therapy: new neuromuscular blocking drugs. *N Engl J Med*. 1995;332:1691–1699, with permission.

mean onset time of paralysis for SCh was 39 ± 13 seconds, and for rocuronium was 44 ± 15 seconds, which was neither statistically nor clinically significant. The dose of rocuronium is critical to the success of rapid intubation. The correct dose of rocuronium for RSI is 1.0 mg per kg, not 0.6 mg per kg as is commonly recommended. The duration for the 1.0 mg per kg dose is 46 minutes.[10,12,13]

- **What is the correct dose of SCh for RSI?** Intubating conditions are directly related to the dose of SCh used, with excellent intubating conditions in more than 80% of patients receiving 1.5 mg per kg or more of SCh.[1] Increasing the dose of SCh from 0.5 to 2 mg per kg increases the duration of action only from 5.2 to 7.5 minutes, reinforcing the notion that the half-life of SCh in vivo is about 1 minute, as shown by Kato et al.[14] There is sufficient evidence that decreasing doses of SCh produce inferior intubating conditions. Therefore, we firmly recommend 1.5 mg per kg of SCh for emergent RSI.
- **What is the correct dose of rocuronium for RSI?** 1.0 mg per kg is the optimal dose of rocuronium for RSI.[8,15]
- **SCh use in patients with open eye injuries.** SCh has been linked to an increase in intraocular pressure. However, there has never been a case report of vitreous extrusion following the use of SCh in a patient with an open globe injury.[16] Therefore, we recommend that the NMBA for RSI in patients with open globe injury be selected as for any other patient.
- **Timing of hyperkalemia after significant (>5% body surface area) burns.** Schaner et al.[17] and Gronert et al.[18] found the greatest risk 18 to 66 days postburn in two studies in 1969 and 1975. Viby-Mogensen et al.[19] found dangerous rises in serum potassium as early as 9 days postburn. SCh can be safely used within the first week of a burn, but should be withheld after the first week until clinical healing of the burn wound is complete. We recommend a 5-day postburn cut-off.

- **SCh use in denervation injuries (stroke, Guillain–Barré syndrome, polio, spinal cord trauma, myasthenia gravis, etc.).** Denervation injuries cause a change in the number and function of junctional and extrajunctional ACH receptors at 4 to 5 days postinjury.[20,21] This can result in massive serum potassium increases that can cause cardiac arrest. SCh can be safely used up to 5 days post-denervation begins and then should be avoided until muscle atrophy is complete and the event is no longer dynamic.
- **SCh use in myopathic patients (muscular dystrophy, rhabdomyolysis, crush injuries, prolonged immobility, etc.).** Myopathies cause hyperkalemia by a similar mechanism as denervation, that is, changes in ACH receptor function and density.[22] Congenital myopathies are considered an absolute contraindication to SCh; its use in patients with myopathies can result in rhabdomyolysis and resuscitation-resistant hyperkalemic arrest.[23,24] Hyperkalemia secondary to occult, undiagnosed myopathy must be considered in children who experience cardiac arrest after SCh.[25] When a patient with known rhabdomyolysis is encountered, SCh should be avoided.
- **SCh use in patients with preexisting hyperkalemia.** Few studies to date have examined the risk of SCh administration in hyperkalemic patients.[26] In a meta-analysis, Thapa and Brull[27] identified four controlled studies of patients with and without renal failure, and there were no cases in which serum potassium increased by more than 0.5 mEq per L. The largest series, involving more than 40,000 patients undergoing general anesthesia, identified 38 adults and children with hyperkalemia (5.6 to 7.6 mEq per L) at the time they received SCh. None of these patients had an adverse event, and the authors calculated that the maximum likelihood of an adverse event related to SCh in hyperkalemic patients is 7.9%.[26] The long-held dogma to avoid SCh in any patient with renal failure is not valid, and SCh's independence of renal excretion makes it an excellent agent to consider when renal function is impaired.[28,29] We recommend that when hyperkalemia is present, or believed to be present (e.g., patient with end-stage renal disease), and the ECG shows stigmata of hyperkalemia (peaked T waves or increased QRS duration), an alternative agent, such as rocuronium, should be used for RSI. Otherwise, renal failure, or nominal hyperkalemia (i.e., without ECG changes), is not a contraindication to SCh.
- **SCh use in patients with severe (especially intra-abdominal) infections.** Patients with intra-abdominal infections lasting longer than 1 week are susceptible to SCh-induced hyperkalemia.[30] SCh-induced hyperkalemia risk increases with increasing severity of infection.[31]
- **Treatment for SCh-induced MH.** Discontinue any anesthetic use. Dantrolene, 2.5 mg per kg IV, is the recommended therapy, and it can be repeated every 5 minutes to a total dose of 10 mg per kg.[32] In a review of 21 patients with presumed MH, 11 patients immediately treated with dantrolene survived, and 3 of 4 patients who did not receive treatment until 24 hours later died (6 patients were excluded because of insufficient evidence that MH was the cause of decompensation).[33]
- **Sugammadex evidence.** The molecular shape of sugammadex allows it to encapsulate rocuronium and reverse neuromuscular blockade.[34] Early studies demonstrate safe and effective reversal of rocuronium neuromuscular blockade in <2 minutes.[35–37]

REFERENCES

1. Naguib M, Samarkandi AH, El-Din ME, et al. The dose of succinylcholine required for excellent endotracheal intubating conditions. *Anesth Analg.* 2006;102:151–155.
2. Sagarin MJ, Chiang V, Sakles JC, et al. Rapid sequence intubation for pediatric emergency airway management. *Pediatr Emerg Care.* 2002;18:417–423.
3. Tayal VS, Riggs RW, Marx JA, et al. Rapid-sequence intubation at an emergency medicine residency: success rate and adverse events during a two-year period. *Acad Emerg Med.* 1999;6:31–37.
4. Sakles JC, Laurin EG, Rantapaa AA, et al. Airway management in the emergency department: a one-year study of 610 tracheal intubations. *Ann Emerg Med.* 1998;31:325–332.

5. Li J, Murphy-Lavoie H, Bugas C, et al. Complications of emergency intubation with and without paralysis. *Am J Emerg Med*. 1999;17:141–143.

6. Gnauck K, Lungo JB, Scalzo A, et al. Emergency intubation of the pediatric medical patient: use of anesthetic agents in the emergency department. *Ann Emerg Med*. 1994;23:1242–1247.

7. Magorian T. Comparison of rocuronium, succinylcholine, and vecuronium for rapid-sequence induction of anesthesia in adult patients. *Anesthesiology*. 1993;79:913–918.

8. Laurin EG, Sakles JC, Panacek EA, et al. A comparison of succinylcholine and rocuronium for rapid-sequence intubation of emergency department patients. *Acad Emerg Med*. 2000;7:1362–1369.

9. Mazurek A, Rae B, Hann S, et al. Rocuronium versus succinylcholine: are they equally effective during rapid-sequence induction of anesthesia? *Anesth Analg*. 1998;87:1259–1262.

10. Andrews J, Kumar N, van den Brom RH, et al. A large simple randomized trial of rocuronium versus succinylcholine in rapid-sequence induction of anaesthesia along with propofol. *Acta Anaesthesiol Scand*. 1999;43:4–8.

11. Perry JJ, Lee JS, Sillberg VA, et al. Rocuronium versus succinylcholine for rapid sequence induction intubation. *Cochrane Database Syst Rev*. 2008;(2):CD002788.

12. McCourt KC, Salmela L, Mirakhur RK, et al. Comparison of rocuronium and suxamethonium for use during rapid sequence induction of anaesthesia. *Anaesthesia*. 1998;53:867–871.

13. Cheng CA, Aun CS, Gin T. Comparison of rocuronium and suxamethonium for rapid tracheal intubation in children. *Paediatr Anaesth*. 2002;12:140–145.

14. Kato M, Shiratori T, Yamamuro M, et al. Comparison between in vivo and in vitro pharmacokinetics of succinylcholine in humans. *J Anesth*. 1999;13:189–192.

15. Kirkegaard-Nielsen H, Caldwell JE, Berry PD. Rapid tracheal intubation with rocuronium: a probability approach to determining dose. *Anesthesiology*. 1999;91:131–136.

16. Vachon CA, Warner DO, Bacon DR. Succinylcholine and the open globe. Tracing the teaching. *Anesthesiology*. 2003;99:220–223.

17. Schaner PJ, Brown RL, Kirksey TD, et al. Succinylcholine-induced hyperkalemia in burned patients I. *Anesth Analg*. 1969;48:764–770.

18. Gronert GA, Dotin LN, Ritchey CR, et al. Succinylcholine-induced hyperkalemia in burned patients II. *Anesth Analg*. 1969;48:958–962.

19. Viby-Mogensen J, Hanel HK, Hansen E, et al. Serum cholinesterase activity in burned patients. II: Anaesthesia, suxamethonium and hyperkalaemia. *Acta Anaesthesiol Scand*. 1975;19:169–179.

20. Martyn JA, White DA, Gronert GA, et al. Up-and-down regulation of skeletal muscle acetylcholine receptors. Effects on neuromuscular blockers. *Anesthesiology*. 1992;76:822–843.

21. Gronert GA, Lambert EH, Theye RA. The response of denervated skeletal muscle to succinylcholine. *Anesthesiology*. 1973;39:13–22.

22. Gronert GA, Theye RA. Pathophysiology of hyperkalemia induced by succinylcholine. *Anesthesiology*. 1975;43:89–99.

23. Gronert GA. Cardiac arrest after succinylcholine: mortality greater with rhabdomyolysis than receptor upregulation. *Anesthesiology*. 2001;94:523–529.

24. Smith CL, Bush GH. Anaesthesia and progressive muscular dystrophy. *Br J Anaesth*. 1985;57:1113–1118.

25. Larach MG, Rosenberg H, Gronert GA, et al. Hyperkalemic cardiac arrest during anesthesia in infants and children with occult myopathies. *Clin Pediatr*. 1997;36:9–16.

26. Schow AJ, Lubarsky DA, Olson RP, et al. Can succinylcholine be used safely in hyperkalemic patients? *Anesth Analg*. 2002;95:119–122, table of contents.

27. Thapa S, Brull SJ. Succinylcholine-induced hyperkalemia in patients with renal failure: an old question revisited. *Anesth Analg*. 2000;91:237–241.

28. Powell DR, Miller R. The effect of repeated doses of succinylcholine on serum potassium in patients with renal failure. *Anesth Analg*. 1975;54:746–748.

29. Koide M, Waud BE. Serum potassium concentrations after succinylcholine in patients with renal failure. *Anesthesiology*. 1972;36:142–145.

30. Kohlschutter B, Baur H, Roth F. Suxamethonium-induced hyperkalaemia in patients with severe intra-abdominal infections. *Br J Anaesth*. 1976;48:557–562.

31. Khan TZ, Khan RM. Changes in serum potassium following succinylcholine in patients with infections. *Anesth Analg*. 1983;62:327–331.

32. Gronert GA, Antognini JF, Pessah IN. Malignant hyperthermia. In: Miller RD, ed. *Anesthesia*. 5th ed. Philadelphia, PA: Churchill-Livingstone; 2000:1033–1050.

33. Kolb ME, Horne ML, Martz R. Dantrolene in human malignant hyperthermia. *Anesthesiology*. 1982;56:254–262.

34. Sacan O, White PF, Tufanogullari B, et al. Sugammadex reversal of rocuronium-induced neuromuscular blockade: a comparison with neostigmine-glycopyrrolate and edrophonium-atropine. *Anesth Analg*. 2007;104:569–574.

35. Suy K, Morias K, Cammu G, et al. Effective reversal of moderate rocuronium- or vecuronium-induced neuromuscular block with sugammadex, a selective relaxant binding agent. *Anesthesiology*. 2007;106:283–288.

36. Groudine SB, Soto R, Lien C, et al. A randomized, dose-finding, phase II study of the selective relaxant binding drug, sugammadex, capable of safely reversing profound rocuronium-induced neuromuscular block. *Anesth Analg*. 2007;104:555–562.

37. Sparr HJ, Vermeyen KM, Beaufort AM, et al. Early reversal of profound rocuronium-induced neuromuscular blockade by sugammadex in a randomized multicenter study: efficacy, safety, and pharmacokinetics. *Anesthesiology*. 2007;106:935–943

23

Anesthesia and Sedation for Awake Intubation

Alan C. Heffner • Peter M.C. DeBlieux

INTRODUCTION

Humans protect their airway at virtually any cost. In fact, it is generally impossible to even glimpse the glottis with a laryngoscope in a fully awake and aware patient. The "awake" methods of endoscopy referred to in the difficult airway algorithm are rarely performed without pharmacologic assistance. Even in patients who are unaware because of their illness, sensibilities must be attenuated by a combination of local anesthesia and systemic sedation in order to facilitate diagnostic and therapeutic airway endoscopy.

Focusing on emergency airway management, the "awake" intubation is frequently indicated in situations where abnormal airway anatomy or difficult laryngoscopy is suspected. As a general rule, local anesthesia is first optimized in order to limit potential untoward effects of systemic sedation. In uncooperative or decompensating patients, however, sedation may dominate over local anesthesia.

DESCRIPTION

Awake laryngoscopy has two main roles, both of which apply to patients with anticipated difficult intubation: (1) to determine whether intubation is feasible, thus facilitating a decision regarding the use of neuromuscular blockade to complete the procedure, and (2) to intubate, particularly in circumstances when the patient's airway is deteriorating (i.e., the dynamic airway) as in angioedema, upper airway burns or trauma.

An awake look intended to determine the feasibility of nasal or oral intubation can be accomplished in two ways. A flexible endoscope (e.g., flexible fiberoptic or video bronchoscope or nasopharyngoscope) is inserted through the nostril to evaluate periglottic anatomy in patients with neck disease or acute injury to determine if nasal intubation or orotracheal intubation is feasible. This can be performed quickly with topical nasal anesthesia and minimal, if any, sedation.

The second approach engages a standard or video laryngoscope to perform laryngoscopy, with the intention of confirming glottic visualization. Awake rigid laryngoscopy is more stimulating and requires greater degrees of local anesthesia and sedation than does its flexible endoscopy counterpart. Concentrated local anesthesia of the mouth, oro- and hypopharynx facilitates the procedure and minimizes the dose of systemic sedation required. If the glottis is adequately visualized, the airway manager may either proceed with awake intubation, or may withdraw the laryngoscope and perform rapid sequence intubation (RSI). The approach is dictated by the clinical circumstance.

- If the difficult airway is rapidly dynamic and evolving, then it is advisable to intubate the patient during the awake direct or video laryngoscopy, as the airway may deteriorate significantly within minutes or as a result of laryngoscopic manipulation. If there is reasonable concern that the airway might change, intubation should be attempted on the first good opportunity.
- If the difficult airway is subacute to chronic and is more a confounder to intubation than the primary reason for airway crisis (e.g., fixed cervical or maxillofacial disease), then the goal is to confirm feasibility of intubation. Glottis visualization is followed by laryngoscope withdrawal and proper RSI, with the knowledge that the airway is very unlikely to deteriorate further between steps. Cases of slowly evolving acute disease (e.g., infection and inhalation burn) are reasonable opportunities to take the same approach. Appropriate supplies and drugs are prepared before the first laryngoscopy to minimize the delay to definitive RSI.

INDICATIONS AND CONTRAINDICATIONS

Awake intubation is indicated when the airway manager is not confident that gas exchange will be assured by any or all of the airway techniques if the patient is rendered apneic (see Chapters 2 and 3). Although the difficult airway assessment defines an airway as potentially difficult if it meets any or all of a number of markers (LEMON), the degree of perceived difficulty and the decision whether to use an RSI technique or an awake approach depend both on the patient and experience and judgment of the clinician. Local anesthesia of the upper airway with or without sedation facilitates upper airway endoscopy even when intubation is not anticipated. Common indications include airway examination for foreign body, supraglottitis, hoarseness, stridor, and blunt or penetrating neck injury.

The only contraindication to the use of this strategy is a patient who mandates an immediate airway. Rapidly deteriorating airway situations require immediate management through another means, as there is insufficient time for patient preparation before intervention (see Chapter 3 discussion of the "forced to act" scenario). Adequate time and patient cooperation (usually with the use of anesthesia and sedation) are the most important limitations to awake endoscopy. In addition, copious airway secretions or blood thwart efforts to effectively anesthetize the airway and may obscure the view of flexible endoscopes.

LOCAL ANESTHESIA FACTORS

Local anesthesia of the airway may be produced topically, by injection, or by combining both techniques. The selection of a local anesthetic agent depends on the properties of the agent and how it is supplied (concentration and preparation—aqueous, gel, or ointment). Potent local anesthesia may enable the airway to be visualized with little no sedation. As a general rule, local anesthesia should be optimized before sedation is given to the high-risk patients selected for this technique.

Airway secretions are a barrier to topical anesthetics and are capable of diluting applied agents or washing them away from the intended target region. Antisialogogues are effective adjuncts to reduce secretion production and improve topical anesthesia and endoscopy conditions. The antimuscarinic agent glycopyrrolate (Robinul) is the preferred agent. The greatest drawback is time to effective drying which is 10 to 20 minutes following intravenous (IV) administration (glycopyrrolate 0.01 mg per kg; usual adult dose 0.4 to 0.8 mg IV). Given sufficient time, even if only 10 minutes, it is advisable to administer glycopyrrolate to facilitate local anesthesia of the upper airway.

Lidocaine remains a favored drug for airway anesthesia because of its rapid onset (2 to 5 minutes to peak effect), safety, and widespread availability. Concentrations of 2% (20 mg per ml) to 4% (40 mg per ml) are optimal for topical administration. Addition of epinephrine provides no additional advantage.

Anesthetics applied to mucous membranes undergo rapid systemic absorption. The maximum safe dose of topical anesthetic applied to mucous membranes depends on the method and timing of administration. Although traditional dosage guidelines may be excessively conservative when drugs are administered by aerosol or atomizer, we recommend a maximum lidocaine dose of 4 mg per kg. This dose should be calculated before administration. As always, clinical judgment is required, and meticulous attention to detail is necessary when lidocaine is applied to the airway in order to achieve effective anesthesia without producing toxicity.

Aerosolization of aqueous lidocaine is easy and effective. Gas flow directed nebulizers, as are used for inhalational therapy in asthma, are an effective first step to initiate broad (nasal, oral, and hypopharyngeal) local anesthesia during an emergency airway situation. Four milliliters of lidocaine can be administered over 10 minutes while additional agents and equipment are prepared. Augmentation with additional focused topical application is the norm.

Atomizers produce larger droplets than nebulizers, such that medication rains out in the region local to administration. For topical anesthesia of the upper airway, atomizers are more rapid and effective than nebulizers. The DeVilbiss atomizer (Fig. 23-1) and Mucosal Atomization Device (LMA North America, San Diego, CA) (Fig. 23-2) are two examples of commonly use atomizers.

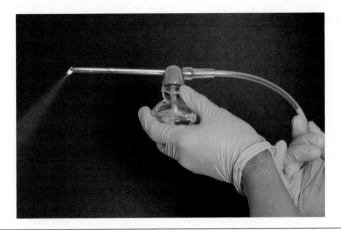

Figure 23-1 ● **De Vilbiss Atomizer.**

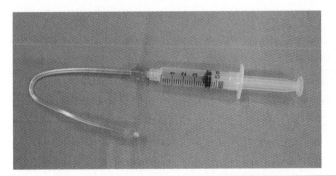

Figure 23-2 ● **Mucosal Atomization Device.**   The syringe forces the local anesthetic solution through the atomizing tip, resulting in a very fine mist, which can be synchronized with the patient's inspiration.

Lidocaine is also available in gel for paste formulas to permit direct local administration. Some combination of these formula applications often is warranted.

Nasal Anesthesia

The nasal mucosa is highly vascular and tends to bleed during manipulation. Topical vasoconstriction improves nasal passage caliber and prevent epistaxis although evidence for this practice is not strong. Phenylephrine (Neo-synephrine) 0.5% or oxymetazoline (Afrin) 0.05% solution is sprayed and sniffed into each nostril 2 to 3 minutes before application of local anesthesia. Cocaine 4% (40 mg per ml) can also be used.

Virtually all local anesthetic agents are effective when used topically in the nose. Cocaine 4% and tetracaine 0.45% are particularly effective because of their tissue penetration and ability to eliminate deep pressure discomfort commonly associated with nasal manipulation. Lidocaine is also effective (discussed previously), although it is associated with burning dysesthesia and produces less deep anesthesia.

Commonly used techniques for focused nasal anesthesia include:

• Nebulize a mixture of 4 ml of 4% lidocaine with 1 ml of 1% phenylephrine.
• Atomize agent directly into the nostril while asking the patient to sniff.
• Inject viscous anesthetic gel (4 ml) into the nares with a small syringe while asking the patient to sniff. The gel can be distributed throughout the nasal passage using a cotton dip applicator or through insertion of a nasopharyngeal airway.

Oral Anesthesia

Topical anesthesia of the oral cavity focuses on the tongue to attenuate the gag response, and to reduce the discomfort associated with manipulation (e.g., grasping the tongue with gauze and pulling it forward to draw the epiglottis forward during endoscopic exam).

- The mouth is best anesthetized topically by having the patient gargle and swish with a 4% aqueous lidocaine solution. Gargling also augments anesthesia of the oro- and hypopharynx.
- "Butter" the tongue base with lidocaine paste, ointment, or gel applied with a tongue depressor. Apply 5 ml of 5% lidocaine evenly to the posterior base of the protruded tongue just as you would apply butter to a piece of toast. Maintain the mouth open and tongue protruded for several minutes to allow the formula to melt down the base of the tongue. Manual control of tongue with gauze while asking the patient to pant "like a dog" is an easy maneuver.
- An atomizer can also be used to spray the structures of the oral cavity.

Oro- and Hypopharyngeal Anesthesia

The major sensory supply to the oro- and hypopharynx is the glossopharyngeal nerve (see Chapter 4). Although cooperative patients can gargle anesthetic to initiate the process, the best way to achieve dense local anesthesia to permit laryngoscopy or awake intubation is through a nerve block at the base of the palatopharyngeal arch (posterior tonsillar pillar; see Fig. 4-4). The following two techniques are commonly used:

- A 23G angled tonsillar needle with 1 cm of exposed needle tip is inserted 0.5 cm behind the midpoint of the posterior tonsillar pillar and directed laterally and slightly posteriorly (Fig. 23-3). Two ml of 2% lidocaine are deposited following a negative aspiration. Although

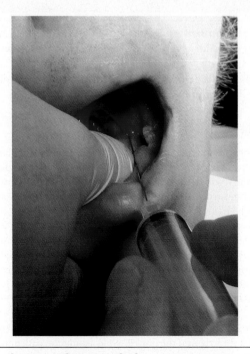

Figure 23-3 ● **Glossopharyngeal Nerve Block.** Insertion point for a 23G angled tonsillar needle.

this block is effective, it is not widely used because of the proximity of the carotid artery and risk of carotid injection in up to 5% of cases.

- Topical technique: The "butter" the tongue technique mentioned earlier provides effective anesthesia for deep hypopharyngeal structures. The ointment liquefies as it warms and runs down the base of the palatopharyngeal arch, penetrates the mucosa, and reaches the glossopharyngeal nerve. Distribution to the valleculae and pyriform recesses provides local anesthesia and blocks the internal branch of the superior laryngeal nerve to provide laryngeal anesthesia.

Laryngeal Anesthesia

The drying imperative does not apply to the larynx. Topical local anesthesia of this structure can be provided using a manual spray device, an atomizer, or nebulizer to spray 4 ml of 4% aqueous lidocaine. Alternatively, one can block the superior laryngeal branch of the vagus nerve (see Fig. 4-6):

- The internal branch of the superior laryngeal nerve can be blocked as it runs just deep to the mucosa in the pyriform recess using Jackson forceps to hold a cotton pledget soaked in 4% lidocaine against the mucosa for 1 minute (Fig. 23-4).
- This block can also be performed using an external approach to the nerve as it perforates the thyrohyoid membrane just below the greater cornu of the hyoid bone. A 21G to 25G needle is passed medially through skin to contact the hyoid bone as posteriorly as possible. The needle is then walked caudad off the hyoid. Resistance may be appreciated as the thyrohyoid membrane is perforated. Following aspiration to rule out entry into the pharyngeal lumen or a vessel, 3 ml 2% lidocaine can be injected. If the hyoid cannot be palpated or if palpation produces undue patient discomfort, then the thyroid cartilage is used as a landmark. The needle is walked cephalad from a point on the thyroid cartilage, about one-third of the distance from the midline to the greater cornu. Complications include intra-arterial injection, hematoma, and airway distortion.

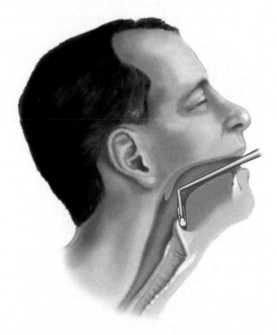

Figure 23-4 ● **Use of Jackson Cross-over Forceps to Perform a Transmucosal Superior Laryngeal Nerve Block.** A cotton pledget, soaked in 4% lidocaine, is held against the mucosa for about 1 minute.

Tracheal Anesthesia

The trachea is best anesthetized topically. Drying is unnecessary. Local anesthetic agent can be sprayed into the trachea through handheld spray devices, atomizer, or nebulizer. Additional anesthetic can be applied through the working channel during fiberoptic endoscopy.

- Tracheal and laryngeal anesthesia can be produced by puncturing the cricothyroid membrane and injecting local anesthetic agent directly into the trachea. A 5-ml syringe containing 3 ml of 4% lidocaine aqueous is attached to a 20G IV catheter-over-needle device. It may be helpful to cut the plastic cannula to 1.5 cm in length to minimize tracheal stimulation and cough. A small area of skin is anesthetized over the cricothyroid membrane using a 25G to 27G needle. The needle-cannula is then inserted into the trachea, while aspirating for air. Once the air column is entered, the plastic cannula is advance over the needle into the trachea. The needle is withdrawn and discarded. Lidocaine is injected at end exhalation with the subsequent inspiration and cough facilitating downward and upward spread of anesthetic.

SEDATION TECHNIQUES

Awake endoscopy during an emergency airway situation frequently relies on some degree of IV titration of systemic sedation to supplement topical anesthesia. Mild to moderate sedation is typically required similar to that used for painful procedures, such as for reduction of a dislocated shoulder or drainage of a deep cutaneous abscess.

A variety of sedative-hypnotic medications may be used, including midazolam, propofol, etomidate, ketamine, and others. Agent selection depends on the clinical situation, medication availability, and airway manager experience with each medication. In general, it is best to achieve sedation for airway examination by the same methods used for other procedures so the airway manager is using familiar agents and doses. Deep anesthesia defeats the fundamental purpose of an awake approach to maintain spontaneous ventilation and active airway protection.

All agents classified as sedative-hypnotics (e.g., benzodiazepines, barbiturates, propofol, and etomidate) cause respiratory depression in a dose-dependent fashion. This is also true of opioids such as fentanyl and morphine, particularly when used in conjunction with sedative-hypnotic agents. Fragile patients with compensated respiratory failure may be rendered critically bradypneic or apneic with relatively small doses of these agents. Sedative and opioid analgesia also produce some degree of muscle relaxation. Patients with upper airway obstruction may progress to complete obstruction if these agents invoke a loss of critical upper airway muscle tone. The operator should always be prepared to proceed directly to a surgical airway (i.e., double setup situation) when sedation and local anesthesia are undertaken on a patient with partial or impending airway obstruction (see Chapter 34).

Ketamine is a unique dissociative agent that maintains muscle tone and spontaneous respirations when used at low to moderate doses. Doses exceeding 1 mg per kg IV may invoke respiratory and cardiovascular depression. Ketamine may also sensitize the larynx to laryngospasm in the face of laryngeal inflammation. The preservation of airway maintenance and spontaneous ventilation are important for this procedure, and ketamine is a preferred agent. Ketamine should be titrated in 10- to 20-mg aliquots IV until the patient can tolerate an awake look. The patient may be dissociated, but ordinarily will continue to breathe spontaneously and maintain patency of the airway. Some authors advocate a combination of ketamine and propofol drawn up in the same syringe to make a concentration of 5 mg per ml of each (5 ml of 10 mg per ml ketamine plus 5 ml of 10 mg per ml of propofol in a 10-ml syringe) titrated 1 to 2 ml at a time. Although this method administers two agents in a fixed combination, it appears to be effective and safe, and the two drugs are compatible in the same syringe. Alternatives include balanced use of a benzodiazepine (e.g., midazolam) and an opioid (e.g., fentanyl), intravenously titrated etomidate, or other agents used for painful, stimulating procedures. All agents require continuous vigilance with respect to airway patency and adequacy of ventilation.

Uncooperative or intoxicated patients may require chemical restraint before and during airway assessment. If hypoxia or severe respiratory distress is the cause of the combative behavior, an awake technique is neither advised nor likely to succeed. Haloperidol, a butyrophenone, is rapid acting such that IV doses of 2 to 5 mg in the adult can be carefully titrated to effect at 3- to 5-minute intervals.

Two additional newer agents show promise for awake endoscopy during emergency situations. Remifentanil is an ultra–short-acting opioid with rapid onset and offset, both measured in tens of seconds rather than minutes. There is a wide range of recommended dosing and I selected a conservative starting dose. An IV bolus of 0.75 mcg/kg may precede the continuous infusion which is generally started at 0.05-0.1 mcg/kg/minute with subsequent titration to effect. Dosing should be calculated on lean body mass and reduced by as much as 50% to 70% in the elderly. Anecdotally, remifentanil infusion appears to attenuate both the gag reflex and laryngeal reflexes, and can facilitate airway anesthesia. It may be particularly useful in patients with hyperactive gag reflexes, and in the presence of excess secretions.

Dexmedetomidine is an IV α_2-agonist indicated for induction of general anesthesia and sedation during critical illness. It possesses desirable properties for awake endoscopy including rapid onset of hypnosis, analgesia, and amnesia without respiratory depression. Typical dosing is 1 mcg per kg IV load over 10 minutes followed by infusion at 0.1 mcg/kg/hour and titrated to effect. Supplemental doses of an alternative agent may be required. Bradycardia and hypotension are uncommon, but important side effects.

SUMMARY

- Effective topical anesthesia of the upper airways is most effective when the drug is applied to dry mucous membranes.
- For mucosal drying, we recommend glycopyrrolate 0.01 mg per kg IV; usual adult dose is 0.4 to 0.8 mg IV
- When time allows, local anesthesia is first optimized in order to limit potential untoward effects of systemic sedation. Uncooperative or rapidly decompensating patients are exceptions where sedation may dominate over local anesthesia.
- The dissociated anesthesia and preserved respiratory drive produced with low to moderate dose IV ketamine (<1 mg per kg) make it a prime agent for awake endoscopy procedures.
- Systemic sedation should be titrated with extreme caution in patients with impending airway obstruction.

EVIDENCE

- **Is there any evidence for the use of ketamine and propofol together?** "Ketofol," the combination of ketamine and propofol, for procedural sedation has emerged over the last decade.[1,2] Fixed dose (1:1 mixture of ketamine 10 mg per ml and propofol 10 mg per ml) single-syringe mixtures are frequently used.[3,4] Although theoretically advantageous to limit dose-related adverse events of each agent, there are little data to support improved efficacy or safety over single agent sedation. There are no specific data for use of this combination in airway management.
- **Can local anesthesia of the upper airway cause airway obstruction?** In the presence of pre-existing airway compromise, topical anesthesia and instrumentation are associated with

airway compromise resulting from dynamic airflow obstruction with or without associated laryngospasm.[5–7] Preparation for immediate surgical airway control is a necessity whenever one applies topical anesthesia or performs instrumentation of an inflamed, compromised airway. In certain cases, awake cricothyrotomy or tracheostomy under local anesthesia is a reasonable option.

- **What is the evidence for dexmedetomidine use during awake airway procedures?** Rapid onset hypnosis and amnesia without accompanying respiratory depression are primary sedation goals during awake airway maneuvers. As anticipated, the favorable pharmacologic profile of dexmedetomidine led to its application in patients with tenuous or difficult airways. Growing case report and trial evidence support the safety and efficacy of dexmedetomidine as the primary and/or sole hypnotic agent to facilitate awake fiberoptic intubation.[8,9]

REFERENCES

1. Mortero RF, Clark LD, Tolan MM, et al. The effects of small dose ketamine on propofol sedation: respiration, postoperative mood, perception, cognition and pain. *Anesth Analg*. 2001;92:1465–1469.

2. Badrinath S, Avramov MN, Shadrick M, et al. The use of a ketamine-propofol combination during monitored anesthesia care. *Anesth Analg*. 2000;90:858–862.

3. Willman EV, Andolfatto G. A prospective evaluation of "ketofol" (ketamine/propofol combination) for procedural sedation and analgesia in the emergency department. *Ann Emerg Med*. 2007;49(1):23–30.

4. Andolfatto G, Willman E. A prospective case series of single syringe ketamine-propofol (Ketofol) for emergency department procedural sedation and analgesia in adults. *Acad Emerg Med*. 2011;18(3):237–245.

5. Ho AM, Chung DC, To EW, et al. Total airway obstruction during local anesthesia in a non-sedated patient with a compromised airway. *Can J Anaesth*. 2004;51(8):838–841.

6. McGuire G, el-Beheiry H. Complete upper airway obstruction during awake fibreoptic intubation in patients with unstable cervical spine fracture. *Can J Anaesth*. 1999;46(2):176–178.

7. Ho AM, Chung DC, Karmakar MK, et al. Dynamic airflow limitation after topical anaesthesia of the upper airway. *Anaesth Intensive Care*. 2006;34(2):211–215.

8. Bergese SD, Candiotti KA, Bokesch PM, et al. A phase IIIb, randomized, double-blind, placebo controlled, multi-center study evaluating the safety and efficacy of dexmedetomidine for sedation during awake fiberoptic intubation. *Am J Ther*. 2010;17(6):586–595.

9. Bergese SD, Patrick Bender S, McSweeney TD, et al. A comparative study of dexmedetomidine with midazolam and midazolam alone for sedation during elective awake fiberoptic intubation. *J Clin Anesth*. 2010;22(1):35–40.

24

Differentiating Aspects of the Pediatric Airway

Robert C. Luten • Nathan W. Mick

THE CLINICAL CHALLENGE

Airway management in the pediatric population presents many potential challenges, including age-related drug dosing and equipment sizing, anatomical variation that continuously evolves as development proceeds from infancy to adolescence, and the performance anxiety that invariably accompanies the resuscitation of a critically ill child. Clinical competence in managing the airway of a critically ill or injured child requires an appreciation of age- and size-related factors, and a degree of familiarity and comfort with the fundamental approach to pediatric airway emergencies.

The principles of airway management in children and adults are the same. Medications used to facilitate intubation, the need for alternative airway management techniques, and the basic approach to performing the procedure are similar whether the patient is 8 or 80 years of age. There are, however, a few important differences that must be considered in emergency airway management situations. These differences are most exaggerated in the first 2 years of life, after which the pediatric airway gradually develops more adult-like features.

APPROACH TO THE PEDIATRIC PATIENT

General Issues

A recent review of the pediatric resuscitation process attempted to define elements of the mental (cognitive) burden of providers, when dealing with the unique aspects of critically ill children compared with adults. Age- and size-related variables unique to children introduce the need for more complex, nonautomatic, or knowledge-based mental activities, such as calculating drug doses and selecting equipment. The concentration required to undertake these activities while under stress may subtract from other important mental activity such as assessment, evaluation, prioritization, and synthesis of information, referred to in the resuscitative process as critical thinking activities. The cumulative effect of these factors leads to inevitable time delays and a corresponding increase in the potential for decision-making errors in the pediatric resuscitative process. This is in sharp contrast to adult resuscitation, where drug doses, equipment sizing, and physiologic parameters are usually familiar to the provider, leading to more automatic-type decisions that free the adult provider's attention for critical thinking. In children, drug doses are based on weight and may vary by an order of magnitude depending on age (i.e., 3-kg neonate vs. a 30-kg 8-year-old vs. a 100-kg adolescent). The use of resuscitation aids in pediatric resuscitation significantly reduces the cognitive load (and error) related to drug dosing calculations and equipment selection by relegating these activities to a lower order of mental function (referred to as "automatic" or "rule based"). The results are reduced error, attenuation of psychological stress, and an increase in critical thinking time. Table 24-1 is a length-based, color-coded equipment reference chart (Broselow–Luten-based "resuscitation guide") for pediatric airway management that eliminates error-prone strategies based on age and weight. Both equipment and drug dosing information are included in the Broselow–Luten system and can be accessed by a single length measurement or patient weight. This system is also available as part of a robust online resource (www.ebroselow.com).

Specific Issues

Anatomical and functional issues

The approach to the child with airway obstruction (the most common form of a difficult pediatric airway) incorporates several unique features of the pediatric anatomy.

1. Children obstruct more readily than adults do and the pediatric airway is especially susceptible to airway obstruction resulting from swelling. See Table 26-4 that outlines the effect of 1-mm edema on airway resistance in the infant (4-mm airway diameter) versus the adult (8-mm

TABLE 24-1
Equipment Selection

	Pink[a]	Red	Purple	Yellow	White	Blue	Orange	Green
Length (cm)-based pediatric equipment chart								
Weight (kg)	6–7	8–9	10–11	12–14	15–18	19–23	23–31	31–41
Length (cm)	60.75–67.75	67.75–75.25	75.25–85	85–98.25	98.25–110.75	110.75–122.5	122.5–137.5	137.5–155
ETT size (mm)	3.5	3.5	4.0	4.5	5.0	5.5	6.0 cuff	6.5 cuff
Lip-to-tip length (mm)	10–10.5	10.5–11	11–12	12.5–13.5	14–15	15.5–16.5	17–18	18.5–19.5
Laryngoscope size+blade	1 straight	1 straight	1 straight	2 straight	2 straight	2 straight or curved	2 straight or curved	3 straight or curved
Suction catheter	8F	8F	8F	8–10F	10F	10F	10F	12F
Stylet	6F	6F	10F	10F	10F	10F	14F	14F
Oral airway (mm)	50	50	60	60	60	70	80	80
Nasopharyngeal airway	14F	14F	18F	20F	22F	24F	26F	30F
Bag/valve device	Infant	Infant	Child	Child	Child	Child	Child/adult	Adult
Oxygen mask	Newborn	Newborn	Pediatric	Pediatric	Pediatric	Pediatric	Adult	Adult
Vascular access	22–24/23–25	22–24/23–25	20–22/23–25	18–22/21–23	18–22/21–23	18–20/21–22	18–20/21–22	16–20/18–21
Catheter/butterfly	Intraosseous	Intraosseous	Intraosseous	Intraosseous	Intraosseous	Intraosseous	Intraosseous	Intraosseous
NG tube	5–8F	5–8F	8–10F	10F	10–12F	12–14F	14–18F	18F

(continued)

TABLE 24-1
Equipment Selection (continued)

	Pink[a]	Red	Purple	Yellow	White	Blue	Orange	Green
Urinary catheter	5–8F	5–8F	8–10F	10F	10–12F	10–12F	12F	12F
Chest tube	10–12F	10–12F	16–20F	20–24F	20–24F	24–32F	24–32F	32–40F
BP cuff	Newborn/infant	Newborn/infant	Infant/child	Child	Child	Child	Child/adult	Adult
LMA[b]	1.5	1.5	2	2	2	2–2.5	2.5	3

Directions for use: (1) measure patient length with centimeter tape or with a Broselow tape; (2) using measured length in centimeters or Broselow tape measurement, access appropriate equipment column; (3) column for ETTs, oral and nasopharyngeal airways, and LMAs; always select one size smaller and one size larger than recommended size.

[a]For infants smaller than the pink zone, but not preterm, use the same equipment as the pink zone.

[b]Based on manufacturer's weight-based guidelines:

Mask size	Patient size (kg)
1	≤5
1.5	5–10
2	10–20
2.5	20–30
3	>30

Permission to reproduce with modification from Luten RC, Wears RL, Broselow J, et al. Managing the unique size related issues of pediatric resuscitation: reducing cognitive load with resuscitation aids. *Ann Emerg Med.* 1992;21:900–904.

airway diameter). Nebulized racemic epinephrine causes local vasoconstriction and can reduce mucosal swelling and edema to some extent. For diseases such as croup, where the anatomical site of swelling occurs at the level of the cricoid ring, the narrowest part of the pediatric airway, racemic epinephrine can have dramatic results. Disorders located in areas with greater airway caliber, such as the supraglottic swelling of epiglottitis or the retropharyngeal swelling of an abscess, rarely produce findings as dramatic. In these latter examples, especially in epiglottitis, efforts to force a nebulized medication on a child may agitate the child, leading to increased airflow velocity and dynamic upper airway obstruction.

2. Noxious interventions can lead to dynamic airway obstruction and precipitate respiratory arrest, leading to the admonition to "leave them alone." The work of breathing in the crying child increases 32-fold, elevating the threat of dynamic airway obstruction and hence the principle of maintaining children in a quiet, comfortable environment during evaluation and management for upper airway obstruction (Fig. 24-1A–C).

3. Bag-mask ventilation (BMV) may be of particular value in the child who has arrested from upper airway obstruction. Note in Figure 24-1C that efforts by the patient to alleviate the obstruction may actually exacerbate it, as increased inspiratory effort creates increased negative extrathoracic pressure, leading to collapse of the malleable extrathoracic trachea. The application of positive pressure through BMV causes the opposite effect by stenting the airway open and relieving the dynamic component of obstruction (Fig. 24-1C,D). This mechanism explains the recommendation to try BMV as a temporizing measure, even if the patient arrests from obstruction. There have been numerous case reports of children with epiglottitis successfully resuscitated utilizing BMV.

4. Apart from differences related to size, there are certain anatomical peculiarities of the pediatric airway. These differences are most pronounced in children <2 years of age, whereas children >8 years of age are similar to adults anatomically and the 2- to 8-year-old period is one of transition. The glottic opening is situated at the level of the first cervical vertebra (C-1) in infancy. This level transitions to the level of C-3 to C-4 by age 7 and to the level of C-5 to C-6 in the adult. Thus, the glottic opening tends to be higher and more anterior in children as opposed to adults. The size of the tongue with respect to the oral cavity is larger in children, particularly infants. The epiglottis is also proportionately larger in a child making efforts to visualize the airway with curved blade by insertion of the blade tip into the vallecula and lifting the epiglottis out of the way more difficult. Thus a straight blade, which is used to directly lift the epiglottis up, is recommended in children younger than 3 years (Table 24-2).

Blind nasotracheal intubation is relatively contraindicated in children younger than 10 years for at least two reasons: Children have large tonsils and adenoids that may bleed significantly when traumatized, and the angle between the epiglottis and the laryngeal opening is more acute than that in the adult, making successful cannulation of the trachea difficult.

Children possess a small cricothyroid membrane and in children younger than 3 to 4 years, it is virtually nonexistent. For this reason, needle cricothyrotomy may be difficult, and surgical cricothyrotomy is virtually impossible and contraindicated in infants and small children up to 10 years of age.

Although younger children possess a relatively high, anterior airway with the attendant difficulties in visualization of the glottic aperture, this anatomical pattern is consistent from one child to another, so this difficulty can be anticipated. The adult airway is subject to more variation and age-related disorders leading to a difficult airway (e.g., rheumatoid arthritis, obesity, etc.). Children are predictably "different" not "difficult." Figure 24-2 demonstrates anatomical differences particular to children.

Physiologic issues

There are two important physiologic differences between children and adults that impact airway management (Box 24-1). Children have a basal oxygen consumption that is approximately twice that of adults. Coupled with a proportionally smaller functional residual capacity (FRC) to body weight ratio these factors result in more rapid desaturation in children compared with adults given

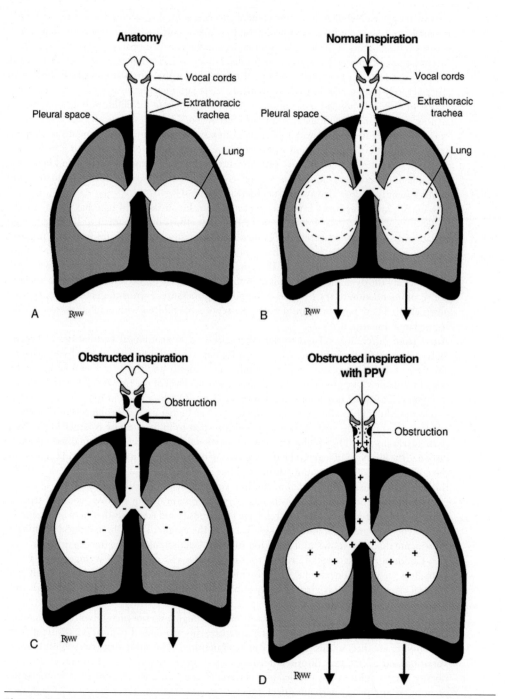

Figure 24-1 ● **Intra- and Extrathoracic Trachea and the Dynamic Changes that Occur in the Presence of Upper Airway Obstruction.** **A:** Normal anatomy. **B:** The changes that occur with normal inspiration; that is, dynamic collapsing of the upper airway associated with the negative pressure of inspiration on the extrathoracic trachea. **C:** Exaggeration of the collapse secondary to superimposed obstruction at the subglottic area. **D:** Positive-pressure ventilation (PPV) stents the collapse/obstruction versus the patient's own inspiratory efforts, which increase the obstruction. (Adapted from Cote CJ, Ryan JF, Todres ID, et al., eds. *A Practice of Anesthesia for Infants and Children.* 2nd ed. Philadelphia, PA: WB Saunders; 1993, with permission.)

TABLE 24-2
Anatomical Differences between Adults and Children

Anatomy	Clinical significance
Large intraoral tongue occupying relatively large portion of the oral cavity and proportionally larger epiglottis	Straight blade preferred over curved to push distensible anatomy out of the way to visualize the larynx and elevate the epiglottis
High tracheal opening: C-1 in infancy vs. C-3 to C-4 at age 7, C-5 to C-6 in the adult	High anterior airway position of the glottic opening compared with that in adults
Large occiput that may cause flexion of the airway, large tongue that easily collapses against the posterior pharynx	Sniffing position is preferred. The larger occiput actually elevates the head into the sniffing position in most infants and children. A towel may be required under shoulders to elevate torso relative to head in small infants
Cricoid ring is the narrowest portion of the trachea as compared with the vocal cords in the adult	Uncuffed tubes provide adequate seal because they fit snugly at the level of the cricoid ring. Correct tube size essential because variable expansion cuffed tubes not used
Consistent anatomical variations with age with fewer abnormal variations related to body habitus, arthritis, chronic disease	Younger than 2 y, high anterior; 2–8 y, transition; and older than 8 y, small adult
Large tonsils and adenoids may bleed; more acute angle between epiglottis and laryngeal opening results in nasotracheal intubation attempt failures	Blind nasotracheal intubation not indicated in children; nasotracheal intubation failure
Small cricothyroid membrane landmark, surgical cricothyrotomy impossible in infants and small children	Needle cricothyrotomy recommended and the landmark is the anterior surface of the trachea, not the cricoid membrane

an equivalent duration of preoxygenation. The clinician must anticipate and communicate this possibility to the staff and be prepared to provide supplemental oxygen by BMV if the patient's oxygen saturation drops below 90%.

Drug Dosage and Selection

The dose of succinylcholine (SCh) in children is different from that in adults. SCh is rapidly metabolized by plasma esterases and distributed to extracellular water. Children have a larger volume of extracellular fluid water relative to adults: at birth, 45%; at age 2 months, approximately 30%; at age 6 years, 20%; and at adulthood, 16% to 18%. The recommended dose of SCh, therefore, is higher on a per kilogram basis in children than in adults (2 vs. 1.5 mg per kg). All drug dosage determinations are most appropriately and safely done using resuscitation aids such as the Broselow–Luten system previously described.

In 1993, the U.S. Food and Drug Administration (FDA), in conjunction with pharmaceutical companies, revised the package labeling for SCh in the wake of reports of hyperkalemic cardiac arrest following the administration of SCh to patients with previously undiagnosed neuromuscular disease. Initially, it stated that SCh was contraindicated for elective anesthesia in pediatric patients because of this concern, although the wording was subsequently altered to embrace a risk–benefit analysis when deciding to use SCh in children. However, both the initial advisory warning and the revised warning continue to recommend SCh for emergency or full-stomach intubation in children. Pediatric drug doses are provided in Table 24-3.

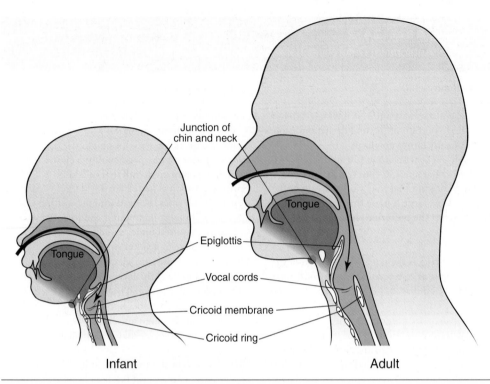

Figure 24-2 ● The anatomical differences particular to children are (1) higher, more anterior position of the glottic opening (note the relationship of the vocal cords to the chin/neck junction); (2) relatively larger tongue in the infant, which lies between the mouth and glottic opening; (3) relatively larger and more floppy epiglottis in the child; (4) the cricoid ring is the narrowest portion of the pediatric airway versus the vocal cords in the adult; (5) position and size of the cricothyroid membrane in the infant; (6) sharper, more difficult angle for blind nasotracheal intubation; and (7) larger relative size of the occiput in the infant.

Equipment Selection

Table 24-1 references length-based recommendations for emergency equipment in pediatric patients. Appropriately sized equipment can be chosen with a centimeter length measurement or with a Broselow tape.

A word of caution with respect to the storage of airway management equipment for children: Despite best efforts (e.g., equipment lists or periodic checks), it is not uncommon for newborn equipment to be mixed in with or placed in proximity to the smallest pediatric equipment. This practice may lead to newborn equipment being used in older children for whom it may not function properly or may, in fact, be dangerous. Examples include the no. 0 laryngoscope blade, which is too short to allow visualization of the airway; the 250-cc newborn BMV, which provides inadequate ventilation

---

Box 24-1. Physiologic Differences

Physiologic difference	Significance
Basal O_2 consumption is twice adult values (>6 ml/kg/min). Proportionally smaller FRC as compared with adults	Shortened period of protection from hypoxia for equivalent preoxygenation time as compared with adults. Infants and small children often require BMV while maintaining cricoid pressure to avoid hypoxia

TABLE 24-3
Drugs—Pediatric Considerations

Drug	Dosage	Pediatric-specific comments
Premedications		
Atropine	0.02 mg/kg	An option <1 y of age
Lidocaine	1.5 mg/kg IV	Head injury, asthma, older than 10 y
Fentanyl	1–3 µg/kg IV	In head injury, older than 10 y
Induction agents		
Midazolam	0.3 mg/kg IV	Use 0.1 mg/kg if hypotensive
Thiopental	3–5 mg/kg IV	Lower dose to 1 mg/kg or delete if perfusion poor
Etomidate	0.3 mg/kg IV	
Ketamine	2 mg/kg IV, 4 mg/kg IM	
Propofol	2–3 mg/kg IV	
Paralytics		
SCh	2 mg/kg IV	Have atropine drawn up and ready
Pan/vecuronium	0.2 mg/kg IV	May increase to 0.3 mg/kg of vecuronium for RSI (0.1 mg/kg for maintenance of paralysis)
Rocuronium	1.0 mg/kg IV	For RSI

volumes; and various other equipment, such as oral airways that can cause airway obstruction if too small, or a curved laryngoscope blade that may not reach and pick up the relatively large epiglottis, or effectively remove the large tongue from the laryngoscopic view of the airway (see Table 24-4).

1. **Endotracheal tubes**

   The correct endotracheal tube (ETT) size for the patient can be determined by a length measurement and by referring to the equipment selection chart. The formula (16 + age in years)/4 is also a reasonably accurate method of determining the correct tube size. However, the formula cannot be used in children younger than 1 year and is only useful if an accurate age is known, which cannot always be determined in an emergency. Uncuffed ETTs are recommended in the younger pediatric age groups, and cuffed tubes are used for size 5.5 mm and up (Fig. 24-3). The admonition to avoid cuffed tubes is historical and in the past, there was an unacceptably high rate of subglottic stenosis resulting from failure to carefully monitor cuff pressures. Newer ETT make it easier to monitor cuff pressures and can be safely used in children, provided clinicians recognize the following fact: A cuffed tube adds 0.5 mm to the internal diameter (ID) so a smaller than predicted tube may be required. The cuffed tube should be placed with the cuff deflated initially and inflated with the minimum volume of air needed to effect an adequate seal.

   When intubating a young child, there is a tendency to insert the ETT too far, usually into the right mainstem bronchus. Various formulas can be used to determine the correct insertion distance (e.g., tube size times 3; age/2 + 10). For the example, a 3.5-mm ID tube should be inserted 3.5 × 3 = 10.5 cm at the lip. Alternatively, a length-based chart can be used. We recommend placing a piece of tape on the tube at the appropriate lip-to-tip centimeter line which serves as a constant reminder of the correct position of the tip of the ET tube in the intubated patient.

2. **Tube securing devices**

   An all too frequent complication following intubation is inadvertent extubation. ETTs must be secured at the mouth. Head and neck movement, particularly extension which translates into movement of the tube up and potentially out of the trachea, should be minimized.

TABLE 24-4
Dangerous Equipment

Equipment	Problem
No. 0 or no. 00 laryngoscope ETT blades	Valuable time can be lost trying to visualize the glottic opening if mistaken for a no. 1 blade
Curved no. 1 laryngoscope blades	Straight blades are preferred because of the following: • The epiglottis is picked up directly, not indirectly, by compressing the hyoepiglottic ligament in the vallecula • The tongue and mandibular anatomy are more easily elevated from the field of vision
250-cc BMV	Cannot generate adequate tidal volumes
Cuffed ET tubes <5.0 mm	If leak pressures are not monitored, ischemia of the tracheal mucosa may develop with the potential for scarring and stenosis
Oral airways <50 mm	Unless appropriate size oral airways are used, they may act to increase, rather than relieve, obstruction
Any *other* equipment too small	Sizing is critical to function!

Note: Only appropriate size is functional. Frequently, very small sizes are placed in the pediatric area without attention to appropriateness of size. This can greatly contribute to a failed airway outcome.

A cervical collar placed after intubation prevents flexion and extension and therefore can help prevent ETT dislodgement (Fig. 24-4). The ETT is traditionally secured by taping the tube to the cheek, although various commercial devices are also available.

3. **Oxygen masks**

   The simple rebreather mask used for most patients provides a maximum of 35% to 60% oxygen and requires a flow rate of 6 to 10 L per minute. A non-rebreather mask can provide approximately 70% oxygen in children if a flow rate of 10 to 12 L per minute is used. For emergency airway management, and particularly for preoxygenation for rapid sequence intubation (RSI), the pediatric non-rebreather mask is preferable. Adult non-rebreather masks can be used for older children but are too large to be used for infants and small children and will entrain significant amounts of "room" air. Properly configured bag-mask systems (i.e., those that have a one-way expiratory valves [e.g., "duck bill"] and small dead space) are capable of delivering oxygen concentrations >90%, if correctly used. The spontaneously breathing patient closes the duck-billed expiratory valve on inspiration, and on expiration, the expired carbon dioxide (CO_2) is vented through the valve into the atmosphere. Adult type units tend not to be used in infants and small children because of dead space considerations and size-related awkwardness leading some to prefer pediatric non-rebreather masks.

4. **Oral airways**

   Oral airways should only be used in children who are unconscious. In the conscious or semi-conscious child, these airways can incite vomiting. Oral airways can be selected based on the Broselow tape measurement or can be approximated by selecting an oral airway that fits the distance from the angle of the mouth to the tragus of the ear.

5. **Nasopharyngeal airways**

   Nasopharyngeal airways are helpful in the obtunded but responsive child. The correctly sized nasopharyngeal airway is the largest one that comfortably fits in the naris but does not produce blanching of the nasal skin. The correct length is from the tip of the nose to the tragus of the ear and usually corresponds to the nasopharyngeal airway with the correct diameter. Care must be taken to suction these airways regularly to avoid blockage.

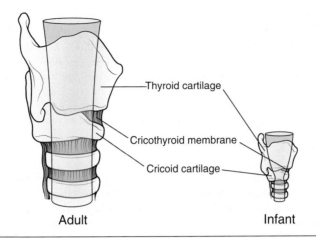

Figure 24-3 ● Airway Shape.   Note the position of the narrowest portion of the pediatric airway, which is at the cricoid ring, creating a funnel shape, versus the cylindrical shape seen in the adult, where the vocal cords form the narrowest portion. This is the rationale for using the uncuffed tube in the child; it fits snugly, unlike the cuffed tube used in the adult, which is inflated once the tube passes the cords to produce a snug fit. (Modified with permission from Cote CJ, Todres ID. The pediatric airway. In: Cote CJ, Ryan JF, Todres ID, et al., eds. *A Practice of Anesthesia for Infants and Children*. 2nd ed. Philadelphia, PA: WB Saunders; 1993.)

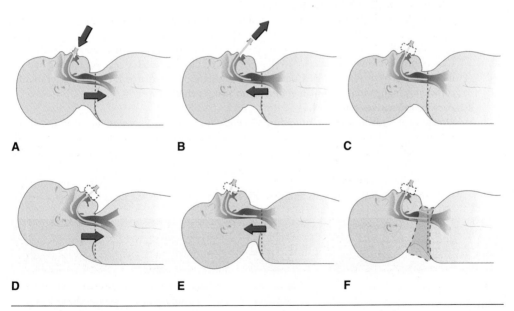

Figure 24-4 ● Securing the ET Tube.   **A:** Unsecured tube sliding in/down. **B:** Unsecured tube sliding out/up. **C:** Tube secured to prevent in/out, up/down movement. **D:** Secured tube moving down and in as head flexes. **E:** Secured tube moving up/out as head extends. **F:** Neck movement prevented by cervical collar, thus preventing tube movement in the trachea.

6. **Nasogastric tubes**

BMV may lead to insufflation of the stomach, hindering full diaphragmatic excursion and preventing effective ventilation. A nasogastric (NG) tube should be placed soon after intubation to decompress the stomach in any patient who has undergone BMV and requires ongoing mechanical ventilation postintubation. Often in such patients, the abdomen is distended or tense, making the problem obvious, but other times it is difficult to identify the difference between this and the normally protuberant abdomen of the young child. Difficulty in ventilation that is felt be related to reduced compliance should prompt the placement of an NG tube. Length-based systems identify the appropriate NG tube size.

7. **BMV equipment**

For emergency airway management, the self-inflating bag is preferred by most over the anesthesia ventilation bag mostly based on familiarity. These bag-mask units should have an oxygen reservoir so that at 10 to 15 L of oxygen flow, one can provide a FiO_2 of 90% to 95%. The smallest bag that should be used is 450 ml. Neonatal bags that are smaller (250 ml) do not provide effective tidal volume even for small infants. Many of the pediatric BMV devices have a positive-pressure relief (pop-off) valve. The pop-off valve may be set by the manufacturer to open at anywhere between 20 and 45 cm of water pressure (CWP), depending on whether the bag unit is intended for infants or small children (respectively) and is used to prevent barotrauma. Emergency airway management often requires higher peak airway pressures, so the bag should be configured without a pop-off valve or with a pop-off valve that can be closed. Practically, it is a good practice to store the BMV device with the pop-off valve closed so that initial attempts to ventilate the patient can achieve sufficient peak airway pressure to achieve ventilation. Chapter 25 discusses this issue in more detail and offers suggestions to prevent its occurrence.

8. **End-tidal CO_2 ($ETCO_2$) detectors**

Colorimetric $ETCO_2$ detectors are as useful in children as in adults. A pediatric size exists for children weighing <15 kg while the adult model should be used for children weighing >15 kg. If an adult-sized $ETCO_2$ device is used inappropriately for a small child, there may be insufficient CO_2 volumes to cause the detector to change color, resulting in a false-negative reading and removal of a correctly placed tube. Conversely, the resistance in a pediatric $ETCO_2$ detector may be sufficiently high to make ventilation difficult in a larger child.

9. **Airway alternatives (Table 24-5)**

Orotracheal intubation is the procedure of choice for emergency airway management of the pediatric patient, including those patients with potential cervical spine injury where RSI with in-line manual stabilization is preferred. Nasotracheal intubation is relatively contraindicated in children.

Cricothyrotomy is the preferred emergency surgical airway in adults. The cricothyroid space emerges as one ages and is really only accessible after the age of 10 years. "Needle

TABLE 24-5
Alternatives for Airway Support

BMV	May be the most reliable temporizing measure in children. Equipment selection, adjuncts, and good technique are essential
Orotracheal intubation (usually with RSI)	Still the procedure of choice for emergent airway in potential cervical spine injury and most other circumstances
Needle cricothyrotomy	Recommended as last resort in infants and children, but data lacking
Laryngeal mask	Viable alternative
Blind nasotracheal intubation	Not indicated for children younger than 10 y
GlideScope	Well studied in adults, a potential alternative in children

cricothyrotomy" in children younger than 8 to 10 years is the term used when one accesses the airway in a percutaneous manner in young children even though it is recognized that the point of entry into the airway is often the trachea as opposed to the cricothyroid space.

Other devices that may be of use in failed airway management in young children are laryngeal mask airways (LMAs) and the GlideScope. LMAs are made for even newborns and young infants and may be useful as a temporizing measure when direct laryngoscopy proves difficult. The GlideScope is supplied in sizes appropriate for pediatric patients, although currently the penetration of this technology to all clinical settings has not occurred. The Combitube is easy to insert, but currently there are no models for pediatric patients <48 in tall. These and other adjuncts are discussed in Chapter 25.

INITIATION OF MECHANICAL VENTILATION

In emergency pediatrics, two modes of ventilation are used. Pressure-limited ventilation is the mode used for newborns and small infants while volume-limited ventilation is used for older children and adults. One can arbitrarily set 10 kg as the weight below which pressure-limited ventilators should be used, although volume-limited ventilators have been used effectively in smaller children. Generally speaking, the younger the child is, the more rapid the ventilatory rate. The initial ventilatory rate in infants is typically set between 20 and 25 per minute. Inspiratory/expiratory ratios are set at 1:2, and the typical peak inspiratory pressure (PIP) at initiation of ventilation is between 15 and 20 CWP. These initial settings in a pressure-controlled ventilation mode will usually give a tidal volume of 8 to 12 ml per kg. These initial settings are adjusted according to subsequent clinical evaluation and chest rise. Positive end-expiratory pressure should also be set at 3 to 5 cm of water and FiO_2 at 1.0. The Broselow–Luten length-based system also provides guidance for approximate starting tidal volumes, ventilator rates, and inspiratory times.

Once initial settings have been established, it is critical that the patient be quickly reevaluated and adjustments made, particularly as pulmonary compliance, airways resistance, and leak volumes change with time, precluding adequate ventilation with the initial settings of pressure-controlled ventilation. Clinical evaluation of ventilatory adequacy is more important than formulae to ensure adequate ventilation. Once adjustments are made and the patient appears clinically to be ventilated and oxygenating, blood gas determinations, or continuous pulse oximetry and $ETCO_2$ monitoring, should be used for confirmation and to guide additional adjustments (Table 24-6 and Box 24-2).

RSI TECHNIQUES FOR CHILDREN

The procedure of RSI in children is essentially the same procedure as in adults with a few important differences outlined as follows:

1. Preparation
   • Use resuscitation aids that address age- and size-related issues in drug dosing and equipment selection (e.g., Broselow–Luten tape).
2. Preoxygenation
   • Be meticulous. Children desaturate more rapidly than adults do.
3. Pretreatment
   • None. Atropine is optional but may be considered for infants <1 year of age.
4. Paralysis with induction
   • Induction agent selection as for adult: dose by length or weight.
   • SCh 2 mg per kg IV or rocuronium 1 mg per kg.
   • Anticipate desaturation; bag ventilate if oxygen saturation (SpO_2) is <90%.

5. Protection and positioning
   • Optional: apply Sellick maneuver.
6. Placement with proof
   • Confirm tube placement with $ETCO_2$ as for adult.
7. Postintubation management
   Ventilation guidelines are mentioned above. In almost all cases, children who are intubated and mechanically ventilated should be sedated and paralyzed in the emergency department to prevent deleterious rises in intracranial or intrathoracic pressures and inadvertent ETT dislodgement.

EVIDENCE

• **When is "a kid a kid" from the standpoint of airway management?** The phrase "kids are different" has long been used to bring attention to the unique differences between children and adults. From an airway management perspective, those differences are most pronounced in the first 2 years of life, after which there is a gradual transition, both anatomically and physiologically, to adulthood. For simplicity's sake, and because many children requiring airway management cannot be weighed, we define "children" as patients who fit on the Broselow tape. Those who do not are considered adults for dosing, equipment selection, and other recommendations. Children who are larger than the last zone on the tape are usually at least 80 lb (36 kg), at least 5 ft tall (>150 cm or approximately 60 in), and at least 10 years old.

TABLE 24-6
Initiation of Mechanical Ventilation

I. Initial settings		
Ventilator type	Pressure limited	Volume limited
Respiratory rate	20–25/min	12–20/min, by age
Positive end-expiratory pressure (cm H_2O)	3–5	3–5
FiO_2	1.0 (100%)	1.0 (100%)
Inspiratory time	≥0.6 s	≥0.6 s
Inspiratory/expiratory ratio	1:2	1:2
Pressure/volume settings	For pressure ventilation, start with PIP of 15–20 cm H_2O. Assess chest rise and adjust to higher pressures as needed. For volume ventilation, start with tidal volumes of 8–12 ml/kg. Start at lower volumes and increase to a PIP of 20–30 cm H_2O. *These are initial setting guidelines only. Assess chest rise and adjust accordingly*	
II. Evaluate clinically and make adjustments	Most patients will be ventilated with volume-cycled ventilators. Poor chest rise, poor color, and decreased breath sounds require *higher* tidal volume. Check for pneumothorax or blocked tube. Ensure that tube size and position are optimal and leaks are not present. For patients ventilated with pressure-cycled ventilators, these findings may indicate the need to increase the PIP	
III. Laboratory information	Arterial blood gas should be performed approximately 10–15 min after settings are stabilized. Additional samples may be necessary after each ventilator adjustment, unless ventilatory status is monitored by $ETCO_2$ and SpO_2	

Box 24-2. Emergency Pediatric Airway Management—Practical Considerations

---

Anatomical
- Anticipate high anterior glottic opening
- Do not hyperextend the neck
- Uncuffed tubes are used in children younger than 8 y
- Use straight blades in young children

Physiologic
- Anticipate desaturation

Drug dosage and equipment selection
- Use length-based system. Do *not* use memory or do calculations
- NG tube is an important airway adjunct in infants
- Stock pediatric non-rebreather masks

Airway alternatives for failed or difficult airway
- Surgical cricothyrotomy—contraindicated until age 10 y
- Blind nasotracheal intubation—contraindicated until age 10 y
- Combitube—only if >4 ft tall
- Needle cricothyrotomy—acceptable

- **What are the particular barriers to successful airway management in children?** Time delay and error are associated with the management of children in emergency situations.[1] Pediatric emergencies are complicated by the fact that children vary in size, creating logistical difficulties, especially with respect to drug dosing and equipment selection. This mental burden (or "cognitive load") can be reduced by the use of resuscitation aids which save time and reduce errors. A review analyzed the effect of these variables on the mental burden in the resuscitative process and demonstrated how resuscitation aids can help mitigate their effect.[2] Simulated emergency patient encounters have confirmed that the Broselow–Luten color-coded emergency system reduces time delay and errors by eliminating the cognitive burden associated with these situations.[3]

  To the extent that the process can be simplified (e.g., limiting the number of recommended medications, reducing the complexity and number of decisions required), time is freed up for critical thinking that can then be dedicated to the priorities of airway management. The management of children in extremis can be stressful, and as such, RSI should be kept simple and uncomplicated to reduce this stress.

- **Should I use a nondepolarizing relaxant to defasciculate before using SCh in children?** Defasciculation has been recommended in past editions of this text to attenuate the rise in intracranial pressure (ICP) seen in patients with intracranial pathology. Rapid and atraumatic tracheal intubation is the primary goal for all head-injured trauma patients and minimizing the complexity of RSI by eliminating the defasciculation step contributes positively to this intent. Our view is that the SCh-induced increase in ICP in this setting is not clinically relevant, and that even if there is a modest increase in ICP with SCh, the consequences of poor airway and ventilatory management outweigh any potential benefit. Hypoxia, hypercarbia, the noxious stimulation associated with laryngoscopy, delay in securing airway, and aspiration are much more deleterious than any proven benefit from defasciculation. Defasciculation therapy is therefore not recommended in the emergency setting, and the ICP concerns are not a significant contraindication to SCh.

- **Should atropine be used as a premedication for RSI in children?** The evidence does not support atropine as a universal premedication in children; however, it is an issue that is difficult to definitively resolve based on current literature. Traditionally, atropine has been used to prevent the bradycardia associated with a single dose of SCh in children, a rare, but serious event. A few recent studies failed to show a difference in response to SCh with or without atropine in children,[4,5] with similar numbers in the atropine- and non–atropine-treated groups developing transient, self-limited decreases in heart rate. The absence of evidence of benefit, however, should not be construed as "proof" when dealing with uncommon events. Atropine also has significant, but rare side effects including paradoxical bradycardia if incorrectly dosed.[6] For these reasons, atropine as a "routine" premedication for pediatric RSI is not recommended.

Atropine may have a role when manipulating the airway of infants younger than 1 year because of their disproportionate predominance in vagal tone, coupled with a relatively greater dependency on heart rate for cardiac output.[7] However, most bradycardic episodes are because of hypoxia or are a transient, vagally mediated reflex response that resolves spontaneously. It is better to treat the hypoxia or the reflex if it occurs.

In an effort to keep the process of RSI in children as simple as possible, we are not recommending the routine use of atropine. In special circumstances, such as with infants younger than 1 year (3, 4, and 5 kg, and pink or red zones on the Braselow–Luten tape and airway card), atropine can be considered optional.

- **Should opioids be used as pretreatment medications in children?** There is excellent evidence that premedication with synthetic opioids before direct laryngoscopy and tracheal intubation attenuates the increase in ICP, intraocular pressure, mean arterial pressure, myocardial oxygen consumption, and pulmonary artery pressure caused by this noxious stimulus. The attenuation of the reflex sympathetic response to laryngoscopy and intubation conferred by pretreatment with an opioid is dose dependent and generally requires 3 to 5 minutes for peak effect (fentanyl). During this time, the side effects of a narcotic can be significant (respiratory depression, cough, hypotension, and stiff chest). RSI in an emergency is usually a life-threatening cardiorespiratory event that already has created a stress-induced increase in catechols. For this reason, and because the dosing and administration of small doses of opioids in children is fraught with the potential for overdose, we do not routinely recommend use of opioids *in children* and place more emphasis on induction of general anesthesia and rapid onset of muscle relaxation to create ideal intubating conditions.

- **Should lidocaine be used as a pretreatment medication in children?** Lidocaine has been recommended for children with presumed elevation of ICP (usually resulting from head trauma) to prevent further rises in ICP related to laryngoscopy and intubation.[8] Most of the data for this recommendation, however, is extrapolated from adult studies and nontraumatic elevated ICP situations.

There are no data to support or refute the use of lidocaine in children to prevent or mitigate the reflex bronchospasm related to airway manipulation. Studies related to the use of lidocaine in children to blunt the sympathetic response to intubation are inconsistent.[9,10] We therefore do not recommend the use of lidocaine pretreatment for children younger than 10 years undergoing RSI.

- **SCh versus rocuronium as a paralytic in children—which is the preferred agent?** In the 1990s, the FDA warned against the use of SCh in children following case reports of hyperkalemic cardiac arrest following the administration of SCh to patients with undiagnosed neuromuscular disease. The pediatric anesthesia community at that time challenged the FDA decision on the basis of the risk versus benefit in patients requiring emergency intubation, leading to a modification of their position to a "caution." There is no body of evidence that specifically addresses the relative risks and benefits of SCh versus rocuronium in children to guide recommendations.

Currently, SCh remains the agent of choice for emergency full-stomach intubations.[11,12] Although rocuronium is preferred in pediatrics by some practitioners, for simplicity's sake, we recommend SCh as first-line treatment for adults and children.

- **Are cuffed ETTs contraindicated in pediatric emergency airway management?** The issue of whether cuffed ETTs are safe or required in children younger than 8 to 10 years has been debated for some time because of the anatomical and functional seal afforded by the subglottic area. Two studies have addressed this issue.[13,14] Deakers et al.[13] studied 282 patients intubated in the operating room, emergency department, or ICU. In their observational prospective, nonrandomized study, they found no difference in postextubation stridor, the need for reintubation, or long-term upper airway complications. Khine et al.[14] compared the incidence of postextubation croup, inadequate ventilation, anaesthetic gases leaking into the environment, and the requirement for a tube change resulting from air leak. In this study, of children younger than 8 years, the authors found no difference in croup, more attempts at intubation with uncuffed tubes, less gas flow required with cuffed tubes, or less gas leakage into the environment.

Even though it may seem that the use of cuffed tubes in younger children does not result in any postextubation sequelae, it must be made clear that these studies monitored cuff inflation pressures, a practice that is uncommonly performed in emergency intubations. For this reason, it seems reasonable to recommend the use of uncuffed ETTs to avoid excessive tracheal mucosal pressure with the potential sequelae of scarring and stenosis. However, for some patients in whom high mean airway pressures are expected, such as those with acute respiratory diseases and asthma, the placement of a cuffed tube with the cuff initially deflated, and inflated if necessary, may be appropriate. The most recent Pediatric Advanced Life Support standards[15] recommend cuffed tubes, but with the qualifier *only if leak pressures are monitored.*

- **Why do children desaturate more quickly than adults with comparable degrees of preoxygenation?** An infant uses 6 ml of oxygen/kg/minute as compared with the adult who uses 3 ml/kg/minute. The FRC reduction in an apneic child is far greater than in the apneic adult. This is because of the differences in the elastic forces of the chest wall and the lung. In children, the chest wall is more compliant, and the lung elastic recoil is less than in adults. An analysis of these forces reveals that if they are brought into equilibrium as in the apneic patient, a value of FRC around 10% of total lung capacity is predicted instead of the observed value of slightly <40%. These same factors also reduce the FRC in the spontaneously breathing patient, albeit to a lesser degree. FRC is further reduced with the induction of anesthesia and by the supine position. The clinical implication of the decreased effective FRC combined with increased oxygen consumption is that the preoxygenated, paralyzed infant has a disproportionately smaller store of intrapulmonary oxygen to draw on as compared with the adult. Pulmonary pathology in critically ill patients may further reduce the ability to preoxygenate. It is therefore critical that these factors be considered when preoxygenating a pediatric patient. BMV with cricoid pressure may be required to maintain oxygen saturation above 90% during RSI, especially if multiple attempts are required or the child has a disorder that compromises the ability to preoxygenate.[16,17]

REFERENCES

1. Oakley P. Inaccuracy and delay in decision making in pediatric resuscitation, and a proposed reference chart to reduce error. *Br Med J.* 1988;297:817–819.

2. Luten R, Wears R, Broselow J, et al. Managing the unique size related issues of pediatric resuscitation: reducing cognitive load with resuscitation aids. *Acad Emerg Med.* 2002;9:840–847.

3. Shah AN, Frush KS. Reduction in error severity associated with use of a pediatric medication dosing system: a crossover trial. Presented at the AAP 2001 National Conference and Exhibition, Section on Critical Care; October 2001; San Francisco, CA.

4. McAuliffe G, Bisonnette B, Boutin C. Should the routine use of atropine before succinylcholine in children be reconsidered? *Can J Anaesth.* 1995;42:724–729.

5. Fleming B, McCollough M, Henderson SO. Myth: atropine should be administered before succinylcholine for neonatal and pediatric intubation. *CJEM.* 2005;7:114–117.

6. Tsou CH, Chiang CE, Kao T, et al. Atropine-triggered idiopathic ventricular tachycardia in an asymptomatic pediatric patient. *Can J Anaesth.* 2004;51:856–857.

7. Rothrock SG, Pagane J. Pediatric rapid sequence intubation incidence of reflex bradycardia and effects of pretreatment with atropine. *Pediatr Emerg Care*. 2005;21:637–638.

8. Zaritsky AL, Nadkarni VM, Hickey RW, et al. *PALS Provider Manual*. Dallas, TX: American Heart Association; 2002.

9. Splinter WM. Intravenous lidocaine does not attenuate the haemodynamic response of children to laryngoscopy and tracheal intubation. *Can J Anaesth*. 1990;37(pt 1):440–443.

10. Tanaka K. Effects of intravenous injections of lidocaine on hemodynamics and catecholamine levels during endotracheal intubation in infants and children [in Japanese]. *Aichi Gakuin Daigaku Shigakkai Shi*. 1989;27:345–358.

11. Robinson AL, Jerwood DC, Stokes MA. Routine suxamethonium in children: a regional survey of current usage. *Anaesthesia*. 1996;51:874–878.

12. Weir PS. Anaesthesia for appendicectomy in childhood: a survey of practice in Northern Ireland. *Ulster Med J*. 1997;66:34–37.

13. Deakers TW, Reynolds G, Stretton M, et al. Cuffed endotracheal tubes in pediatric intensive care. *J Pediatr*. 1994;125:57–62.

14. Khine HH, Corddry DH, Kettrick RG, et al. Comparison of cuffed and uncuffed endotracheal tubes in young children during general anesthesia. *Anesthesiology*. 1997;86:627–631.

15. American Heart Association. Pediatric advanced life support. *Circulation*. 2005;112:IV-167–IV-187.

16. Angostoni E, Mead J. Statics of the respiratory system. In: Fenn WO, Rahn H, eds. *Handbook of Physiology*. Washington, DC: American Physiologic Society; 1964.

17. Lumb A. Elastic forces and lung volumes. In: James E. ed. *Nunn's Applied Respiratory Physiology*. 5th ed. Oxford, England: Butterworth-Heineman; 2000:51–53.

25

Pediatric Airway Techniques

Robert C. Luten • Steven A. Godwin

INTRODUCTION

For the most part, the airway devices and techniques used in older children and adolescents are no different from those used in adults. The same cannot be said of small children (younger than 3 years) and infants (younger than 1 year), mostly related to two factors: the airway anatomy in these age groups is substantially different from the adult form, and some of the commonly used rescue devices are not available in pediatric sizes (e.g., Combitube). We limit our discussion to those rescue devices that are available for the pediatric population *and* that have evidence of successful use in children.

Mastering these techniques is straightforward and necessary if one is to manage the emergent pediatric airway. The following discussion describes the appropriate use of the various airway modalities in pediatrics, with emphasis on age appropriateness.

TECHNIQUES USED IN ALL CHILDREN

Bag-mask ventilation and endotracheal intubation

Refer to Chapters 9 and 12 for a detailed description of bag-mask ventilation (BMV) and endotracheal intubation. As in adults, oral and nasopharyngeal airways are important adjuncts to BMV, especially in small children in whom the tongue is relatively large in relation to the volume of the oral cavity. Recommendations and the rationale for the use of specific equipment (curved or straight blades, cuffed vs. uncuffed tubes) are described in Chapter 24. Use of size-appropriate equipment for pediatric airway management is critical to success, even in the most experienced hands. Proper BMV technique is particularly important in pediatric patients because the indication for intervention is most often primarily related to a respiratory disorder, and the child is likely to be hypoxic. In addition, pediatric patients are subject to more rapid oxyhemoglobin desaturation, so that BMV with cricoid pressure (Sellick maneuver) applied is frequently required during the preoxygenation and paralysis phases of rapid sequence intubation. Pediatric BMV requires smaller tidal volumes, higher rates, and size-specific equipment. The pediatric airway is particularly amenable to positive-pressure ventilation, even in the presence of upper airway obstruction (see Chapters 24 and 26).

Tips for successful BMV ventilation in children

Although BMV in the pediatric population fails infrequently, attention to detail remains critical to success: the mask seal must be adequate, the airway open, and the rate and volume of ventilation appropriate to the patient's age. Two errors of technique tend to occur. First, there is a tendency in the excitement of the situation to press the mask portion of the unit downward in an attempt to obtain a tight seal, resulting in neck flexion and upper airway obstruction. The head should be extended slightly rather than flexed thereby relieving, rather than producing, obstruction caused by the tongue and the relaxed pharyngeal anatomy (Fig. 25-1).

Second, there is a tendency to bag at an excessive rate. The cadence for bagging should permit adequate time for exhalation (actually repeating the words "squeeze, release, release" is helpful to assure adequate cadence). Textbooks recommend faster rates for smaller children. From a practical point of view, however, this cadence can be used for all ages. Always place an oral airway in the unconscious child before ventilating with a bag and mask because the pediatric tongue is large relative to the size of the oropharynx and is more prone to obstruct the upper airway.

The positioning described in the previous paragraph is usually obtained while applying the one-handed, C-grip technique to the mask. The thumb and index finger support the mask from the bridge of the nose to the cleft of the chin, avoiding the eyes. The bony prominences of the chin are lifted up by the rest of the fingers, placing the head in mild extension to form the sniffing position. Care is taken to avoid pressure on the airway anteriorly to prevent collapsing and obstructing the pliable trachea.

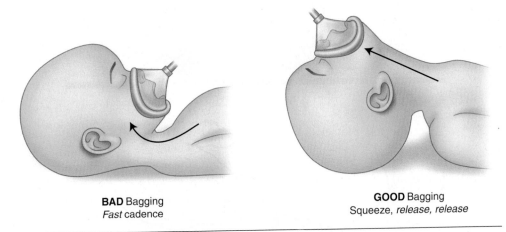

BAD Bagging
Fast cadence

GOOD Bagging
Squeeze, *release, release*

Figure 25-1 ● A: *BAD* Bagging. *Fast cadence.* B: *GOOD* Bagging. Squeeze, *release, release.* Part A demonstrates the flexed position causing obstruction, whereas Part B demonstrates extended position which relieves obstruction.

The two-handed technique can also be used. By opening the jaw slightly and pulling it forward, an obstruction may be relieved. The jaw can be moved further forward after opening the mouth slightly ("translating the mandible" forward; see Chapter 9), while using the thenar eminences of the palm to seal the mask on the face. A second provider squeezes the bag. If ventilation is not immediately facilitated with these maneuvers, positioning should be reassessed and a nasopharyngeal airway be placed to supplement the oropharyngeal airway.

Tips for succesful endotracheal intubation in children

Preintubation

1. Position correctly: Proper positioning of the patient is key to prevent obstruction and provide optimal alignment of the axes of the airway. Optimal alignment of the laryngeal, pharyngeal, and oral axes in adults usually requires elevation of the occiput to flex the neck on the torso and extend the head at the atlanto-occipital joint. Because of the larger relative size of the occiput in small children, elevation of the occiput is usually unnecessary, and extension of the head may actually cause obstruction. Slight anterior displacement of the atlanto-occipital junction is all that is needed (i.e., pulling up on the chin to create the sniffing position). In small infants, elevation of the shoulders with a towel may be needed to counteract the effect of the large occiput that causes the head to flex forward on the chest. As a general rule, once correctly positioned, the external auditory canal should lie just anterior to the shoulders. Whether this position requires support beneath the occiput (older child/adult), the shoulders (small infant), or no support (small child) (Fig. 25-2A) can be determined using this rule of thumb. These are guidelines only, and each individual patient is different. A quick trial to find the optimal position may be of use. Figure 25-2B demonstrates the most common position for intubating the small child, the so-called sniffing position, and how this is achieved in a child of this size.

   Even with optimal positioning, external manipulation of the airway (e.g., backward, upward (cephalad), and rightward pressure maneuver) may increase visualization of the glottis. This may be especially helpful in small children who have anterior airways, and trauma patients who cannot be optimally aligned.

2. Mark lip-to-tip distance with tape: The endotracheal tube (ETT) has centimeter markings along its length. The lip-to-tip distance is the the distance from the lip to a point half way between the vocal cords and the carina (i.e., midtrachea), which represents ideal positioning of the ETT in the trachea. Before a pediatric intubation, the ETT should be marked clearly with

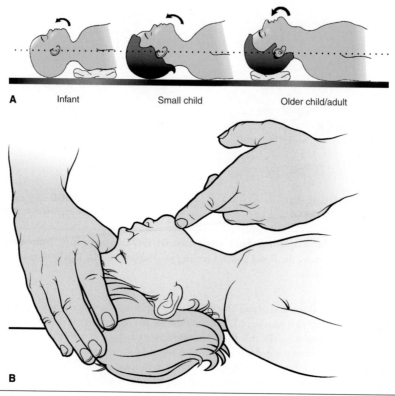

Figure 25-2 ● **A:** Clinical determination of optimal airway alignment, using a line passing through the external auditory canal and anterior to the shoulder **B:** Application of the line to determine optimal position. In this small child, the occiput obviates the need for head support, yet the occiput is not so large as to require support of the shoulders. Note that a line traversing the external auditory canal will pass anterior to the shoulders. With only slight extension of the head on the atlanto-occipital joint, the sniffing position is achieved.

tape at the appropriate lip-to-tip distance. This will serve to orient the intubator to the correct ETT insertion depth for this patient.

Always select one tube size larger and one tube size smaller than the predicted tube size. Note all three tubes are taped at the same predicted lip-to-tip distance. The lip-to-tip distance is constant for a given patient and does not change if a smaller tube or larger tube is used.

As a rule of thumb, three times the chosen ETT size is used to estimate the lip-to-tip distance; for example, for a 3.5-mm ETT, the lip-to-tip distance would be 10.5 cm. Should a smaller tube actually be used because of a traumatized, narrowed glottic opening, recalculation of the lip-to-tip distance using the smaller diameter would result in an incorrect distance.

Direct Laryngoscopy

1. Look up and not more deeply: The pediatric airway lies higher in the neck than the adult airway. When doing direct laryngoscopy, the visual line of sight angle must be adjusted so that the intubator can *look up* to see the glottic opening. Physicians who rarely intubate children, and who fail to make this adjustment, may have trouble visualizing the glottic opening in children.

2. Use a stylet: The pediatric ETT is smaller and more pliable than the larger adult tubes. Therefore, a stylet should be used for all pediatric intubations.

3. Enter from the side: As in the adult, passing the ETT down the center of one's line of sight obliterates the target (the glottis). Entering from the side of the mouth with the ETT permits one to keep the target in view at all times. This maneuver is probably more important in children than in adults as the field of view is smaller in children.

4. Use the maxilla to stabilize your hand after passing the ETT: The thumb of the right hand naturally contacts the mandible during this procedure. It should be stabilized and maintained in that position, holding the tube to prevent movement until it is secured.

Postintubation

Inadvertent extubation is a frequent, but entirely avoidable, complication. ETTs must be secured at the lip to prevent in and out slippage, and head movement, which translates to ETT movement, must also be prevented. Flexion of the neck causes the tube to move further down into the airway, whereas neck extension causes the tube to move up and out of the trachea. This effect is most marked in the younger child with a proportionally larger occiput. Securing the ETT at the lip is traditionally done by taping the tube to the maxilla to prevent the tube from slipping in or out. Adequate securing of the ETT with tape requires experience. An alternative to taping is the application of various commercial ETT holder devices.

Application of a cervical collar prevents the flexion and extension movements of the neck and maintains ETT position in the trachea, preventing inadvertent extubation.

BMV and cricoid pressure

Although the value of cricoid pressure in preventing aspiration during intubation is dubious, cricoid pressure prevents gastric insufflation with BMV, even with ventilation pressures >40 cm H_2O. This is especially important in infants, in whom gastric distention may compromise ventilation and increase the risk of aspiration.

Positive-pressure relief valves (also known as "pop-off" valves)—the good and the bad

A pop-off valve is designed to prevent the delivery of excessive pressure to the lower airway and limit the risk of barotrauma. These valves are incorporated in infant and pediatric resuscitation bags by most manufacturers. The relief valve opens at a preset peak airway pressure (usually 20 to 45 cm water pressure) limiting the peak pressure that can be delivered to the lungs. However, in the face of upper airway obstruction, increased airway resistance, or decreased pulmonary compliance, higher pressures may be required. In situations such as these, the operator should disable the valve.

In addition to the pop-off valve, many manufacturers incorporate manometers into the unit so that one can monitor peak airway pressures as they perform BMV. A leak at the site of the manometer port may interfere with one's ability to achieve airway pressures sufficient to effect adequate gas exchange.

Even though troubleshooting inadequate BMV starts with evaluating the adequacy of mask seal and assessing airway patency, the performance of a "leak test" immediately before beginning BMV will establish the status of the pop-off valve and test for a leak at the manometer site (or other parts of the unit). The leak test is performed by removing the mask from the bag, occluding the mask port with the palm of one hand, and squeezing the bag with the other hand. If the bag remains tight, no escape of gas, or "leak," has occurred. If the bag does not remain tight, gas is escaping from the system somewhere, most commonly from the pop-off valve or the manometer port, although other causes of the leak may be present. The pressure leakage from an open manometer port occurs immediately on compressing the bag as opposed to the open pop-off valve, which vents only once the preset pressure is exceeded. The amount of volume lost will vary, depending on the size of the leak. This test is also useful for screening adult bags for malfunctions and leaks. After a negative test (i.e., the bag remains tight with squeezing), the port occluding palm hand should be released, and the bag squeezed to confirm that gas escapes properly from the inspiratory limb of the bag.

Laryngeal mask airways

The laryngeal mask airway (LMA) is a safe and effective airway management device for children undergoing general anesthesia and is considered a rescue option in the event of a failed airway in children and infants. Placement of the LMA in children is a relatively easily learned skill, particularly if the correct size of mask is chosen. The LMA has also been used successfully in difficult pediatric airways and should be considered as an alternative device for emergency airway management in these patients (e.g., Pierre Robin deformity). As in the adult, difficult pediatric intubations have also been facilitated by the use of the LMA in combination with such devices as the bronchoscope.

The LMA has a few important associated complications, which are especially prevalent in smaller infants, including partial airway obstruction by the epiglottis, loss of adequate seal with patient movement, and air leakage with positive-pressure ventilation. To avoid obstruction by the epiglottis in these younger children and infants, some authors have suggested a rotational placement technique in which the mask is inserted through the oral cavity "upside-down" and then rotated 180° as it is advanced into the hypopharynx. The LMA is contraindicated in the pediatric patient or adult with intact protective airway reflexes, and, therefore, is not suitable for awake airway management unless the patient is adequately sedated and the airway is topically anesthetized. LMA use is also contraindicated if foreign body aspiration is present or suspected because it may aggravate an already desperate situation and is likely to fail to provide adequate ventilation and oxygenation because the obstruction is distal to the device. The LMA comes in multiple sizes to accommodate children from neonate to adolescent.

Needle cricothyrotomy

Although virtually every textbook chapter, article, or lecture on pediatric airway management refers to the technique of needle cricothyrotomy as the recommended last-resort rescue procedure, there is little literature to support its use and safety. Few of the "experts" who write about needle cricothyrotomy have experience performing the procedure on live humans. Newer devices, such as the LMA and others, may further reduce the rare need for needle cricothyrotomy, but nevertheless, any clinician who manages pediatric emergencies as part of his or her practice must be familiar with the procedure and its indications, and must have the appropriate equipment readily accessible in the emergency department.

Needle cricothyrotomy is indicated as a life-saving, last-resort procedure children younger than 8 to 10 years who present or progress to the "can't intubate, can't oxygenate" scenario and whose obstruction is proximal to glottic opening. The classic indication is epiglottitis where BMV and intubation are judged to have failed (although true failure of BMV is rare in epiglottitis, and failure is more often caused by a failure of technique than by a truly insurmountable obstruction). Other indications include facial trauma, angioedema, and other conditions that preclude access to the glottic opening from above. Needle cricothyrotomy is rarely helpful in patients who have aspirated a foreign body that cannot be visualized by direct laryngoscopy because these foreign bodies are usually in the lower airway. It would also be of questionable value in the patient with croup because the obstruction is subglottic. In these patients, the obstruction is more likely to be bypassed by an ETT introduced orally into the trachea with a stylet, than blindly by needle cricothyrotomy.

Various commercially available needles are also available for percutaneous needle cricothyrotomy as well (Table 25-1). The simplest equipment, appropriate for use in infants, consists of the following:

- 14G over-the-needle catheter
- 3.0-mm ETT adapter
- 3- or 5-ml syringe

It is a good practice to preassemble the kit, place it in a clear bag, seal the bag, and tape it in an accessible place in the resuscitation area.

TABLE 25-1
Recommended Commercial Catheters

These catheters are available commercially and can be used as an option:

Jet ventilation catheter (Ravussin). Sizes 13G and 14G, not the 16G catheter. Although listed as jet ventilation catheters, we recommend them only for use with bag-mask ventilation. http://www.hospitecnica.com.mx/productos/VBMventilator%20jet.pdf

6F Cook Emergency Transtracheal Airway Catheters. They are available in two sizes, 5 and 7.5 cm. We only recommend the 5-cm catheter. http://www.cookmedical.com/cc/dataSheet. do?id=1307

Procedure

Place the child in the supine position with the head extended over a towel under the shoulder. This forces the trachea anteriorly such that it is easily palpable and can be stabilized with two fingers of one hand. The key to success is strict immobilization of the trachea throughout the procedure. The following statement appears in many textbooks describing this procedure: "Carefully palpate the cricothyroid membrane." In reality, it is difficult to do this in an infant and is not essential. Indeed, in smaller children, it may be impossible to precisely locate the cricothyroid membrane, so the proximal trachea is often accessed. The priority is an airway and provision of oxygen. Complications from inserting the catheter elsewhere into the trachea besides the cricothyroid membrane are addressed later. Consider the trachea as one would a large vein, and cannulate it with the catheter-over-needle device directed caudad at a 30° angle. Aspirate air to ensure tracheal entry, and then slide the catheter gently off the needle, removing the needle. Attach the 3.0-mm ETT adapter to the hub of the catheter and commence bag ventilation. The provider will note exaggerated resistance to bagging. This is normal and is related to the small diameter of the catheter and the turbulence created by ventilating through it. It is not generally the result of a misplaced catheter or poor lung compliance secondary to pneumothorax. It is helpful to practice BMV through a catheter to experience the feel of the significantly increased resistance. The operator must be vigilant that expiration also occurs by watching for the chest to fall after inspiration, ordinarily through the patient's glottis and not through the catheter.

The required pressures are well above the limits of the pop-off valve; therefore, it must be disabled in order to permit gas flow through the catheter. Jet ventilation has also been advocated, although extreme caution must be exercised to prevent barotrauma. Jet ventilation should be considered only by those familiar with its use and in children older than 5 to 6 years. However, even in this age group, if adequate oxygen saturation can be maintained with bag mask ventilation, this is preferable to jet ventilation. If jet ventilation is used, the ventilator must have a pressure control valve system. Start with low pressure (20), and titrate to adequate chest rise and fall and oxygen saturation, using exceedingly brief bursts of ventilation while observing chest rise, followed by sufficient exhalation time again judged by watching the chest fall. Percutaneous needle ventilation techniques are contraindicated in patients with complete upper airway obstruction.

TECHNIQUES USED IN ADOLESCENTS AND ADULTS

Blind nasotracheal intubation

Nasotracheal intubation in children is uniformly discouraged and is frequently considered contraindicated. This recommendation is based on the fact that the sharp angle of the nasopharynx and pharyngotracheal axis in children precludes a reasonable likelihood of success with this technique when performed blindly. A second reason is that children are at increased risk for hemorrhage because of the preponderance of highly vascular and delicate adenoidal tissue. The direct visualization technique is, however, commonly used in small infants and children for chronic ventilator management in the intensive care unit setting. Using direct visualization with a laryngoscope once the ETT has passed into the oro- and hypopharynx, tracheal placement is aided with Magill forceps. However, this technique is not helpful in emergency airway management. In general, the technique of blind nasotracheal intubation, which is essentially the same as that described for adults has few, if any, primary indications in pediatric emergency airway management, and in any case, is not recommended for patients younger than 10 years.

Combitube

The Combitube represents an excellent, easily learned rescue airway device that is available only for patients of height >48 in, so is of limited application in pediatric emergency airway management.

Surgical cricothyrotomy

The cricothyroid membrane in small infants and children is minimally developed (Fig. 25-3). Surgical or cricothyrotome-based cricothyrotomy should not be attempted in children younger than 10 years, except in extraordinary circumstances. In children younger than 10 years, needle cricothyrotomy with BMV is recommended. As with adults, adolescents may have easily identifiable and accessible anatomy, and, therefore, cricothyrotomy may be a reasonable rescue technique in this age group. Cricothyrotomy using a commercially available kit (Pedi-trake) has not been shown to be successful or even safe. Box 25-1 summarizes recommendations for invasive airway procedures in children.

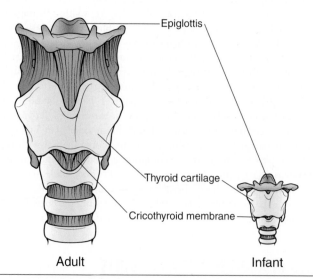

Figure 25-3 ● Cricothyroid Membrane. Comparative size of the adult **(left)** versus pediatric **(right)** cricothyroid membrane. Note that not only is the larynx smaller, but also the actual membrane is smaller proportionately in comparison, involving one-fourth to one-third the anterior tracheal circumference versus two-thirds to three-fourths in the adult. This pediatric drawing is that of a toddler, which accommodates a 4.5-mm ETT.

Box 25-1. Summary Recommendations for Invasive Airway Procedures in Children

---

5 years old
Needle cricothyrotomy and bag ventilation

5–10 years old
Consider needle cricothyrotomy and bag ventilation[a]
Percutaneous Seldinger technique and bag ventilation
(TTJV regulated to low PSI is discouraged unless done by experienced operator)

>10 years
Operator preference
Needle cricothyrotomy with TTJV *or* surgical cricothyrotomy

---

[a]There is less evidence to support this recommendation in this age group; however, it may be the only available option and should be converted to a more definitive airway.

EVIDENCE

- **Does a needle cricothyrotomy with BMV in children provide sufficient oxygenation and ventilation to avoid hypoxia and hypercarbia?** The evidence surrounding pediatric needle cricothyrotomy is based on an animal study by Cote et al.[1] using a 30-kg dog model. Cote was able to demonstrate that dogs representative in size of a 9- to 10-year-old child could be oxygenated through a 12G catheter and 3.0 ETT adapter with a bag for at least 1 hour (the study duration). Rises in $PaCO_2$ levels were noted, but were not believed to be significant because children normally tolerate mild degrees of hypercarbia well.[1]

  One adult retrospective study reported that 48 patients were successfully oxygenated and ventilated using transtracheal ventilation through a 13G intratracheal catheter for up to 360 minutes. Transtracheal jet ventilation (TTJV) was used primarily in 47 of these patients, although 6 patients did receive conventional bagging measures until TTJV circuits could be initiated. During manual transtracheal ventilation, each patient demonstrated increases in $PaCO_2$ on blood gases but maintained PaO_2 values >100 mm Hg.[2]

- **Should the LMA be considered as both a rescue device and an alternative airway in the management of difficult emergency pediatric airways?** Most of the literature regarding the use of LMAs in children has been compiled from the anesthesia experience in the operating room. Therefore, little information is available for the use of the LMA in the acute emergency setting. However, an observational study by Lopez-Gil et al.[3,4] has demonstrated that the skill for placement of the LMA could be rapidly learned by anesthesia residents with a low complication rate. Published case reports have demonstrated success of the LMA in the pediatric patient with difficult airways, including isolated severe retrognathia, Dandy-Walker syndrome, and Pierre Robin syndrome.[5,6]

  At least one prospective study reports a higher incidence of airway obstruction, higher ventilatory pressures, larger inspiratory leaks, and more complications in smaller children (those weighing <10 kg) with LMA use than in the older child. These authors recommend that the risk–benefit should be carefully weighed in younger children before using the LMA with paralysis and positive-pressure ventilation. Importantly, the success rate for placement of the LMA in this study that was performed in elective cases undergoing prolonged ventilation was high at 98%.[7] Although airway managers should be aware of these potential complications, this study is not generalizable to the emergency setting and should not deter providers from implementing this as a *rescue device* in infants or young children with failed airways, or as a planned approach to an infant or young child with an identified difficult airway. In the failed airway situation, the LMA may be a lifesaving bridge, providing effective oxygenation and ventilation until a definitive airway can be secured.

REFERENCES

1. Cote CJ, Eavey RD, Todres ID, et al. Cricothyroid membrane puncture: oxygenation and ventilation in a dog model using an intravenous catheter. *Crit Care Med*. 1988;16:615–619.

2. Ravussin P, Freeman J. A new transtracheal catheter for ventilation and resuscitation. *Can Anaesth Soc J*. 1985;32:60–64.

3. Lopez-Gil M, Brimacombe J, Alvarez M. Safety and efficacy of the laryngeal mask airway: a prospective survey of 1,400 children. *Anaesthesia*. 1996;51:969–972.

4. Lopez-Gil M, Brimacombe J, Cebrian J, et al. Laryneal mask airway in pediatric practice: a prospective study of skill acquisition by anesthesia residents. *Anesthesiology*. 1996;84:807–811.

5. Selim M, Mowafi H, Al-Ghamdi A, et al. Intubation via LMA in pediatric patients with difficult airways. *Can J Anaesth*. 1999;46:891–893.

6. Stocks RM, Egerman R, Thompson JW, et al. Airway management of the severely retrognathic child: use of the laryngeal mask airway. *Ear Nose Throat J*. 2002;81:223–226.

7. Park C, Bahk JH, Ahn WS, et al. The laryngeal mask airway in infants and children. *Can J Anaesth*. 2001;48:413–417.

26

The Difficult Pediatric Airway

Joshua Nagler • Robert C. Luten

OVERVIEW

Age-related anatomic and physiologic differences in the normal infant or small child can make airway management challenging. However, these differences can be anticipated and addressed in most pediatric patients as discussed in Chapter 24. The *difficult* pediatric airway, as in adults, is defined by historical or physical examination attributes that predict challenges with mask ventilation, laryngoscopy, or intubation. In the pediatric population, most of these cases result either from acute insults that modify normal airway anatomy or from known congenital abnormalities. Difficulty revealed only after unsuccessful attempts at airway management, or a *failed* pediatric airway, is rare in children.

The approach to the emergent difficult airway in the adult patient is described in Chapters 2 and 3, which should be read before this chapter. The same concepts of anticipation and planning are also applicable in children. The use of rapid, easy to remember, and sensitive tools to identify patients with potential difficulty is paramount. Children differ from adults, however, with regard to which predictors of difficulty are most common (see Table 26-1). For example, age-dependent features (e.g., beards, and age >55 years) and progressive disease processes (e.g., cervical rheumatoid arthritis) are less applicable in children. However, using LEMON to look for abnormal facial features and assessing for signs of obstructive airway disease will be of high yield (see Table 26-2). The majority of children with difficult airways, however, will present with recognizable disease processes or with known congenital abnormalities associated with airway difficulty. Therefore, this chapter will focus on these common etiologies of difficult pediatric airways and offer management strategies.

COMMON CAUSES OF DIFFICULT AIRWAYS IN CHILDREN

Causes of difficult airways in children can be categorized into four groups:

1. Acute infectious causes
2. Acute noninfectious causes
3. Congenital anomalies
4. No known abnormality, with unexpected difficulty

TABLE 26-1
A Sample Comparison of Pediatric and Adult Risk Factors

A. Risk factors for adult difficult airway usually not present in infants and young children:
  1. Obesity
  2. Decreased neck mobility (not including immobilization following trauma)
  3. Teeth abnormalities
  4. Temporomandibular joint problems
  5. Beards
B. Risk factors for pediatric difficult airway not present in adults:
  1. Small airway caliber susceptible to obstruction from edema or infection
  2. Discomfort secondary to dealing with age- and size-related variables
  3. Discomfort secondary to infrequency of patient encounters

TABLE 26-2
Key Features in Applying the LEMON Assessment in Children

Look	• Gestalt is the most important predictor of airway difficulty in children
	• Presence of dysmorphic features are associated with abnormal airway anatomy and may predict difficulty
	• Small mouth, large tongue, recessed chin, and major facial trauma are usually immediately apparent
Evaluate (3:3:2)	• Has not been tested in children
	• May be difficult to perform in an uncooperative child, or infant with a "pudgy" neck
	• Gross assessment of mouth opening, jaw size, and larynx position may be utilized instead
	• If 3:3:2 assessment is performed, use the child's not the provider's fingers
Mallampati	• Cooperation may be an issue
	• Mixed data in children (see "Evidence" Section)
Obstruction Obesity	• Airway obstruction is a relatively frequent indication for airway management in children
	• Second to the gestalt *Look*, assessing for obstruction is perhaps the most fruitful step in identifying difficulty airways in children
	• A focused, disease-specific history and physical examination (voice change, drooling, stridor, and retractions) can accurately identify children with acute or chronic upper airway obstructive pathology
	• Obesity is a growing epidemic in children, although the impact on the pediatric airway is less significant than in adults
Neck	• Limited positioning in immobilized pediatric trauma patients is similar to adults
	• Intrinsic cervical spine immobility from congenital abnormalities is very rare, and acquired conditions (e.g., ankylosing spondylitis and cervical rheumatoid arthritis) are essentially nonexistent in young children

Difficult Airways Secondary to Acute Infectious Causes

Examples of acute infectious processes that alter an otherwise normal anatomy include the following:

- Epiglottitis
- Croup
- Bacterial tracheitis
- Retropharyngeal abscess
- Ludwig's angina

Epiglottitis is the classic paradigm for an acute infectious process causing a difficult airway. Although disease incidence has declined dramatically since the introduction of the *Haemophilus influenzae* type b (Hib) vaccine, cases continue to be reported secondary to vaccine failures or alternative bacterial etiologies, most commonly gram-positive cocci.[1] Progressive edema and swelling of the epiglottis and surrounding structures can quickly lead to proximal airway obstruction. Despite the rarity of this diagnosis, hospitals should have protocols in place to rapidly summon anesthesia and surgical personnel for any child with a concerning presentation. Agitation of children with epiglottitis can increase turbulent flow and aggravate airway obstruction. Ideally airway evaluation and intervention should occur in the controlled setting of an operating room where equipment and staff are available for rigid bronchoscopy and surgical airway management as needed. However, if a child deteriorates, attempts at bag-mask ventilation (BMV), direct laryngoscopy and endotracheal intubation may be necessary in the emergency department (ED). If these efforts are unsuccessful, needle cricothyrotomy (see Chapter 25) can be life-saving. Epiglottitis represents the prototype indication for an invasive airway, bypassing the proximal obstruction and allowing oxygenation and ventilation through the patent trachea.

Croup is a common reason for children to present to the ED with airway compromise. Although commonly grouped with epiglottitis, croup is usually a clinically distinct entity (see Table 26-3). Respiratory distress is common, as subglottic airway narrowing can have a profound effect on airway resistance on the smaller diameter trachea in children (see Table 26-4). However, croup patients are rarely toxic appearing. Fortunately, patients with croup respond well to nebulized epinephrine and steroids, and intubation is rarely required. If patients present in extremis or medical therapy fails, bagging may be difficult given the increased airway resistance, however visualization during laryngoscopy is not usually affected.

Importantly, if a child with croup is ill enough to require intubation, a smaller endotracheal tube (ETT) should be used because the narrowed subglottis may not accommodate age- or length-predicted ETT size. It is important to remember, however, that the ETT insertion distance (i.e., lip-to-tip distance) is not affected despite using a smaller-sized tube. Therefore, while length-based references such as a Broselow–Luten tape will remain accurate, formulaic calculation based on the tube diameter (i.e., three times ETT size) should be based on the age appropriate sized ETT, not the downsized tube.

Bacterial tracheitis has become a leading cause of respiratory failure from acute upper airway infections.[2] As in croup, inflammation in tracheitis is subglottic, although affected children tend to be older and often more ill appearing. Airway management is similar to croup. Again, visualization is rarely compromised; however, a smaller ETT size should be used. In addition, given the presence of thick purulent secretions within the trachea, patients with tracheitis will require vigilant monitoring for tube obstruction.

Retropharyngeal abscess rarely presents with airway compromise, although it is frequently included in the differential diagnosis of acute life-threatening upper airway obstruction. These patients most commonly present with odynophagia and neck stiffness. Lateral neck films reveal thickening of the retropharyngeal space. Most of these patients respond to antibiotics, although in some patients, drainage in the operating room is required. Rarely, if ever, is it necessary to actively manage the airway of these patients in the ED. If the obstruction is large enough to require emergent airway intervention, it is important to remember that placement of an extraglottic device may not be feasible, and alternative backup approaches should be considered.

Ludwig's angina. is an exceedingly rare pediatric diagnosis and unlikely to require emergency airway management in the ED. If encountered, difficulty with displacement of the tongue into the inflamed submandibular space should be anticipated, and approaches other than direct laryngoscopy should be readily available.

Difficult Airways Secondary to Noninfectious Processes

- Foreign body
- Burns
- Anaphylaxis and angioedema
- Trauma

Foreign body aspiration is perhaps the most feared pediatric airway problem. Therefore, the approach to the child with airway compromise from foreign body aspiration has earned a full discussion in Chapter 27.

Patients with upper airway burns or inhalational injuries can be identified by soot in the mouth, carbonaceous sputum, singed nasal hair, or facial burns. Caustic ingestions may show facial or oropharyngeal mucosal injury. If upper airway edema has already occurred, patients may have drooling, hoarseness, or frank stridor. In contrast to processes like croup that commonly improve with medical therapy, patients with significant mucosal injury or edema predictably worsen over time. Therefore, intubation should occur as early as possible as progressive edema will make visualization

TABLE 26-3
Management of the "Most-Feared" Pediatric Airway Problems

Disease	Pathology and deterioration	Approach	FB removal maneuvers	BMV two-person techniques	Intubation	Needle cricothyrotomy
Epiglottitis	Rapidly progressing disease process affecting the supraglottic structures (epiglottis and aryepiglottic folds). Patients are usually ill-appearing, although they may be in minimal distress Decompensation can occur: 1. When a patient is stimulated or manipulated, leading to dynamic airway obstruction 2. As a result of progressive deterioration over time secondary to fatigue, although the respiratory arrest may occur precipitously	Stable → observe → OR for defin airway Decompensation: BMV → intubation → Failed Airway: needle cricothyroidotomy needle cricothyrotomy Horton	Not indicated	Effective in *most* patients who deteriorate Technique: A two-handed seal, with another rescuer providing sufficient pressure to overcome the obstruction	Usually successful. Use tube size 1 mm smaller. Use stylet. Suction, visualize, press on chest, and look for bubble	The paradigm indication for needle cricothyrotomy *if* BMV and intubation are unsuccessful

(continued)

TABLE 26-3
Management of the "Most-Feared" Pediatric Airway Problems (continued)

Disease	Pathology and deterioration	Approach	FB removal maneuvers	BMV two-person techniques	Intubation	Needle cricothyrotomy
Croup	Slowly progressive (hours to days) disease process affecting the subglottic trachea, causing dynamic inspiratory augmented obstruction. Deterioration is usually progressive rather than sudden and related to respiratory muscle fatigue, although as in the case of epiglottis, the arrest may also occur precipitously	Stridor at rest → racemic epi and steroids Persistent distress → ICU decompensation → BMV → Intubation	Not indicated	Effective. Positive pressure overcomes obstruction by acting as a stent. May require high pressures	Proximal airway normal; therefore, should not be problematic. Consider ETT one size smaller and use stylet	Not indicated because obstruction is distal to cricothyroid membrane
FB aspiration (see Chapter 27)	Patients with aspirated FBs have the potential for decompensation secondary to acute airway obstruction. The level of obstruction may vary from the hypopharynx, above or below the glottis, to the mainstem bronchus	Stable → observe → transfer for removal Decompensation FB removal maneuvers → Direct visualization and removal with Magill forceps → Intubation to force FB distally into mainstem bronchus	Indicated if *appropriate* (i.e., patient completely obstructs)	Should not be used before attempts to remove FB. May be obviated by intubation	Last resort in an effort to push FB distally into mainstem bronchus	Usually not indicated because FB will be distal to the obstruction if other efforts have failed

FB, foreign body; BMV, bag-mask ventilation; OR, operating room; epi, epinephrine; ICU, intensive care unit; ETT, endotracheal tube.

TABLE 26-4 Effect of 1-mm Edema on Airway Resistance		
	Change in cross-sectional area	Change in resistance
Infant	44% decrease	200% increase
Adult	25% decrease	40% increase

These figures reflect the quietly breathing infant or adult. If the child cries, the work of breathing is increased 32-fold. This underscores the principle of maintaining children in a quiet, nonthreatening, and comfortable environment during evaluation and in preparation for management.

and tube passage dramatically more difficult over time (see Table 26-6). Succinylcholine may be used during rapid sequence intubation (RSI) as the risk of hyperkalemia from burns occurs after 5 days. Cuffed ETTs are recommended to accommodate the changes in airway edema over the natural course of recovery.[3] Laryngeal mask airways (LMAs) may not pass easily, and therefore may be less reliable as a rescue device, so surgical airway equipment should be readily available.

Anaphylaxis and angioedema also cause progressive edema in the tongue, supraglottic structures, and the larynx. The goal is always to use aggressive medical therapy to limit progression. However, patients with compromised airways secondary to anaphylactic or anaphylactoid reactions (e.g., angioedema) who do not rapidly respond to medical treatment require early intervention. As with inhalation injuries a backup airway management plan should be immediately available.

Trauma poses unique challenges in the management of the pediatric airway. Facial trauma can impede an effective mask seal, limit mouth opening, or result in blood or secretions in the oropharynx making visualization difficult. Avulsed teeth, blood, vomitus, or other foreign material can obstruct the airway. Expanding hematoma or displaced bony injuries can impede direct laryngoscopy. Primary neck trauma can distort anatomy or injure the larynx and trachea and risk complete airway compromise during intervention. Finally, the risk of cervical spine injury requires maintenance of immobilization, which affects the ability to position the patient for optimal visualization and intubation. Despite these challenges, the majority of pediatric trauma patients who require airway intervention will be managed with RSI and direct laryngoscopy for intubation. Significant trauma may limit the utility of an LMA. Therefore, simultaneous preparation for a surgical airway should be performed as a backup airway plan.

Difficult Airways Secondary to Congenital Anomalies

Patients with difficult airways secondary to congenital anomalies receive the most attention in discussions of difficult airways in pediatrics. However, they are encountered much less frequently than acute insults to airways described previously. The literature concerning these patients usually describes elective situations, managed by experienced pediatric anesthesiology subspecialists in well-equipped operating rooms using elaborate techniques performed under controlled conditions. This information is not relevant to the management of the airway if these children present emergently.

Oftentimes, patients with congenital anomalies presenting to the ED require intubation for reasons unrelated to their difficult airway (e.g., a child with Pierre Robin syndrome with respiratory failure secondary to asthma). The best approach for these patients, time permitting, is to obtain expert subspecialty assistance as early as possible and, as with all patients, to aggressively manage the medical condition to try to obviate the need for invasive airway management.

There are a range of anatomic abnormalities and named syndromes that predict difficulty with pediatric airway management. It is impractical and unnecessary to commit all to memory. Instead, common findings can be categorized into four groups, which can be identified using the

LEMON assessment (see Table 26-2). These include a small chin (micrognathic mandible), a large tongue, a small or limited-opening mouth, and a neck that is either short or immobile.

The micrognathic mandible is the most common anatomical feature in the child rendering intubation difficult. The small mandible reduces the available space (mandibular space) into which the tongue and submandibular tissue must be compressed with the laryngoscope blade to visualize the glottic opening (see Fig. 26-1). A significantly recessed (micrognathic) mandible can be recognized by drawing a line that touches the forehead and maxilla and continues inferiorly (Fig. 26-2). In a patient with grossly normal anatomy, the line also touches the tip of the chin. In the micrognathic patient, a gap between the line and the tip of the chin is observed. A relatively large tongue can have a similar effect, with limited room for displacement given its mass and resultant obstruction of the direct view of the glottis.

Similarly, a mouth that is small or does not open fully can make laryngoscopy difficult. The ability to place appropriately sized equipment into the oral cavity and to create a direct line of sight to the laryngeal structures can be compromised.

Restricted neck movement can also make it challenging to align the oral axis with the pharyngeal and tracheal axes, making sufficient direct visualization possible. A short neck exaggerates the acuity of the angle around the tongue toward the glottis, which can make laryngoscopy and/or passage of an ETT difficult.

In patients with known or newly identified anatomic abnormalities as described above, the difficult airway algorithm should be used. The airway approach in these patients might include an awake (sedated) look to assess the degree to which the mouth can be opened, the tongue can be

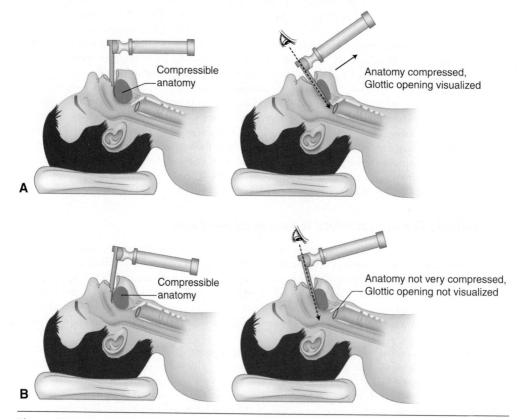

Figure 26-1 ● **A:** A normal-sized mandible provides room for the tongue and associated tissue to be compressed into the mandibular space by the laryngoscope blade, allowing visualization of the glottic opening. **B:** A small mandible cannot easily accommodate the tongue, which therefore remains in the line of sight of the laryngoscopist.

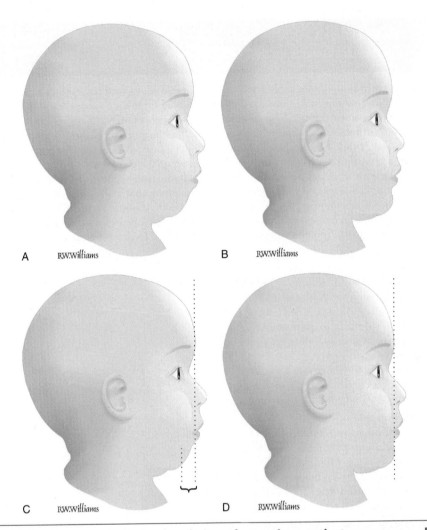

Figure 26-2 ● It may not always be obvious that a given patient possesses a difficult airway. Micrognathia (A) may not be readily apparent unless compared to a normal child. (B) In the normal patient, a line drawn from the forehead, touching the anterior maxilla, also will touch the chin. (D). Failure to do so indicates a degree of micrognathia ©. (Extrapolated from Frankville D. *ASA Refresher Course.* Parkridge, IL: American Society of Anesthesiologists; 2001:126.)

displaced into the mandibular space, or the larynx can be viewed with limited neck positioning. If the awake look suggests passage of an ETT is likely to be difficult, neuromuscular blockade and RSI might be avoided or postponed until backup strategies are in place. Other potential approaches are reviewed throughout this book, and summarized in Table 26-5.

For patients in extremis or in crash situations, the clinician is left with no other options than those used in other patients. Fortunately, even when difficulty is predicted, straightforward approaches such as BMV or endotracheal intubation are usually successful and should remain the mainstay of therapy.

No Known Abnormality, with Unexpected Difficulty

Perhaps the greatest fear for most practitioners is to encounter unexpected difficulty after initiating airway management in a child *without* recognized congenital or acquired abnormalities.

TABLE 26-5
Therapeutic Options for the Difficult Airway

The difficult airway algorithm applies to both children and adults with few exceptions; most notably, blind nasotracheal intubation is contraindicated in children younger than 10 years, as is surgical cricothyrotomy. Most children will not be cooperative with an awake, nonsedated look. Combitube, a useful adjunct in adults, is not manufactured for patients <48 in (122 cm) tall. Otherwise, the same approach and options are recommended for both children and adults, the only difference being that they are required less frequently

There are a variety of airway devices for use in the pediatric patient. However, developing and maintaining competency is challenging with infrequent use, particularly in emergencies and by emergency practitioners. It is therefore probably best to choose a smaller number of options, but aim to gain the maximum experience with them. The following devices and procedures are listed according to appropriateness in different levels of clinical acuity

Crash situation
Noninvasive
    Endotracheal (ET) intubation (infancy to adulthood)
    LMA (infancy to adulthood)
    Combitube (>48 in [122 cm] tall)
    King LT (infancy to adulthood)
    Video laryngoscopy (infancy to adulthood)
Invasive
    Needle cricothyrotomy[a] (<5+ years)
    Seldinger cricothyrotomy[a] (>5 years)
    Surgical cricothyrotomy (>10 years)

Stable situation
  ET intubation (awake) (adolescents to adulthood)
  ET intubation (RSI) (infancy to adulthood)
  LMA (infancy to adulthood)
  Fiberoptic intubation (infancy to adulthood)
  Blind nasotracheal intubation (>10 years)
  Video laryngoscopy (infancy to adulthood)

Stable expectant management patients
All EDs should have a plan in place for managing patients with disorders such as foreign body aspiration, epiglottitis, etc. This usually requires prior agreement of consultants willing to respond immediately to those emergencies

[a]There are no published data to support the best means of ventilation in children following needle cricothyrotomy. Both transtracheal jet ventilation (TTJV) and BMV have been recommended. However, with no clear supporting data, and a high risk of barotraumas and complications related to TTJV, we suggest practitioners utilize BMV with conversion to a more definitive airway as soon as possible. If a cricothyrotomy catheter has been placed (by Seldinger or surgical technique) BMV should be used.

Fortunately, these circumstances are very uncommon. The anesthesia literature suggests that the incidence of *unanticipated* difficult intubation, using large sample sizes from the operating room is vanishlingly low, a refelection of the infrequency of difficult airways, but also of the ability of practitioners to use systematic strategies to effectively identify those patients with difficulty. The management approaches for the *unexpected* pediatric difficult airway are similar to those for the expected difficult airway (see Table 26-5).

TABLE 26-6
Timing of Intervention According to Anticipated Clinical Course

Expectant intervention group: Intervene *only* if deterioration occurs:
1. Assemble subspecialty multidisciplinary team for definitive management:
   Foreign body
   Epiglottitis
2. Obtain subspecialty assistance if deterioration appears likely:
   Para-airway *diagnoses* (diseases such as retropharyngeal or peritonsillar abscess or Ludwig's angina that are usually stable on presentation and deterioration is uncommon)

Early intervention group: Intervene *early* (preventively):
   Burns
   Anaphylaxis: usually responds to medical treatment; anaphylactoid-like reactions such as angioedema respond less reliably to medical treatment
   Trauma

TIMING THE INTERVENTION

As is the case for adults, the anticipated clinical course of the presenting condition becomes a key determinant in the decision whether to actively intervene in the airway or to observe the patient for possible deterioration. Table 26-6 groups disorders from both infectious and noninfectious causes according to timing of intervention based on anticipated clinical course. The expectant intervention group represents patients in whom the intervention itself may be more hazardous than a period of close observation, during which preparation is rapidly undertaken for definitive management. In these children, the airway should be actively managed in the ED only if deterioration occurs. The rationale in these cases is that intervention is best done in a controlled environment by a multidisciplinary team with expertise in the management of difficult airways. Treatment in less than ideal conditions may lead to untoward outcomes.

The signs and symptoms of impending airway obstruction in children are important indicators that guide the approach to the early intervention group. These disorders, if left to expectant treatment, have a greater potential for deterioration. An example, as discussed above, is the burn or caustic ingestion patient who is beginning to develop a raspy voice. This symptom may herald deterioration, although the degree and pace of progression cannot be predicted. However, it must be assumed that progression to the point of obstruction is possible, in which case intubation will be extremely difficult if not impossible. For this reason, intervention earlier rather than later is recommended. Patients with compromised airways secondary to anaphylactic or anaphylactoid reactions (e.g., angioedema) who do not respond immediately to medical treatment similarly require early intervention.

SUMMARY

- Effective pediatric airway management is focused on anticipating and planning for difficulties.
- The systematic approach to identify the difficult airway in adults can also be used in children. In general, looking for obvious abnormalities (L of LEMON) and evaluating for upper airway obstruction (O) are the highest yield features of the LEMON assessment, when applied to children.
- Most difficult pediatric airways are related to acute insults to otherwise normal anatomy, or to known congenital abnormalities. Unexpected difficulty in children is very rare.
- Pattern recognition is important to the appropriate management of the common presentations of acute infectious and noninfectious compromise airway emergencies.

- Management of children with difficult airways should follow the difficult airway algorithm, just as with adults. The vast majority of patients will still be managed with RSI and direct laryngoscopy.

EVIDENCE

- **What is the incidence of difficult and failed airways in children?** Although definitions and contexts vary, pediatric data demonstrate the rarity of difficult airways in children. Using a database of nearly 9,000 children being endotracheally intubated *in the operating room* at a tertiary care children's hospital where referral bias predicts more complex patients, the incidence of difficult airways was just 0.42%.[1] Importantly, even for those with difficult airways, there were no mask ventilation failures or need for surgical airways in this study. Another large database study of over 24,000 pediatric general anesthesia cases found a similarly low incidence.[2] The only published pediatric data *from the ED* setting includes 156 patients, in which <1% required a surgical airway secondary to failed intubation.[3] These data were collected in the late 1990s, and one might expect that with the more widespread availability of video laryngoscopy and other advanced airway devices, this might be even less frequent today.
- **How reliable is the Mallampati scoring system in children?** Many studies have evaluated the accuracy of the original and modified Mallampati tests in predicting difficulty airways in adults.[4] However data are limited in children. In a single published study of 476 patients from newborns to 16 years of age, the predictive sensitivity of Mallampati testing was only 0.162. Importantly, of 16 patients with a poor view on laryngoscopy, 12 (75%) had Mallampati class 1 or 2 airways and therefore were not predicted to be difficult.[5] Although a lack of cooperation in infants and young children may contribute to the poor predictive value in the pediatric population, a tongue blade was used as needed in this study population to facilitate mouth opening and maximal tongue excursion. The concept of evaluating the size of a child's tongue relative to his/her oral cavity remains important, even if this specific classification schema has limited supporting data in pediatrics.
- **Have clinical tools to predict difficult airways in children been validated?** The predictive merits of individual anthropomorphic measurements (e.g., hyomandibular, thyromental, mandibular, and interdental lengths) and systematic clinical evaluation are confined to adults and have not been well tested in children. However, despite a paucity of data, logic and anecdotal experience support that global assessment for features that might predict airway difficulty is important and should be routinely performed.

REFERENCES

1. Tong DC, Beus J, Litman RS. The Children's Hospital of Philadelphia Difficult Airway Registry. *Anesthesiology*. 2007;107:A1637.

2. Murat I, Constant I, Maud'huy H. Perioperative anaesthetic morbidity in children: a database of 24,165 anaesthetics over a 30-month period. Paediatr Anaesth 2004;14:158-66.

3. Sagarin MJ, Chiang V, Sakles JC, et al. Rapid sequence intubation for pediatric emergency airway management. *Pediatr Emerg Care*. 2002;18:417–423.

4. Lee A, Fan LT, Gin T, et al. A systematic review (meta-analysis) of the accuracy of the Mallampati tests to predict the difficult airway. *Anesth Analg*. 2006;102:1867–1878.

5. Kopp VJ, Bailey A, Calhoun PE, et al. Utility of the Mallampati classification for predicting difficult intubation in pediatric patients. *Anesthesiology*. 1995;83:A1147.

27

Foreign Body in the Pediatric Airway

Robert C. Luten • Joshua Nagler

BACKGROUND

Foreign body aspiration (FBA) is a common cause of morbidity and mortality in children. More than 17,000 children are seen in emergency departments each year for choking-related episodes, with >150 deaths per year. The age group most at risk is 1 to 3 years of age. These children may choke on food substances given their incomplete dentition, immature swallowing coordination, and tendency toward distraction during meals. In addition, infants and toddlers are newly adapted to walking and have a tendency to put everything in their mouths. This increases their risk of unwitnessed choking events. Older children more commonly aspirate things such as pins and pen caps, which they are holding in their mouths.

PRESENTATION

Children who have aspirated foreign material may present acutely following a *witnessed or reported* event. Families commonly report a choking or gagging episode. Such an event, followed by sudden onset of coughing with unilateral wheezing or decreased aeration represents the classic diagnostic triad for FBA in the mainstem or lower bronchi. When the foreign body becomes lodged more proximally, partial upper airway obstruction can lead to hoarseness or stridor. Complete obstruction of the trachea or larynx can occur either from mechanical blockage or from induced laryngospasm. The mortality with complete laryngeal obstruction approaches 50%.

Many children have *unwitnessed* aspiration events. Infants are preverbal and young children may not recognize the need to tell their parents. As a result, respiratory symptoms may be incorrectly attributed to illnesses such as asthma or croup. Subsequent recurrent pulmonary infections may lead to the delayed diagnosis of chronic FBA. This can occur weeks to months after the aspiration event.

For the purpose of this chapter, we will focus only on acute airway management in the context of known or suspected FBA.

TECHNIQUE

The approach to the management of FBA will differ depending on whether the obstruction is partial or complete, and the level of consciousness of the child.

Partial Airway Obstruction

Children with FBA who have the ability to cough, cry, or speak are demonstrating adequate air exchange, and therefore have incomplete airway obstruction. Beyond infancy, children will naturally hold themselves in a position that maximizes airway patency. In addition, they possess a reflexive cough, which is the most effective means of clearing the airway. These patients, therefore, should be managed "expectantly." That is, no attempts at relief maneuvers should be attempted to avoid dislodgement of the foreign body to a location that aggravates the degree of obstruction.

Resources should be summoned to provide removal in the operating room setting whenever possible. If an operating room or pediatric expert resources are unavailable, an alternative plan must be initiated. Appropriately sized equipment should be gathered for foreign body removal, as well as for more definitive airway management in the event that the child progresses to complete airway obstruction (discussed below).

Attempts at removal of the foreign body for children with partial airway obstruction are rarely performed in the emergency department. Children are unlikely to cooperate with efforts to remove an airway foreign body even with effective topical anesthesia. Furthermore, unintentionally placing a laryngoscope blade too deeply in small children will risk placing direct pressure on the foreign body which can further obstruct the airway. Therefore, in most cases, the child should be allowed to continue to attempt to clear the foreign body reflexively as long as possible, or until an operating room is available. Only when the patient is showing signs of tiring or progression toward complete obstruction, should attempts at removal be made. In such circumstances, sedation with ketamine titrated intravenously to effect if possible (or 4 mg per kg IM if not) reliably produces dissociative sedation while maintaining respiratory drive and airway reflexes. Once sedated, the laryngoscope is methodically inserted a small distance at a time, while attempting to identify any supraglottic foreign body.

If the patient progresses to complete obstruction, either because of unavoidable progression or as a result of attempts at removal, immediate intervention is required.

Complete Airway Obstruction

The loss of the ability to phonate in an awake child with a suspected FBA indicates complete airway obstruction. Chest wall movement will persist with attempted respiratory efforts; however, no sounds will be heard on inspiration or expiration. Conscious children will appear scared, although infants will not reliably place their hands to their neck to signify choking as older children or adults will. Instead, they will often raise clenched fists above their heads with eyes wide open as an expression of distress.

Pediatric Basic Life Support (BLS) techniques should be used immediately in the conscious patient with complete airway obstruction from FBA. The goal is to generate intrathoracic pressure to expel the foreign body from the airway. In infants, this is most safely attempted with the child in a head down position, using repeated cycles of back blows and chest compressions, five per cycle. Subdiaphragmatic abdominal thrusts (the Heimlich maneuver) are not recommended in infants because of the risk of accidental injury to the relatively large liver protruding beneath the costal margin. In children older than 1 year, the Heimlich maneuver is recommended, just as with adults. These initial maneuvers should be repeated until either the foreign body is expelled or the patient becomes unresponsive.

There is no role for attempting instrumentation to remove the foreign body in a conscious child. With complete obstruction of the airway, rapid oxygen desaturation will render the patient unconscious within 1 or 2 minutes, at which point attempts at removal can be made. For the child who presents unconscious, the oropharynx should first be examined for a visible foreign body. If something is seen, it should be removed directly. If no foreign material is seen, a blind oropharyngeal finger sweep should **not** be performed. In the emergency department, the immediate maneuver is direct laryngoscopy for possible foreign body visualization and removal. This is exactly analogous to the adult patient (see Chapter 40). The administration of a neuromuscular blocking agent is not indicated for the initial attempt. Only if children have clenched teeth or other signs of muscle activity will it be necessary to use a rapid onset neuromuscular blocking agent. If the foreign body can be identified under direct laryngoscopy, it should be removed using Magill or alligator forceps, or other available instruments. Care must be taken to avoid advancing the foreign body to a position where it becomes more tightly lodged or to a location where it is no longer retrievable. Similarly, organic material may be friable and should be grasped gently to avoid creating smaller fragments that can fall deeper into the tracheobronchial tree.

If the foreign body cannot be retrieved during laryngoscopy or expelled by blind maneuvers, attempts should be made to advance the foreign material distally into either mainstem bronchus using an endotracheal tube. The child should be intubated and the endotracheal tube inserted as deeply as possible, advancing the obstructing material with it. The tube should then be withdrawn to the standard "lip-to-tip" distance provided by the Broselow–Luten tape or other formulas. At this point, ventilation of the unobstructed lung is attempted (see Fig. 27-1). High resistance following this maneuver may result from soft material such as food substances becoming lodged within the endotracheal tube, preventing easy passage of air. If this occurs, replacement of the endotracheal tube using the appropriate insertion depth provides the most effective means to ventilate the patient through the patent mainstem bronchi.

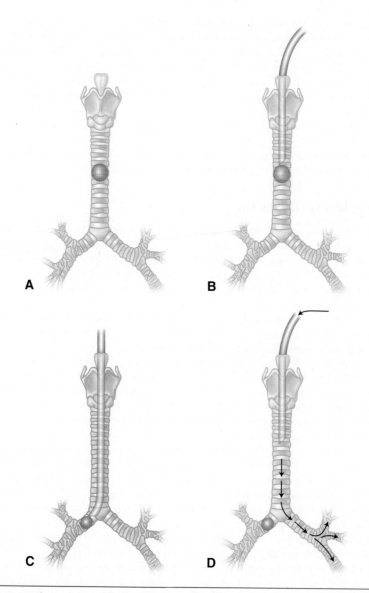

Figure 27-1 ● Advancing a foreign body lodged in the trachea. A. Foreign body lodged in the trachea. B. Endotracheal tube may meet resistance at the level of the foreign body. C. Endotracheal tube is advanced to push the foreign body into a mainstem bronchus D. Endotracheal tube is pulled back to the appropriate "lip to tip" distance, and the unobstructed lung is ventilated.

A percutaneous approach (e.g., needle cricothyrotomy) is rarely indicated in FBA. Details of this approach are provided in Chapter 25. Needle cricothyrotomy will only be successful if the needle entry site is distal to the obstruction (e.g., a foreign body just below the vocal cords at the cricoid ring). If the foreign body cannot be visualized during attempts at direct laryngoscopy, it is unlikely that a percutaneous approach will be distal to the object, rendering the procedure ineffective. Ventilation strategies following percutaneous airway techniques are reviewed in Chapter 25. In patients with complete airway obstruction, it is important to remember that no air can exit through the glottis into the pharynx. The only means for exhalation is through the narrow lumen of the catheter, therefore the risk of barotrauma increases following each delivered breath.

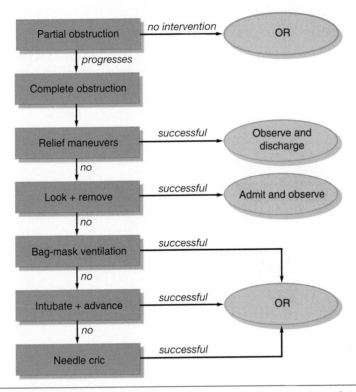

Figure 27-2 ● Stepwise Approach for the Management of an Aspirated Foreign Body.

Both forced intubation and needle cricothyrotomy are temporizing measures designed to reestablish some degree of oxygenation and ventilation. When successful, the patient can then be taken to the operating room for removal of the foreign body with a bronchoscope or by thoracotomy as needed.

An overview of the stepwise approach to managing FBA in children is presented in Figure 27-2. The same for adults is seen in Figure 40-1 in Chapter 40.

TIPS AND PEARLS

1. Many aspiration events in children are unwitnessed, and young children are incapable of verbalizing what has happened. Consider aspiration in any infant/toddler with acute onset of respiratory distress.
2. The safest removal of a foreign body from a pediatric airway occurs in the operating room. Recruit necessary personnel and resources as early as possible.
3. Reflexive cough is likely to be the most successful mechanism for clearing a foreign body from a partially obstructed airway. Avoid interfering with an alert child who is sitting in a position of comfort and coughing.
4. In the emergency department, if there is high suspicion for obstruction from FBA, direct laryngoscopy for possible direct removal should be attempted before positive-pressure breaths to avoid advancing the foreign body to an unreachable position.
5. Avoid the Heimlich maneuver in children <1 year of age to prevent inadvertent injury to the liver.
6. Needle cricothyrotomy is unlikely to be successful in any child in whom the foreign body cannot be visualized above or immediately below the glottis, and therefore should not be attempted in these patients.

EVIDENCE

- **How common is FBA in children and what do they aspirate?** More than 17,000 children are seen in emergency departments each year for choking-related episodes, with >150 deaths per year.[1,2] Younger children typically choke on food items; older children more commonly aspirate things such as pins and pen caps, which they are holding in their mouths.[3]

REFERENCES

1. Nonfatal choking-related episodes among children—United States, 2001. *MMWR Morb Mortal Wkly Rep*. 2002;51:945–948.

2. National Safety Council. Injury Facts. 2008 ed. Chicago, IL: National Safety Council; 2008. https://www.usw12775.org/uploads/InjuryFacts08Ed.pdf

3. Steen KH, Zimmermann T. Tracheobronchial aspiration of foreign bodies in children: a study of 94 cases. *Laryngoscope*. 1990;100:525–530.

28

Approach to the EMS Airway

Frederick H. Ellinger, Jr. • Richard D. Zane • Michael F. Murphy

THE CLINICAL CHALLENGE

Most of the principles of prehospital airway management are similar to those in the emergency department (ED), with the obvious exception that the prehospital environment is necessarily austere. Patient care must often be provided in awkward circumstances such as in private homes, in stairwells, in the seat of a damaged automobile, or on the street, where lighting and position are often not ideal. Local protocols, regional and topographic differences in transport time, the availability or unavailability of neuromuscular blocking agents, limited and varied equipment, limited backup, and mandatory transport of the patient all introduce issues that are not only different from those in the ED, but also different from one prehospital system to another.

The environment of care is "error prone." Strategies designed to minimize error must do so reproducibly in a time-sensitive fashion. Clear definitions and simple evaluation and management memory tools, including mnemonics and algorithms, represent such strategies. Identifying the difficult airway, managing the failed airway, and performing a cricothyrotomy are no different prehospital than they are in-hospital. Thus, the "thinking" and "doing" in the prehospital environment is identical to that which occurs in an ED or operating room (OR).

DELEGATED MEDICAL ACTS AND STANDARDIZED MEDICAL PROTOCOLS

In most North American systems, prehospital care providers perform delegated medical acts based on preestablished, standardized medical protocols. Although protocols ought to reflect best clinical evidence, they are limited from a practical perspective by cost, training, competency maintenance, space constraints, and medical director knowledge of the prehospital setting or individual comfort level.

The equipment available to providers in the field is driven by the protocols approved by the emergency medical services (EMS) system, EMS unit medical director, or medical advisory committee. The type and range of equipment available for managing the *difficult airway* in the prehospital setting is limited compared with most EDs and ORs. Even basic equipment such as the Eschmann introducer (bougie), laryngoscope blades, and endotracheal tubes in an array of types and sizes may be limited in availability. Similarly, the choice of alternate intubating devices, such as the intubating laryngeal mask airway (ILMA or LMA Fastrach) and rescue devices will vary from system to system.

Regardless of the array of devices available, consummate bag-mask ventilation (BMV) technique (including two-handed mask hold requiring two providers if available or necessary) is essential to the prehospital care provider, particularly where the airway is predicted to be difficult and the transport time is relatively brief.

CONTROVERSIES IN PREHOSPITAL AIRWAY MANAGEMENT

Inadequate ventilation and oxygenation have been identified as primary contributors to preventable mortality, both in hospital and out of hospital. It would seem intuitive that successful endotracheal intubation (ETI) ought to mitigate these deaths, and because of this thinking, ETI became the gold standard in prehospital airway management. However, there is considerable controversy as to whether patients requiring ETI should have tracheal intubation performed in the field or deferred until hospital arrival. There is ample evidence that ETI is not a benign intervention in the hands of inexperienced personnel, who use the technique infrequently. Studies have identified that intubation in the field may delay transport to higher echelons of care, injure airways, and lead to worse outcomes.

The *Recommended Guidelines for Uniform Reporting of Data from Out-of-Hospital Airway Management* identifies four methods constituting "advanced airway management": direct oral laryngoscopy and intubation, nasotracheal intubation (NTI), oral rescue techniques (e.g., BMV, LMA, and Combitube), and surgical rescue techniques (transtracheal jet ventilation and cricothyrotomy). These four methods may each be modified by five variables:

1. Oral approach: no facilitating sedative drugs or paralytics
2. Nasal approach: no facilitating sedative drugs or paralytics
3. Sedation-facilitated intubation (including "nonparalytic rapid sequence intubation (RSI)")
4. RSI (i.e., the use of neuromuscular blockade ± induction agents)
5. Other intubation technique (e.g., digital and lighted stylet)

The *actual* number of alternatives available in an EMS system is limited by protocols, training, equipment, and medical direction.

Various LMAs, the King LT airway, and the Combitube (see Chapters 10 and 11) have been introduced successfully in the prehospital care setting as alternatives to ETI for the cardiac arrest (or deeply comatose) patient by basic life support (BLS) providers. These devices also are used for rescue in the setting of failed intubation by advanced life support (ALS) or critical care providers. In some EMS systems, noninvasive ventilation is used as an alternative to ETI for patients in respiratory failure, particularly from chronic obstructive pulmonary disease or acute heart failure.

APPROACH TO THE AIRWAY

The following are the most significant changes in the approach to airway management in EMS over the last decade:

- The emergence of extraglottic devices (EGDs) as first-choice alternatives to BMV in unresponsive patients for BLS providers
- Rapid sequence airway (RSA) which includes the use of induction agents +/– paralytics with the intent of placing a "rescue" EGD instead of endotracheal tube is emerging as a viable option for airway management in limited-access situations or when ETI is predicted to be difficult
- The use of EGDs *instead of* ETI by ALS urban ground ambulance services in unresponsive patients
- The emergence of "nonparalytic RSI" as an alternative to "paralytic RSI" in which a full or tailored dose of an induction agent, but no neuromuscular blocking agent is administered
- Controversy regarding whether ETI is of benefit in ground ambulance ALS EMS services
- Apparent improved outcomes with RSI versus non-RSI methods of intubation in air medical transport systems
- The use of high-fidelity human patient simulation training to improve performance

Factors contributing to improved RSI success rates for prehospital providers have also been identified:

- High-quality initial and ongoing airway management training
- Intense medical oversight and quality management programs
- Frequent exposure to patients in need of active airway management

Improved outcomes for services using RSI are contingent on three factors:

1. Knowing how to correctly perform RSI
2. Being able to identify those patients in whom RSI should not be performed (i.e., identifying the difficult airway [see Chapter 2])
3. Being able to rescue the airway in the event that intubation is unsuccessful and BMV fails

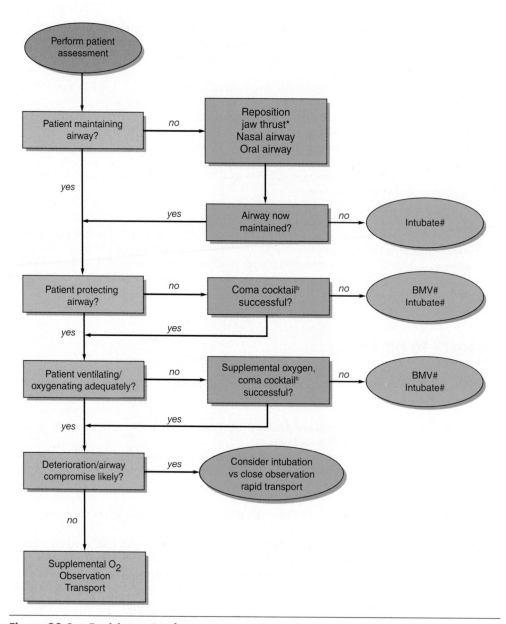

Figure 28-1 ● Decision to Intubate. [a]Caution in trauma; [b]naloxone, glucose; #Or extra-glottic device as per protocol; BMV bag-mask ventilation.

The decision to intubate the patient in the prehospital setting is based on the same principles as those applied in the ED (see Chapter 1). A prehospital algorithm for the decision to intubate is shown in Figure 28-1.

TECHNIQUE

If the patient is not maintaining his or her own airway, the stepwise approach to opening the airway and performing BMV is as described in Chapter 9. In most circumstances, BMV in this setting should be followed by ETI as soon as adequate preparations have been made, and provided the provider is trained and credentialed to intubate. If BMV is unsuccessful, despite careful attention to proper technique, then immediate intubation or placement of an alternate airway device, such as a Combitube, King LT, or LMA, is indicated (see Chapters 10, 11, and 29). As mentioned previously, in Approach to the Airway, there is a school of thought emerging that the use of an EGD may leapfrog ahead of BMV as the first-line technique. This is based on the relative ease of use and high ventilation success rates seen with EGDs relative to the more difficult technique of BMV.

After a patent airway has been established, the next evaluation should determine whether the patient is protecting the airway from aspiration (see Chapter 1). If a "coma cocktail" is unsuccessful in reversing the patient's coma sufficient to permit self-protection of the airway, then active airway management is indicated.

If the patient is maintaining and protecting the airway, assessment of ventilation and oxygenation are made as described in Chapter 1. Similarly, the anticipated clinical course, particularly with respect to likelihood of deterioration, is assessed. Decision-making follows the principles outlined in Chapter 1.

Once a decision to intubate is made, the next step is to choose the best method for intubation. The choice will depend on whether the airway is determined to be difficult, whether neuromuscular blockade is permitted, and the particular protocols related to airway adjuncts and rescue devices, including cricothyrotomy.

Oral intubation employing direct laryngoscopy is the usual method. In the case of the agonal, unresponsive patient, management proceeds exactly as described in Chapter 3 as a crash airway. The crash airway algorithm is no different in EMS than it is in the ED. In some settings, medication-assisted intubation will include both induction (sedative) agent and neuromuscular blockade. In other settings, where neuromuscular blockade is not permitted, medication-assisted intubation will be done with a sedative hypnotic agent. In either case, medication-assisted intubation may be preferable to blind NTI, even in the clenched jaw patient.

If the patient is conscious and combative and requires intubation, then medication-assisted intubation is indicated. At the outset, though, the benefits and risks of intubation should be weighed against the benefits and risks of rapid transport without intubation. Combative or uncooperative behavior is a relative contraindication to blind NTI because of the increased risk of complications in attempting to insert the tube in a patient who is resisting. If the patient is not frankly comatose and is not uncooperative or combative, then assessment must be made as to whether the patient would tolerate laryngoscopy. If the patient is sufficiently cooperative or sufficiently obtunded to permit oral laryngoscopy without medications, then oral intubation may be attempted. Again, preference is expressed for oral intubation over nasal intubation except in circumstances in which the jaw is clenched, preventing oral access. Even in such cases, oral intubation with medication generally is preferable to blind NTI.

Blind NTI is discussed in detail in Chapter 17. In general, although blind NTI has been widely used in prehospital care, it has declined in popularity because of the superiority of medication-assisted oral intubation. Even though RSI is clearly the method of choice many prehospital care providers do not have this option, and blind NTI may be preferable or may be the procedure of choice for the individual operator. Details regarding contraindications and cautions related to NTI are discussed in Chapter 17.

Although many devices have been developed that may be useful for airway management in the prehospital setting, providers should become facile with one or perhaps two rescue techniques and devices such as EGDs (Chapter 29).

Failed Intubation

A failed intubation is usually the result of a combination of factors: a challenging situation, anatomic factors leading to difficult laryngoscopy, and/or intubation and operator skill set. Chapter 30 deals with the difficult airway in EMS and the failed intubation. The technique of cricothyrotomy is addressed in Chapter 18; the decision to perform one in the field is addressed in Chapter 30.

RSI: CUSTOMIZED FOR EMS

The use of RSI, neuromuscular blockade, and sedatives is highly variable from one EMS system to another. Even though an ever-growing number of prehospital systems are using neuromuscular blockade to facilitate intubation in the field, many EMS systems have not instituted RSI for myriad reasons. These include the inability to implement intensive training programs, inadequate exposure to maintain skills, short transport times, insufficient medical oversight and quality management systems, and the failure of the literature to consistently identify clear benefits.

Air medical services and specialized transport teams are usually trained and experienced in the use of neuromuscular blockade for intubation and encounter sufficient numbers of cases to maintain skills and knowledge.

A typical prehospital, drug-assisted intubation protocol using neuromuscular blockade is shown in Box 28-1. The sequence is simplified in the prehospital setting because the medication options are usually fewer.

POSTINTUBATION MANAGEMENT

Most commonly in the prehospital environment, after securing an airway, the patient is bag ventilated rather than placed on a mechanical ventilator, although the latter is preferable if available. As interfacility critical care and specialized care transport become more common, transport ventilators permitting postintubation ventilation will become more prevalent in the pre- or interhospital environment. Additional sedation, e.g. with midazolam, may be necessary to facilitate tube tolerance and ventilation during transport.

TIPS AND PEARLS

- Always weigh the risks and benefits of intubation in the prehospital setting against transporting to the ED. In many circumstances, rapid transport might trump active airway management in the field.
- Master BMV. There are few airway emergencies in the prehospital setting that cannot be temporized or managed adequately with proper BMV until the patient can be transported to the hospital, particularly when transport times are short.
- If transport times are long, especially in systems with high rates of trauma, consider introducing paralytic RSI into the prehospital setting. This approach requires a comprehensive program, including quality oversight and skill maintenance.

Box 28-1. Simplified RSI for Prehospital Care

---

1. Prepare equipment, and ensure that the patient is in an appropriate area for intubation
2. Preoxygenate the patient with non-rebreather mask or BMV for at least 3 minutes, if possible
3. Pretreatment drugs—infrequently used. Suggestion: lidocaine 1.5 mg/kg intravenously for head injury and reactive airways disease
4. Paralysis with sedation—administer sedative drug in adequate dose (e.g., etomidate 0.3 mg/kg) and neuromuscular blocking agent (e.g., succinylcholine 1.5 mg/kg)
5. Positioning—wait 20 seconds. Position the patient for optimal laryngoscopy. Perform Sellick Maneuver as per protocol.
6. Placement—45 seconds after drugs are given, intubate. Confirm endotracheal tube placement, secure tube, and transport patient

- Extraglottic devices, such as the LMA, King LT, and Combitube, play an important role in prehospital airway management.
- Confirm intubation by employing End Tidal Carbon Dioxide end-tidal carbon dioxide ($ETCO_2$) and maintain $ETCO_2$ monitoring throughout patient contact. Take note and document the continued presence of $ETCO_2$ with each patient move.
- All prehospital intubations should have the airway reassessed on arrival at the ED. Even though prehospital providers are trained airway managers and are comfortable caring for patients in respiratory distress, up to 25% of prehospital intubations are found to be esophageal on arrival at the ED. Confirmation of endotracheal tube placement with an $ETCO_2$ detector should be a first priority both in the field and on arrival in the ED.
- When an air medical, critical care, or specialized transport team is asked to transport a patient from an outlying facility to a tertiary care facility, and airway management is required for safe transport, it almost always is preferable to secure the airway while still in the sending health care facility as opposed to en route in an ambulance or helicopter.

SUMMARY

It is unclear at present whether ETI by prehospital care providers improves outcome for specific populations. What *is clear* is that active medical direction, intense quality oversight and maintenance of competency programs, and high-quality airway management training are features of EMS systems that have achieved high advanced airway management success rates and improved outcomes. Other issues such as equipment availability, the air versus ground environment, and the logistics associated with rural versus urban critical care transport/EMS suggest that a single, rigid approach to EMS airway management is unlikely to meet the needs of the various systems and patients.

EVIDENCE

- **Should tracheal intubation be performed in the field at all?** There are several dimensions to this controversy:
  - *Trauma victims*: There continues to be skepticism as to whether the intubation of trauma victims in the prehospital care environment improves survival. During the 1980s, it was generally believed that ETI by EMS personnel had the potential to delay transport and was ineffective in improving survival in urban environments, but might be effective in longer transport environments.[1] Many studies with conflicting results populated the literature during the 1990s and early 2000s.[1,2] The lack of clarity led some to speculate that for selected subsets of the trauma patient population, ETI might be of benefit. It seemed logical to analyze patients with acute, severe head injury. Early studies provided no clear direction[2,3] and a large trauma registry study found that prehospital intubation was associated with adverse outcomes after severe head trauma.[2] There was a subset of air medical transport patients in this study that may have benefited from ETI in the field, although an accompanying editorial maintained that this factor reflected a retrospective association rather than causation.[4] In summary, the question as to whether ETI in trauma victims improves outcome is unresolved, although serious questions as to its benefits have been raised.
  - *Cardiac arrest*: In cardiac arrest patients, the issue of efficacy remains unresolved. In fact, one study of hospital cardiac arrest victims showed that patients who received only CPR with chest compressions had comparable survival outcome to those who received chest compression and mouth-to-mouth ventilation.[5] Furthermore, a large prospective before/after study to determine the incremented benefit of introducing ALS (including intubation) into a

previously optimized system did not show a mortality benefit in cardiac arrest patients.[6] The issue as to the effect of oxygenation and ventilation on mortality in cardiac arrest victims in the prehospital arena remains unresolved.

○ *Children*: Early studies showed that tracheal intubation of children by paramedics was associated with higher failure and complication rates than in adults. Subsequent studies have tended to confirm this early finding.[7] The only prospective, pseudorandomized trial to investigate the effectiveness of ground paramedics in performing tracheal intubation in children showed that there was no demonstrable advantage in survival following ETI compared with groups receiving only BMV.[8] This same study revealed concerns about endotracheal tube displacement and lack of recognition that it had occurred. Finally, for a subpopulation of patients in whom ETI might be expected to show a benefit, children with acute severe head injuries, the issue remains unresolved. A pervasive critique of these studies is that the results reflect a deficiency in pediatric ETI training for EMS personnel. In the final analysis, the emergency intubation of children is an uncommon and anxiety-provoking event for most ALS providers. Both factors are likely to increase performance anxiety and failure rates, compared with the intubation of adults.

- **Is there evidence to support RSI by ALS prehospital providers?** The evidence in the EMS literature regarding the use of RSI is generally nonsupportive except in specific circumstances. For ground EMS systems, several recent well-designed studies have consistently shown suboptimal outcomes, or no difference in outcome, in patients suffering acute severe head injury where RSI was used to facilitate ETI.[9,10] Head injury was deliberately chosen in these studies because earlier studies have suggested that optimal oxygenation and ventilation of these patients improves outcomes. Therefore, it was assumed that successful ETI would demonstrate a benefit. There have been attempts to determine the reasons for the poor outcomes associated with RSI in ground EMS services. These explanations have included the following:
  ○ Increased on-scene time (average 15 minutes in one study)[11]
  ○ Lack of adequate training of the paramedics[2]
  ○ Inappropriate hyperventilation and nonrecognition of hypoxia during induction[12]
  ○ Patient paralysis and multiple attempts at intubation[12]

    Despite recent studies showing the lack of efficacy of RSI in the ground EMS systems, a distinct pattern of improved outcomes has emerged in the subpopulation of those patients where air medical transport had been used.[2]

    Some of the evidence based on which important decisions relating to airway management in prehospital care are based is growing and is presented in Chapters 29 and 30. However, several important issues need to be resolved:
  - Are EGDs more effective than BMV in unresponsive patients in the hands of BLS personnel, and do the outcomes reflect that fact?
  - Are the outcomes of unresponsive patients managed with EGDs rather than ETI by ALS personnel improved?
  - How should ALS providers manage the airway in responsive patients that require airway management?
  - Does ETI by ALS personnel improve outcomes generally and in specific subpopulations of patients?
  - What factors are critical to ensuring that RSI is performed safely in EMS?
  - Is there evidence that airway intervention improves outcome (e.g., cardiac arrest)?

- **Is there evidence in the EMS literature to suggest that intubation success rates using "nonparalytic RSI" are as high as with "paralytic RSI"?** It is suggested in the anesthesia literature that the use of an induction agent alone provides poorer intubating conditions than when a neuromuscular blocking agent is coupled with the induction agent. Bozeman et al.[13] compared two groups in a Helicopter EMS (HEMS) system, one using etomidate alone and the other using neuromuscular blockade (RSI group). The view of the larynx (laryngeal view grade) was significantly better in the RSI group, as was the intubation success rate (92% success with paralytic RSI vs. 25% in the nonparalytic RSI group). Sonday et al.,[14] in contrast, found little difference, whereas Kociszewski et al.[15] found that the neuromuscular agent significantly improved the ease and success of intubation over induction alone.

- **Is there any evidence that intubation training of paramedics on high-fidelity patient simulators is as good as training on live patients in the OR?** Hall et al.[16] studied 36 paramedic students who had never intubated before. He randomized them into two groups. Both groups received didactic instruction and manikin training. Then half went to the OR to intubate 15 patients, while the other group received 10 hours of training on a high-fidelity simulator followed by 15 live intubations. Overall success rates, success on first attempt, and complication rates were similar in both groups.

- **Is there any evidence to support the use of Rapid Sequence Airway (RSA)?** RSA was first described in the literature in 2007 by Braude and Richards.[17] In a subsequent case study published by Braude et al.[18], an air medical helicopter EMS crew elected to induce and paralyze a patient with the sole intent to place an LMA-Supreme (LMA-S). This patient had suffered massive facial deformities and presented with an oxygen saturation of 30% following a motor vehicle crash. The patient received etomidate and rocuronium for the procedure. Post-LMA-S placement oxygen saturation rose to 94% and the patient was successfully managed for many hours with the LMA-S in situ. Southard et al.[19] studied the effectiveness and timeliness of RSA versus RSI by a flight crew in simulated trauma patient using a high-fidelity patient simulator. In this study, it was found that the total time to successful RSA was 145 seconds shorter than the total time required for successful RSI. RSA also maintained higher oxygen saturations than RSI. The RSA group had 42% fewer airway attempts than the RSI group and no episodes of "failed airway." Although not well investigated, the use of RSA in certain situations, such as limited access scenarios, may prove useful and safe. The data from Braude and Southard indicates that RSA is quicker to achieve than that of RSI and may reduce the likelihood of failed airway, particularly in the presence of severe trauma and in limited-access situations such as within a helicopter.

- **What systems elements need to be in place for a drug-assisted intubation program to be successful in EMS?** A paucity of reliable data has hindered the reporting and analysis of information related to prehospital airway management. To address this issue, the National Association of EMS Physicians (NAEMSP) published a position statement in 2004 that articulated guidelines for the uniform reporting of data from out-of-hospital airway management.[20] In all, 39 data points were identified. These standards were to be used by EMS agencies "for defining, collecting, and reporting airway management data."

  Subsequent to that, the NAEMSP, the American College of Emergency Physicians and the American College of Surgeons Committee on Trauma published a position statement on the use of medications to assist in ETI.[21] They recommend that a prehospital Drug Assisted Intubation (DAI) program "… should include, at a minimum, the following elements:
  ○ medical direction with concurrent and retrospective oversight supervision
  ○ proper patient selection; to include training and continuing education designed to demonstrate initial and ongoing competence in the procedure (includes supervised DAI experience)
  ○ training in airway management for patients who cannot be intubated to include; competence in the use of backup rescue airway devices in the event of failed DAI
  ○ standardized DAI protocols including the use of sedation and neuromuscular blockade
  ○ resources for drug storage and delivery
  ○ resources for continuous monitoring and recording of heart rate and rhythm, oxygen saturation, and $ETCO_2$, before, during, and after DAI
  ○ continuing quality assurance, quality control, performance review, and when necessary, supplemental training
  ○ research to clarify the role of DAI on improved patient outcome within EMS systems"

  Evidence is beginning to accumulate that this approach leads to successful DAI programs measured as successful placement of endotracheal tubes in the trachea.[22] Whether this leads to improved outcomes is still unclear, with the probable exception of head injured patients managed by critical care transport or HEMS personnel.[23,24]

REFERENCES

1. Ruchholtz S, Waydhas C, Ose C, et al; Working Group on Multiple Trauma of the German Trauma Society. Prehospital intubation in severe thoracic trauma without respiratory insufficiency: a matched-pair analysis based on the Trauma Registry of the German Trauma Society. *J Trauma*. 2002;52:879–886.

2. Wang HE, Peitzman AB, Cassidy LD, et al. Out-of-hospital endotracheal intubation and outcome after traumatic brain injury. *Ann Emerg Med*. 2004;44:439–450.

3. Ochs M, Davis DP, Hoyt DB. Lessons learned during the San Diego paramedic RSI Trial. *J Emerg Med*. 2003;24:343–344.

4. Zink BJ, Maio RF. Out-of-hospital endotracheal intubation in traumatic brain injury: outcomes research provides us with an unexpected outcome. *Ann Emerg Med*. 2004;44:451–453.

5. Hallstrom A, Cobb L, Johnson E, et al. Cardiopulmonary resuscitation by chest compression alone or with mouth-to-mouth ventilation. *N Engl J Med*. 2000;342:1546–1553.

6. Stiell IG, Wells GA, Field B, et al. Advanced cardiac life support in out-of-hospital cardiac arrest. *N Engl J Med*. 2004;351:647–656.

7. Vilke GM, Steen PJ, Smith AM, et al. Out-of-hospital pediatric intubation by paramedics: the San Diego experience. *J Emerg Med*. 2002;22:71–74.

8. Gausche M, Lewis RJ, Stratton SJ, et al. Effect of out-of-hospital pediatric endotracheal intubation on survival and neurological outcome: a controlled clinical trial. *JAMA*. 2000;283:783–790.

9. Davis DP, Hoyt DB, Ochs M, et al. The effect of paramedic rapid sequence intubation on outcome in patients with severe traumatic brain injury. *J Trauma*. 2003;54:444–453.

10. Dunford J, Davis D, Ochs M, et al. Incidence of transient hypoxia and pulse rate reactivity during paramedic rapid sequence intubation. *Ann Emerg Med*. 2003;42:721–728.

11. Ochs M, Davis D, Hoyt D, et al. Paramedic-performed rapid sequence intubation of patients with severe head injuries. *Ann Emerg Med*. 2002;40:159–167.

12. Ma OJ, Atchley RB, Hatley T, et al. Intubation success rates improve for an air medical program after implementing the use of neuromuscular blocking agents. *Am J Emerg Med*. 1998;16:125–127.

13. Bozeman WP, Kleiner DM, Huggett V. A comparison of rapid-sequence intubation and etomidate-only intubation in the prehospital air medical setting. *Prehosp Emerg Care*. 2006;10:8–13.

14. Sonday CJ, Axelband J, Jacoby J, et al. Thiopental vs. etomidate for rapid sequence intubation in aeromedicine. *Prehospital Disaster Med*. 2005;20:324–326.

15. Kociszewski C, Thomas SH, Harrison T, et al. Etomidate versus succinylcholine for intubation in an air medical setting. *Am J Emerg Med*. 2000;18:757–763.

16. Hall RE, Plant JR, Bands CJ, et al. Human patient simulation is effective for teaching paramedic students endotracheal intubation. *Acad Emerg Med*. 2005;12:850–855.

17. Braude D, Richards M. Rapid sequence airway (RSA): a novel approach to prehospital airway management. *Prehosp Emerg Care*. 2007;11:250–252.

18. Braude D, Southard A, Bajema T, et al. Rapid sequence airway using the LMA-Supreme as a primary airway for 9 h in a multi-system trauma patient. *Resuscitation*. 2010;81:1217.

19. Southard A, Braude D, Crandall C. Rapid sequence airway vs rapid sequence intubation in a simulated trauma airway by flight crew. *Resuscitation*. 2010;81:576–578.

20. Wang HE, Domeier RM, Kupas DF, et al. Recommended guidelines for the uniform reporting of data from out of hospital airway management: a position statement from the National Association of EMS Physicians. *Prehosp Emerg Care*. 2004;8:58–72.

21. Drug assisted intubation in the prehospital setting: position statement of the National Association of Emergency Physicians. *Prehosp Emerg Care*. 2006;10:260.

22. Cushman JT, Hettinger AZ, Farney A, et al. Effect of intensive physician oversight on a prehospital rapid-sequence intubation program. *Prehosp Emerg Care*. 2010;14:310–316.

23. Davis DP, Koprowicz KM, Craig D, et al. The relationship between out-of-hospital airway management and outcome among trauma patients with Glasgow Coma Scale scores of 8 or less. *Prehosp Emerg Care*. 2011;15:184–192.

24. Stiell IG, Spaite DW, Field B, et al. Advanced life support for out-of-hospital respiratory distress. *N Engl J Med*. 2007;356:2156–2164.

29

Alternative Devices for EMS Airway Management

Kevin M. Franklin • Michael F. Murphy

INTRODUCTION

Regardless of the location of the patient, airway evaluation and management are the first priority of the health care provider in any emergency setting. The austere environment in which prehospital providers must function (e.g., poor positioning and lighting, disruptive surroundings, and limited assistance) demands that airway care be carried out both thoughtfully and skillfully to ensure the best outcomes.

Every prehospital provider must acquire and maintain the necessary skills to ensure that adequate gas exchange can be assured until arrival at the hospital, regardless of the device used or the technique used.

Endotracheal intubation is a common *advanced* airway procedure used in the prehospital setting. The incidence of difficult intubation in emergency medical services (EMS) is 11%. Studies of prehospital endotracheal intubation have reported success rates from 75% to 96.6%. This highly variable success rate, coupled with the dire consequences of failure, has been the foundation of much discussion concerning how to best manage the airway in the prehospital setting.

The introduction of medication-assisted intubation (e.g., rapid sequence intubation) has led EMS systems to ensure that their advanced providers are trained in the use of alternative airway devices in addition to BMV, in order to rescue the airway should intubation following paralysis and/or sedation fail. The growth of experience with and research in the prehospital use of these airway devices has led EMS medical directors to examine their use as an alternative to endotracheal intubation for advanced providers, and as an alternative to BMV for basic-level providers. In their 2005 guidelines, The European Resuscitation Council recommends that if ventilation cannot be provided through an endotracheal tube, alternative airway devices should be used for ventilation in the management of cardiac arrest. The American Heart Association guidelines are less directive, stating that their use "appears to be safe."

The approach to airway management in EMS is the same as in the ED or the OR. Chapters 1 to 3, provide the framework with which to approach airway management in the prehospital setting. In this chapter, we introduce alternative airway devices available for prehospital use. In 2007, the National Association of EMS Physicians published a position statement on the use of alternative airway devices in the prehospital setting. We discuss the devices available and their prehospital use. For discussion of surgical airways, please refer to Chapter 18.

Simple-to-use devices such as the King LT, laryngeal mask airway (LMA), and the Combitube have been introduced and validated in the prehospital care setting. These devices may be used in two ways: as an alternative to endotracheal intubation in the cardiac arrest (or deeply comatose) patient by basic life support (BLS) providers, or as a rescue device in the setting of failed intubation by advanced life support (ALS) or critical care providers. The actual number of alternative devices available to a specific EMS system is limited by protocols, training, cost and equipment.

All EMS providers who perform advanced airway interventions should also have at least one alternative airway device at their immediate disposal.

An emerging alternative to endotracheal intubation in the respiratory failure patient is prehospital noninvasive ventilation. Several case series have shown continuous positive airway pressure (CPAP) or bi-level ventilation to be feasible and potentially beneficial in the prehospital setting. Further study is necessary to validate its effectiveness and safety.

ALTERNATIVE AIRWAY DEVICES

Bag-Mask Ventilation

Though a difficult technique to master, bag-mask ventilation (BMV) remains an essential skill for any EMS provider (see Chapter 9). Indeed, proper BMV, coupled with oro- and/or nasopharyngeal airways and cricoid pressure, provides adequate minute ventilation in most cases. Cricoid pressure also offers a measure of protection against gastric insufflation and the aspiration of gastric contents. Improper use of BMV, however, can increase the risk of gastric insufflation, regurgitation, and aspiration of stomach contents. This was described by the Australian Anaesthetic Incident Monitoring Study (AIMS) in which mask ventilation was associated with a potential aspiration risk in 66% of patients. In that study, BMV was the designated method of airway management in 72% of patients who aspirated.

Classification of Devices

Chapters 10 and 11 discuss the taxonomy of these devices and how they are used in airway management. Table 29-1 summarizes this taxonomy to facilitate the discussion that follows.

Each device can be considered in four categories:

a. Evidence that it is effective in EMS for
   i. Uncomplicated airway management
   ii. Rescue airway management
b. Whether it is easy to learn, perform, and maintain the skill
c. The cost of the device
d. The availability of pediatric sizes

Most EMS systems have either limited or no ability to resterilize instruments. As a result, disposable variants of alternative airway devices are a much more attractive option. Further, the availability of pediatric sizes may confer an advantage in terms of procurement, training, and skills maintenance.

Supraglottic devices in EMS

Nonintubating LMAs

The LMA is often the rescue device of choice for prehospital systems. Specifically, the LMA has gained traction as a primary airway device in lieu of BMV for BLS providers, and as for rescuing an airway following a failed ETI for ALS providers. The LMA is inserted blindly through the oropharynx, and the skill is fairly easy to acquire. Details regarding the specific devices and related

TABLE 29-1
Taxonomy for Extraglottic devices (EGDs)

	Reusable	Disposable	Pediatric sizes
Supraglottic	LMA Classic	LMA Unique	Yes
	LMA Proseal	LMA Supreme	No
	LMA Flexible	AMBU Variants	Yes
		Solus	No
		Portex	No
		i-gel	Yes
		SLIPA	
Supraglottic intubating	LMA Fastrack	LMA Fastrack Disposable	No
	Cook ILA	Air Q	No
Infraglottic	King LT	Combitube	No
		King LT	Yes
		EasyTube	No

techniques are provided in Chapter 10. In the authors' opinion, the LMA Supreme is the best of the single-use supraglottic variants for EMS use.

Recent research shows some concern for posterior spinal movement during the placement of the LMA, which may be relevant for patients with a spinal cord injury (SCI). The clinical relevance of this finding has not yet been clarified. Thus, caution should be exercised when using the LMA in the setting of a patient with spinal cord injury.

Training and use of the LMA in simulated patients by new paramedics has shown that it can be placed in approximately 34 seconds (removal from package to initiation of first breath). This clearly demonstrates that the LMA can be rapidly deployed in the patient who is failing, while a more definitive airway is prepared.

Intubating LMA variants

Since the introduction of the LMA, modifications to the design, the introduction of other innovative LMA-type extraglottic devices (EGDs) (see Chapter 10), and the provision of single-use devices, have broadened the opportunity for their use in EMS. For instance, the intubating LMA (ILMA) not only permits rescue gas exchange, but also reliably facilitates blind intubation through the device (see Chapter 10).

In the event that the ILMA provides adequate gas exchange in the field and transport times are relatively short, many believe that intubation through the device should not be performed in the field. Instead, the decision as to how best to achieve a definitive airway should be deferred to hospital arrival.

Ambu LMA variants

The Ambu single-use supraglottic devices are reviewed in Chapter 10. The AuraOnce and AuraStraight are probably the second best of the disposable supraglottic devices available at present. The Aura I is specifically designed for use with the Ambu A Scope, rendering it less useful in EMS.

Other devices

A variety of companies supply single-use supraglottic devices that are relatively inexpensive (e.g., Solus and Portex LMA). These devices have similar failings as the LMA Unique, especially "tip roll", and are not as clinically useful as the LMA Supreme and the Ambu EGDs.

Other devices currently being evaluated in the clinical setting include the i-gel, introduced in 2007, and the Supraglottic Airway Laryngopharyngeal Tube (SALT). The i-gel is a noninflatable supraglottic airway that shows some promise in the anesthesia literature but has limited clinical trials and no emergency airway clinical trials to date. Early indications with the SALT device is that while placement is not an issue, intubation aided by the device is suboptimal.

Incorporation of devices such as these into practice with little or no published evidence or supportive expert opinion should be done with extreme caution. As a result, neither device is likely to see much use in the EMS setting.

Retroglottic (infraglottic) device class

Esophageal obturator airway

In the 1970s the esophageal obturator airway was introduced into the prehospital setting as the first extraglottic airway device. When properly positioned, this blindly inserted device placed a cuffed obturator into the esophagus. A facemask was then applied to the device to permit BMV. This device and a subsequent version, the esophageal gastric tube airway, were widely used as both primary and rescue airway devices. Many complications were reported, however, including esophageal rupture, aspiration, and inadvertent tracheal occlusion by the obturator. Because of its complication profile, difficulty in placement, and failure to provide adequate gas exchange, such devices are no longer part of the EMS airway armamentarium.

Esophageal tracheal Combitube

The esophageal tracheal Combitube (ETC; see Chapter 11) is a blindly inserted, double-lumen tube with balloon cuffs that are positioned below (esophageal) and above (hypo-pharyngeal) the glottis, permitting ventilation through periglottic fenestrations located between the proximal and distal cuffs. Ventilation is also possible if the device is inadvertently inserted into the trachea (<5% of insertions; see Chapter 11). The ETC has become a common alternative airway device used in EMS as both a primary and a rescue airway device in adult patients because of its ease of placement, the preferred neutral cervical positioning for placement in trauma patients, and a perceived benefit of the cuffed esophageal tube in the unfasted patient. In a 6-year study of urban/suburban EMS use of the ETC training required only 6 hours of didactic and manikin practice to achieve an 89.4% successful placement rate. No difference in return of spontaneous circulation (ROSC), survival to admission or survival to discharge was noted between the two devices in a population of 5,822 patients. Complications associated with the use of the ETC include aspiration, pneumothorax, pneumomediastinum, airway injuries, and esophageal lacerations and perforations. Some authors recommend inserting the device using a laryngoscope in an attempt to prevent trauma to the airway.

King LT airway (laryngeal tube airway in Europe)

The King LT, approved for use in the United States in 2003, has been introduced into the armamentarium of airway devices available to prehospital providers. See Chapter 11 for a detailed description of this device and a discussion of the evidence with respect to its use.

Kluger and Short evaluated aspiration in the AIMS database, and determined that the LMA was utilized in 63 of 240 reported cases of potential aspiration. This was compared to BMV and ETI, which prevented aspiration by a mere 39%. The frequency of potential aspiration in the ETI group, however, was significantly less. There are no studies evaluating the outcome for patients with spinal cord injury SCI for either the ETC or the King LT, so no recommendations or benefits of these other devices can be assumed with relation to safety in the SCI patient.

CPAP in EMS

Noninvasive ventilatory support (NVS) is addressed in detail in Chapter 6. NVS, specifically CPAP, is slowly becoming more common in the out-of-hospital setting, especially in both ground and air critical care transport. CPAP is most useful in treating patients who require minimal to moderate additional ventilatory support, such as those with congestive heart failure or an exacerbation of chronic obstructive pulmonary disease.

SUMMARY

Airway management in EMS is undergoing tremendous change. The effect of endotracheal intubation on outcome is seriously questioned. BMV is a difficult skill to teach, learn, and maintain. In contrast, EGDs are notable for their simplicity. The EGD technique is easy to teach, learn, and maintain. Thus, EGDs have demonstrated their superiority to BMV as a first rescue from a failed intubation by advanced EMS personnel.

TIPS AND PEARLS

- EGDs are here to stay in EMS (basic and advanced). In fact, within a decade EGDs will supplant BMV as first-line airway management in the apneic or failing patient. All EMS practitioners should become familiar with with the indications, contraindications, and proper technique for the use of each device.
- Be meticulous in learning the technique of insertion. Correct technique is critical to effective ventilation and oxygenation with these devices.
- Slick marketing does not equate to "evidence" or define the true role for a device. Even devices that look like they should work often do not. Rely on evidence and expert opinion; not the sales force for a particular device.

EVIDENCE

- **Is there a statement that identifies the most appropriate airway management devices for prehospital care providers?** In 2007, the National Association of EMS Physicians published a position statement on the use of alternative airways in the prehospital setting.[1] All EMS providers who practice advanced airway interventions should have access to and training for at least one blind placement device. Such a device may be used either as an alternative to ETI, or as a rescue device, in the case of a failed ETI.
- **How easy is it to learn how to use these devices?**
  BMV
  Despite the fact that it is often difficult to adequately ventilate patients with a BMV in the controlled environment of a hospital, it still remains the most commonly used emergency ventilation device in both the hospital and the prehospital setting. As early as 1986, Cummins et al.[2] reported that maintenance of an adequate mask seal is difficult and often requires more than one person to be effective. Such a luxury is rarely available in the prehospital setting. A study of emergency nurses reported a 25% skill retention rate 6 months after training.[3]
  Supraglottic Airways
  The LMA has been found to be relatively easy to place by paramedics and other allied health professionals in both adult and pediatric patients.[4,5] Although median insertion times were longer with the LMA as compared to BMV (30 vs. 4 seconds), this was not considered to represent a clinically significant difference.[6] In 2000, in a manikin study of the ILMA, Levitan et al.[7] reported a 97% success rate, with a mean time to ventilation of 18 seconds and a mean time to intubation of 17 seconds in a variety of providers, including medical nonintubators and nonmedical personnel after a 60-minute training session. Dries et al.[8] reported similar ease of use in the aeromedical setting. In a review of the Proseal LMA studies (PLMA), insertion success rates have ranged between 90% and 100%; However, studies included in this review did not incorporate the prehospital environment.[9]
  Retroglottic Airways
  Successful placement of the ETC in the prehospital setting as a primary airway device is reported to be 71% to 98%, and 64% to 100% as a rescue airway.[10–12] In a retrospective analysis of ETC placement for failed endotracheal intubation in the prehospital setting, Calkins et al[11] reported a success rate of 70%, with 16% of placements being tracheal. A significantly better success rate for the ETC was published by Cady and Pirrallo.[12] Over a 6 year period the ETC was (placed successfully by EMT-B's) 89.4% of the time. (860 ETC attempts). The King LT has also been shown to be relatively easy to place. In a study by Russi et al.,[14] paramedics with no previous exposure or training were able to place the King LT with 100% success in simulated trauma and medical cases. There are no reports of complications employing the King LT in prehospital care.
- **Although these devices** *provide* **an adequate airway, do they** *protect* **the airway?**

Supraglottic Airways

Although definitive airway protection from regurgitation and aspiration must never be assumed when using an LMA, rates of aspiration in the anesthesia literature have been reported to be as low as 0.02%, likely related to the fasted state of operative patients.[15] Stone et al.,[16] examined 713 cardiac arrest patients undergoing assisted ventilation, and reported a lower incidence of regurgitation with the LMA than with BMV (LMA 3.5%, BMV 12.4%, respectively). In the study by Kluger and Short[17] that evaluated aspiration in the AIMS database, the LMA was the airway being utilized in 63 of the 133 reported cases of aspiration.

Retroglottic Airways

In Quebec, where ETC is performed as a basic-level procedure for all cardiac arrests, Vézina et al.[18] reported an aspiration rate of 17%. Although it is generally believed that the esophageal balloon confers an element of protection against aspiration, there is good evidence that the risk of aspiration with use of the ETC is at least equal to that of the LMA. There is no literature on the aspiration rate with the King LT to permit comparisons or compute risk.

- **Can these devices be used in trauma patients?** Use of the LMA in the management of prehospital trauma patients has undergone limited study. There are conflicting reports on the safe use of the LMA in patients with cervical spine trauma. Keller et al.,[19] used pressure sensors attached to the vertebrae in a stable cadaveric cervical spine model and reported unacceptable posterior vertebral displacement when an LMA was used. However, Brimacombe and Berry,[20] in a fluoroscopically assessed cadaveric model using a destabilized cervical spine, reported no difference in displacement between the LMA and direct laryngoscopy. In a difficult trauma airway algorithm developed by Ollerton et al.,[21] they found that placement of an LMA can be performed both effectively and safely. No such studies exist for either ETC or the King LT, so no recommendations or benefits of these other devices can be assumed with relation to safety in the SCI patient.

    In a study of 420 head trauma patients, the Combitube was used as a rescue airway when endotracheal intubation was unsuccessful (15% of all cases). ETC insertion and ventilation were successful at a rate of 95% when used as a rescue airway.[22]

- **Are there certain situations where I should use a specific device over another?** The majority of the literature addressing the use of EGDs in the prehospital environment concerns the ETC. There is a paucity of data specific to the prehospital environment related to other devices permitting one to be guided to scientifically with respect to device selection. However, most experts agree that systems ought to (1) seriously evaluate whether to promote EGD-based ventilation as a first-line device in unresponsive, apneic patients and relegate BMV to a subsidiary role[23]; and (2) ensure that ALS providers have proficiency and the immediate availability of an EGD in the event that neither BMV nor endotracheal intubation is possible, particularly if medications are used to facilitate airway management.

- **How does the ETC compare to ETI in EMS in terms of outcome?** The only published study on this issue by Cady et al.[24] found that compared with initial paramedic ETI, initial EMT-B ETC placement was not associated with patient survival after out-of-hospital cardiac arrest.

REFERENCES

1. Guyette FX, Greenwood MJ, Neubecker D, et al. Alternate airways in the prehospital setting (resource document to NAEMSP position statement). *Prehosp Emerg Care*. 2007;11:56–61.

2. Cummins RO, Austin D, Graves JR, et al. Ventilation skills of emergency medical technicians: a teaching challenge for emergency medicine. *Ann Emerg Med*. 1986;15:1187–1192.

3. De Regge M, Vogels C, Monsieurs KG, et al. Retention of ventilation skills of emergency nurses after training with the SMART BAG compared to a standard bag-valve-mask. *Resuscitation*. 2006;68:379–384.

4. Deakin CD, Peters R, Tomlinson P, et al. Securing the prehospital airway: a comparison of laryngeal mask insertion and endotracheal intubation by UK paramedics. *Emerg Med J*. 2005;22:64–67.

5. Martin P, Cyna A, Hunter W, et al. Training nursing staff in airway management for resuscitation: a clinical comparison of the face mask and laryngeal mask. *Anaesthesia*. 1993;48:33–37.

6. Guyette FX, Roth KR, LaCovey DC, et al. Feasibility of laryngeal mask airway use by prehospital personnel in simulated pediatric respiratory arrest. *Prehosp Emerg Care*. 2007;11:245–249.

7. Levitan RM, Ochroch EA, Stuart S, et al. Use of the intubating laryngeal mask airway by medical and nonmedical personnel. *Am J Emerg Med*. 2000;18:12–16.

8. Dries D, Frascone R, Molinari P, et al. Does the ILMA make sense in HEMS? *Air Med J*. 2001;20:35–37.

9. Cook TM, Lee G, Nolan JP. The ProSeal laryngeal mask airway: a review of the literature. *Can J Anaesth*. 2005;52:739–760.

10. Atherton GL, Johnson JC. Ability of paramedics to use the Combitube in prehospital cardiac arrest. *Ann Emerg Med*. 1993;22:1263–1268.

11. Calkins TR, Miller K, Langdorf MI. Success and complication rates with prehospital placement of an esophageal-tracheal Combitube as a rescue airway. *Prehospital Disaster Med*. 2006;1(suppl 2):97–100.

12. Cady CE, Pirrallo RG. The effect of Combitube use on paramedic experience in endotracheal intubation. *Am J Emerg Med*. 2005;23:868–871.

13. Rabitsch W, Schellongowski P, Staudinger T, et al. Comparison of a conventional tracheal airway with the Combitube in an urban emergency medical services system run by physicians. *Resuscitation*. 2003;57:27–32.

14. Russi CS, Wilcox CL, House HR. The laryngeal tube device: a simple and timely adjunct to airway management. *Am J Emerg Med*. 2007;25:263–267.

15. Brimacombe J, Berry A. The incidence of aspiration associated with the laryngeal mask airway—a meta-analysis of published literature. *J Clin Anesth*. 1995;7:297–305.

16. Stone BJ, Chantler PJ, Baskett PJ. The incidence of regurgitation during cardiopulmonary resuscitation: a comparison between the bag valve mask and laryngeal mask airway. *Resuscitation*. 1998;38:3–6.

17. Kluger MT, Short TG. Aspiration during anaesthesia: a review of 133 cases from the Australian Anaesthetic Incident Monitoring Study (AIMS). *Anaesthesia*. 1999;54:19–26.

18. Vézina MC, Trépanier CA, Nicole PC, et al. Complications associated with the esophageal-tracheal Combitube in the pre-hospital setting. *Can J Anaesth*. 2007;54:124–128.

19. Keller C, Brimacombe J, Keller K. Pressures exerted against the cervical spine by the standard and intubating laryngeal mask airway. *Anesth Analg*. 1999;89:1296–1300.

20. Brimacombe J, Berry A. Laryngeal mask airway insertion. *Anesthesiology*. 1993;48:670–671.

21. Ollerton JE, Parr MJA, Harrison K, et al. Potential cervical spine injury and difficult airway management for emergency intubation of trauma adults in the emergency department—a systematic review. *Emerg Med J*. 2006;23:3–11.

22. Davis DP, Valentine C, Ochs M, et al. The Combitube as a salvage airway device for paramedic rapid sequence intubation. *Ann Emerg Med*. 2003;42:697–704.

23. Petrar S, Murphy MF, Hung OR. Is a seismic shift in EMS airway management coming? A closer look at oxygenation, ventilation, intubation and alternative airways. *JEMS*. 2009;34:54–59.

24. Cady CE, Weaver MD, Pirallo RG, et al. Effect of emergency medical technician–placed Combitubes on outcomes after out-of-hospital cardiopulmonary arrest. *Prehosp Emerg Care*. 2009;13:495–499.

30

Difficult and Failed Airway Management in EMS

Jan L. Eichel • Mary Beth Skarote • Michael F. Murphy

THE CLINICAL CHALLENGE

The prehospital environment presents an array of unique circumstances to the airway practitioner: The scene is often chaotic and may pose hazards to the emergency medical services (EMS) personnel (e.g., flood, fire, radiation, electrical wires, toxic environment, etc.). In addition, access to the patient and the airway may be challenging because of a variety of factors related to extrication and patient or paramedic position. Even with the patient on a stretcher in an ambulance or helicopter, positioning for airway management may be difficult. In fact, some would argue that all airway management in the field is difficult, particularly if more than basic maneuvers are to be used.

Environmental conditions faced by EMS providers are uncontrollable: both the darkness of night and bright sunlight of day present unique difficulties. Dark environments may hinder the preintubation airway assessment and obscure nonverbal communications among personnel that are inherent in complex rescue environments. Alternatively, bright sunlight is likely to interfere with laryngoscopic visualization of the larynx. Weather conditions, scenes of violence, tactical rescue, large crowds, equipment limitations, well-meaning bystanders, lack of knowledgeable assistants, and other factors conspire to enhance the degree of difficulty posed to the EMS airway manager.

Identifying a difficult airway and managing a failed airway are both technical skills that are no different in the out-of-hospital environment than they are in-hospital. Thus, the cognitive and technical skills required of prehospital practitioners are comparable to those practicing in emergency departments (EDs), operating rooms (ORs) and other in-hospital venues, differences in available equipment and backup not-with-standing.

FACTORS SPECIFIC TO THE OUT-OF-HOSPITAL DIFFICULT AIRWAY

There are two interrelated considerations governing management of the difficult airway in the prehospital environment: time factors and anatomical factors.

Time Factors

When is it better to wait?

Although all emergency airway management situations share this feature, identification of a difficult airway might influence the provider either to be more or less likely to intubate the patient before transport. Consider, for example, the following two cases, each with an anticipated 10-minute transport time:

- A 40-year-old, 80-kg man with sudden collapse, Glasgow Coma Scale 6, with no swallowing reflex, normal respiratory pattern with O_2 saturations of 99%, and severe ankylosing spondylitis.
- A 40-year-old, 80-kg man extricated from a house fire, with stridor, O_2 saturations of 70%, and evidence of upper airway burns.

Both patients have clear indications for securing the airway, although the decision making, particularly with respect to urgency, should be quite different.

In the first case, if the patient is not deteriorating further, it often is best to defer intubation to the ED, where a more formal and controlled neuroprotective RSI can be performed and there are additional options, such as flexible endoscopy, for this difficult airway. The patient's respiratory status, and his or her oxygen saturation, are adequate. Training must emphasize that preservation of vital functions equates to gas exchange, and does not necessarily equate to endotracheal intubation. Additionally, the patient has a chronic difficult airway, one that will not become increasingly difficult if intubation is delayed. The provider and system medical directors must be wary of the *technical imperative*—that operators generally will perform an authorized procedure more often than it is required or indicated. In fact, there is growing evidence that in certain situations, prehospital intubation may not improve outcomes, and may even lead to worse outcomes, and may even lead to worse outcomes.

In the second case, the operator is forced to actively manage the airway despite predicted difficulty with laryngoscopy. Even a brief delay, such as a 10-minute transport, allows time for further deterioration, increasing the threat to the patient and making intubation progressively more difficult. The decision to intubate here is clear, and the provider must proceed deliberately down the EMS Difficult Airway Algorithm (Fig. 30-1).

Anatomic Factors

Predicting the difficult airway

The preintubation airway assessment is essential to identify patients likely to present difficulties for laryngoscopy, bag-mask-ventilation (BMV), extraglottic device (EGD) placement, or cricothyrotomy based on a focused examination of external anatomic features (see Chapter 2). This evaluation permits one to make appropriate airway management plans (Plans A, B, and C) that are most likely to be successful.

The patient with acceptable oxygen saturations and a short transport time displaying predictors of difficult laryngoscopy might be better served by a timely transport to the nearest ED, where

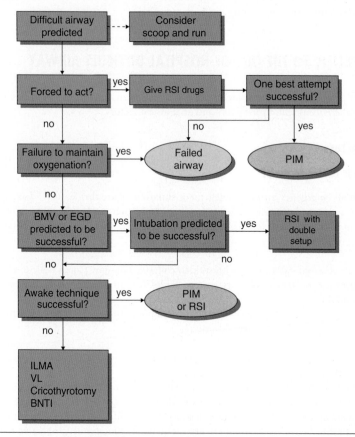

Figure 30-1 ● The EMS Difficult Airway Algorithm. See discussion of the Difficult Airway Algorithm in Chapter 3 for explanation. RSI, rapid sequence intubation or other medication-assisted intubation technique; PIM, post-intubation management; EGD, extra-glottic device; ILMA, intubating laryngeal mask airway; VL, video laryngoscopy; BNTI, blind nasal tracheal intubation.

there are more resources and skilled personnel. This is particularly the case when the difficult airway is chronic or stable, and is not the reason the patient requires intubation. For example, consider the 40-year-old patient above, who had experienced sudden collapse. Suppose that the anticipated transport time is not 10 minutes, but 20 minutes. Suppose also that preintubation assessment identifies that the patient has had head and neck surgery and radiation for cancer, and has limited mouth opening, neck scarring, and some distortion of anatomy. The difficult airway here is stable and will not worsen during transport to an ED, thus making even more compelling the decision to defer intubation until after ED arrival. This extends the window of time that is "acceptable" for transport without intubation because the risk/benefit ratio argues in favor of taking the patient, unintubated, to the ED. This is in stark contrast to the second patient described above with upper airway burns and stridor. Consider this patient in the context of a 5-minute transport time. Here, regardless of how short the transport time is, the likelihood of imminent deterioration both compels intubation and argues for undertaking this at the earliest opportunity. Thus, both the nature and the "stability" of the difficult airway become key factors in the "intubate versus transport" decision. This has been identified as 'context sensitive' airway management.

APPLYING THE EMS DIFFICULT AIRWAY ALGORITHM

When intubation of a difficult airway is required, the EMS Difficult Airway Algorithm (Fig. 30-1) directs one to weigh carefully the RSI (or other medication-assisted intubation) versus "awake" intubation decision. The thought process is identical to that described in Chapter 3. At any point after initiation, if the chosen method is unsuccessful, and oxygenation cannot be maintained, one should move promptly to the failed airway algorithm (Chapter 3). In situations where difficulty is predicted, and airway management is urgently indicated, securing help using on-scene personnel is advisable.

The most difficult airways encountered in the prehospital setting often are those arising in the context of multisystem trauma. The patient may not be able to follow commands or answer questions related to difficult airway assessment, and injuries may be occult. Facial fractures may impede an effective mask seal but may not be readily apparent in a cursory examination. The front portion of the cervical collar might conceal significant injuries to the patient's anterior neck; without opening the collar, the operator has little or no chance of identifying the injuries. Neck mobility may be one factor that the provider has some control over. The immobilization of the cervical spine is known to provide a grade 3 Cormack lehane (C-L) view on direct laryngoscopy approximately 50% of the time. In anticipation of this, the intubator should ready a gum elastic bougie (GEB), if available, or should preferentially a video laryngoscope or optical device, like the Airtraq (see Chapters 13 and 14). When the laryngeal view with immobilization prohibits intubation, the provider must relax immobilization in small increments to permit visualization and intubation. Controlled and cautious cervical spine motion in this circumstance, where the integrity of the spinal column is uncertain, presents less risk to the patient than does failure to assure gas exchange.

Detailed assessment for difficult airway markers is conducted as described in Chapter 2. If a difficult airway is identified, the EMS difficult airway algorithm guides the approach to airway management in the prehospital patient (Fig. 30-1).

The major differences between the difficult airway algorithm pictured in Figure 30-1 and that presented in Chapter 3 are as follows:

- A "scoop and run" option is offered once a difficult airway is predicted. This represents a decision to "scoop and run" to the nearest appropriate receiving center, or to divert the transport to such a center. Such a decision is based on the urgency of the need for emergency airway management, the assessed difficulty, the estimated time required for transport, and available equipment. It requires judgment on the part of requires judgment on the part of the operator. The benefit of transport to a higher level of care is weighed against the risk of delaying airway management for that period of time. Conversely, the benefit of immediate intubation on the scene is weighed against the risk

of undertaking management of a difficult airway in a suboptimal environment with less equipment and back up available.
- The EMS algorithm allows for a variety of system-specific approaches to medication-assisted intubation, whereas the algorithm in Chapter 3 specifies RSI.
- The options once a failed awake intubation has occurred are limited to the use of an EGD, video laryngoscopy, blind nasal intubation, and surgical airway. In Chapter 3, there is the additional option of flexible endoscopy, which is not available in the out-of-hospital environment.

Nevertheless, the thought processes in the two algorithms are identical.

The "forced to act" situation is a particular scenario, and is discussed in depth in Chapter 3. Similar principles apply here as in the ED or hospital environment. As discussed earlier, transport time also should be considered when determining whether it is appropriate to perform a drug-assisted intubation. Again, in many settings, especially urban systems with short transport times, transport to the ED may be preferable to struggling with a difficult airway in the prehospital setting.

Enhancement of the devices available, particularly video laryngoscopy, or even simple adjuncts, such as GEB, may increase first attempt success rates, particularly in the immobilized patient.

THE FAILED AIRWAY IN EMS

The definitions of the failed airway are essentially the same in the EMS environment as those presented in Chapters 2 and 3: failure to maintain oxygenation by any means and failure to intubate on three attempts. Two clinical situations are presented: cannot intubate, can oxygenate: *have time*; cannot intubate, cannot oxygenate: *have no time*. This latter circumstance is often referred to using the abbreviation CICO.

The failed airway algorithm is used as described in Chapter 3. However, decisions at any point are influenced by the devices available to EMS providers, and the skills that they are permitted to perform, as specified by protocol (see Chapter 28).

Although limited resources are available in the field, the use of a second, experienced provider should always be given immediate consideration when the airway is identified as very difficult. The second operator may assist with initial airway management and be designated to attempt placement of an EGD in the case of CICO, while the first operator prepares for the cricothyrotomy. In rare cases, for example, in a patient with lacerations through the soft tissues of the oropharynx and a disrupted upper airway, the airway may best be secured by immediate cricothyrotomy if field protocols permit, and the provider is appropriately trained.

Not infrequently, the prehospital provider will be faced with a failed intubation. A failed intubation is usually multifactorial; the result of an anatomically challenging patient, time pressures, equipment limitations, and, often, provider experience and judgment.

AIRWAY RESCUE

Traditionally, BMV has been the primary rescue device for failed intubation in the out-of-hospital setting, although practice is evolving as more experience is gained with EGDs. Nonetheless, prehospital providers must be expert at BMV using both one-handed and two-handed mask hold techniques, supplemented by oral and nasopharyngeal airways. If BMV is inadequate at providing effective gas exchange, the patient should be repositioned, the jaw thrust maneuver should be applied fully, oral and nasal airways should be placed (if not already), a two-handed technique should be used to seal the mask to the patient, and any other steps should be taken that the operator determines might be helpful (see Chapter 9). A subjective sense that BMV is inadequate or failing should motivate the prompt placement of an EGD. Meticulous BMV and rapid transport might be the appropriate action, however, if oxygenation is adequate and intubation appears difficult or impossible.

If intubation is unsuccessful, it is important to attempt to determine why. Chapter 12 describes the sequence of steps involved in successful direct laryngoscopy. Repositioning the head and neck, backward upward rightward pressure on the thyroid cartilage, a change in blade size or type, or even a change in operator may help.

When laryngoscopy fails and no appropriate rescue devices are available, digital or tactile intubation may be an option in experienced hands (Chapter 17). Although true indications are exceedingly rare, digital intubation requires no specialized equipment and obviates the need to visualize the glottis, or to reposition the head and neck. Some EMS systems permit cricothyrotomy to be performed in the prehospital setting. If this is the case, adequate training and skill maintenance are important. Cricothyrotomy in the field should be an exceedingly rare event. Cricothyrotomy accounts only for approximately 1% of all ED intubations; the incidence among out-of-hospital intubations should be even lower. Performance of a cricothyrotomy, or the identification and attempted rescue of any failed airway, should be subject to quality review.

TIPS AND PEARLS

- In the prehospital environment the use of two providers for the identified difficult airway may prove to be the best use of limited personnel, saving time and preventing complications for patients.
- If possible, have a GEB readily available, particularly for patients in spinal immobilization.
- If manual in-line stabilization of the C-Spine is preventing intubation, ask the individual providing the immobilization to "give me a centimeter" and do so centimeter by centimeter until the ETT can be passed.
- The life of the patient is of paramount importance. Do not delay recognizing intubation failure, and transitioning to an EGD or BMV.
- Monitor end tidal carbon dioxide continuously to detect inadvertent tube dislodgement.
- Avoid the use of neuromuscular blocking agents or potent sedative agents unless you are confident in your ability to provide ongoing, effective gas exchange.

EVIDENCE

- **Is there any evidence that experienced prehospital providers perform better than less experienced ones?** There is, and it is related specifically to the number of airways managed. Garza et al.[1] found that the number of patients in whom intubation was attempted per paramedic was significantly correlated with the intubation success rate. Months of experience per paramedic had no significant correlation with intubation success rate. The investigators also found that paramedics frequently operate under poor environmental conditions and encounter significant distractions while attempting to perform endotracheal intubation.[2]

  Wang et al.[3] found that greater numbers of intubations per practitioner increased success rates. Perhaps the more important finding in this study, however, was that as the experience level of the practitioner increased, the numbers of intubations performed decreased. The implication is that more experience permitted practitioners to use alternative methods, perhaps, because they were able to predict intubation difficulty.
- **Is there evidence that the GEB enhances intubation success rates in EMS?** Evidence specific to EMS does not exist. However, there is ample evidence that success rates and time to in-

tubate are enhanced by this simple device in the hands of anesthesiologists and emergency physicians.[4,5]

- **How common is the difficult and failed airway in EMS?** The incidence of the difficult airway in the OR setting is 1.1% to 3.8% with the failed intubation occurring at 0.13% to 0.3% of cases (see also Chapter 2).[6] So, it is not uncommon to see a difficult airway even in the OR. The incidence of difficult intubation in EMS, where equipment and support are limited, and patients cannot be deferred based on a "preanesthetic" assessment, is 3 to 10 times that seen in the OR, at 11%.[7] Studies of prehospital endotracheal intubation have reported failed intubation rates from 3.4% to 25%.[8,9] It is this variation that has called into question the advisability of prehospital care personnel performing endotracheal intubation in general, and RSI in particular (see Chapter 28).

REFERENCES

1. Garza AG, Gratton MC, Coontz D, et al. Effect of paramedic experience on orotracheal intubation success rates. *J Emerg Med*. 2003;25:251–256.

2. Garza AG, Gratton MC, McElroy J, et al. Environmental factors encountered during out-of-hospital intubation attempts. *Prehosp Emerg Care*. 2008;12:286–289.

3. Wang HE, Abo BN, Lave JR, et al. How would minimum experience standards affect the distribution of out-of-hospital endotracheal intubations? *Ann Emerg Med*. 2007;50:246–252.

4. Tomek S. Bougie it! The gum elastic bougie is a viable adjunct for the difficult endotracheal intubation. *EMS World*. 2011;40(1):26–30, 32.

5. Gataure PS, Vaughan RS, Latto IP. Simulated difficult intubation: comparison of the gum elastic bougie and the stylet. *Anaesthesia*. 1996;51:935–938.

6. Crosby ET, Cooper RM, Douglas MJ, et al. The unanticipated difficult airway with recommendations for management. *Can J Anaesth*. 1998;45:757–776.

7. Adnet F, Jouriles NJ, Le Toumelin P, et al. Survey of out-of-hospital emergency intubations in the French prehospital medical system: a multicenter study. *Ann Emerg Med*. 1998;32:454–460.

8. Jacobs LM, Berrizbeitia LD, Bennett B, et al. Endotracheal intubation in the prehospital phase of emergency medical care. *JAMA*. 1983;250:2175–2177.

9. Krisanda TJ, Eitel DR, Hess D, et al. An analysis of invasive airway management in a suburban emergency medical services system. *Prehospital Disaster Med*. 1992;7:121–126.

31

The Trauma Patient

Michael A. Gibbs • Michael G. Gonzalez • Ron M. Walls

THE CLINICAL CHALLENGE

Effective airway management is a cornerstone of resuscitation of the critically injured patient. Although the nature and timing of airway intervention is influenced by assessment and prioritization of multiple injuries, the fundamental principles of trauma airway management are no different from those applied to management of the airway in other complex medical situations. A consistent approach and a reproducible thought process will maximize success.

Whether a trauma patient requires intubation depends on myriad factors that reach well beyond the airway. The indications for intubation discussed in Chapter 1 include failure of the patient's ability to maintain or protect the airway, as in traumatic coma. In such cases, the need for intubation is clear. Failure of ventilation or oxygenation is less common. The former often is related to intoxicants, head injury, or direct chest injury, such as pneumo- or hemo-thorax. The latter also may arise from direct chest trauma, but also from pulmonary edema caused by diffuse capillary injury in the lung from shock, referred to as "shock lung" or acute respiratory distress syndrome. The most common indication for intubation in trauma, however, also is the most challenging. This is the "anticipated clinical course" indication, wherein multiple injuries, hemodynamic instability, need for painful procedures, likelihood of deterioration, need for surgery, combative behavior, and other considerations lead to a decision to intubate, even though the airway itself, oxygenation, and ventilation are adequate.

In the National Emergency Airway Registry (NEAR) database, the top three primary indications for intubation are head injury (39%), direct airway injury (17%), and multisystem trauma (14%).

APPROACH TO THE AIRWAY

Although many trauma intubations turn out to be straightforward, all should be considered at least potentially difficult. A targeted patient assessment should be performed with the aim of answering two fundamental questions. First: Will the procedure be difficult? Systematic use of the difficult airway mnemonics (Chapter 2) will help answer this question. Second: Will physiology suffer? This question prompts the clinician to anticipate predictable changes in physiology that may occur before, during, or immediately following intubation, as a result of the injuries present, the procedure, or the patient's premorbid condition.

Assessment of Difficulty

Application of the difficult airway mnemonics (LEMON, MOANS, SMART, and RODS) allows the clinician to rapidly identify the difficult airway at the bedside. It is worth noting that the LEMON mnemonic, originally published in the first edition of this manual, in 2000, is recommended as the airway assessment tool of choice in the current (eighth) version of ATLS. The mnemonics are provided in detail in Chapter 2, but are adapted here specifically for the trauma airway:

1. *L*: Look externally. Injury to the face, mouth, or neck may distort anatomy or limit access, making the process of intubation difficult or impossible. The integrity of the mask seal may be impaired by facial hair, external bleeding, preexisting physiognomy, or anatomical disruption (*M*OANS). Injury to the anterior neck, such as by a clothesline mechanism or hematoma, may preclude successful cricothyrotomy (*SM*ART) or extraglottic device (EGD) placement (RO*D*S).
2. *E*: Evaluate 3-3-2. In blunt trauma, the cervical spine is immobilized, and a cervical collar is usually in place at the time that airway decisions must be made. A cervical collar is not particularly effective at limiting cervical spine movement during intubation, but greatly impairs mouth opening, limiting both laryngoscopy and insertion of an EGD (*R*ODS). The front portion of the collar should be opened to facilitate the primary survey and removed entirely during intubation. Other injuries, such as mandibular fractures, may either facilitate or impair oral access, and mouth opening should be assessed as carefully as possible.

3. *M*: Mallampati. The trauma patient is rarely able to cooperate with a formal Mallampati assessment, but the airway manager should open the patient's mouth as widely as possible and inspect the oral cavity for access, using a tongue blade, or the laryngoscope blade, which has the advantage of illumination. At this time, potential hemorrhage or disruption of the upper airway may also be evident (RO*D*S). It is important to refrain from "checking the gag reflex" during mouth opening, as this adds no useful information and may precipitate vomiting.

4. *O*: Obstruction, Obesity. Obstruction, usually by hemorrhage or hematoma, can interfere with laryngoscopy, BMV (M*O*ANS), or EGD placement (R*O*DS). Obesity in the trauma patient presents the same challenges as for the nontrauma patient.

5. *N*: Neck mobility. All patients suffering blunt trauma require in-line stabilization of the cervical spine during airway management. By definition, in-line stabilization significantly impairs the ability to place the patient in the sniffing position and as a result, direct visualization of the glottis will be predictably difficult. When in-line stabilization is required, other measures to improve glottic visualization (e.g., Backward, upward (cephalad), and rightward pressure [BURP] maneuver, and video laryngoscopy) or to achieve airway rescue (e.g., Bougie, EGD, and surgical technique) should be prepared for as part of the overall airway management plan. Two areas of controversy are related to the need for spinal immobilization in patients suffering cranial gunshot wounds and in those suffering penetrating wounds to the neck. In the former group, there is sound evidence that the amount of force delivered by a gunshot wound to the head or face in and of itself is insufficient to fracture the spine. In both groups, decision making should be guided by the neurologic examination. Simply stated, a normal neurologic examination is an indication that the neck can be gently moved to optimize visualization of the airway. A neurologic deficit suggestive of cervical spinal cord injury mandates in-line stabilization.

Special Clinical Considerations

The trauma airway is one of the most challenging clinical circumstances in emergency care. It requires knowledge of a panoply of techniques, guided by a reproducible approach (the airway algorithms), sound judgment, and technical expertise. In this section, we describe the considerations unique to several high-risk scenarios (see Table 31-1).

A—Injury to the airway

Here, the very condition that mandates intubation may also render it much more difficult and prone to failure. Direct airway injury may be the result of

- Maxillofacial trauma
- Blunt or penetrating anterior neck trauma
- Smoke inhalation

TABLE 31-1 The "ABC'S" of the Trauma Airway	
A	• Is there an injury to the Airway?
B	• Is there traumatic Brain injury?
C	• Is there a significant Chest injury?
	• Is there a risk of Cervical spine injury?
S	• Is the patient in Shock?

In cases of distorted anatomy, the approach must be one that minimizes the potential for catastrophic deterioration. Airway disruption may be marginal or significant, real or potential. In either case, the guiding principle is to secure the threatened airway early, while more options are preserved, and the patient's stability permits a more deliberate approach. Careful decisions guided by the airway algorithms will need to be made about the use (or not) of neuromuscular blockade, the primary method of airway management, and the airway rescue plan. The importance of mobilizing resources (equipment and personnel), strong leadership, and effective communication with the entire team cannot be overemphasized.

As for any other anatomically distorted airway, application of the difficult airway algorithm will often lead to a decision to perform an awake intubation. In patients with signs of significant airway compromise (e.g., stridor, respiratory distress, and voice distortion), both the urgency of the intubation and the risk of using neuromuscular blockade are high. When symptoms are more modest, there is more time to plan and execute the airway intervention, but in neither case is delay advisable. The patient's oxygenation should be assessed (i.e., "Is there time?"), and it should be determined if RSI is advisable, possibly under a double setup, even though the airway is difficult (see Chapter 3). This will depend on the clinician's confidence about the likelihood of success of oxygenation using a bag and mask or an EGD, and intubation by direct or video laryngoscopy. Often, an airway not amenable to direct laryngoscope can be managed using a video laryngoscope. When airway management is required immediately, RSI (preferably using a video laryngoscope) with a double setup may be used, but when time permits and the airway is not obscured by blood, the best approach often is awake intubation using a flexible endoscope technique with sedation and topical anesthesia (see Chapter 15). This permits both examination of the airway and careful navigation through the injured area, even when the airway itself has been violated. This is especially true if a tracheal injury is suspected, as no other method of intubation allows the airway to be visualized both above and below the glottis. When the airway is disrupted, the endotracheal tube used should be as small as is reasonable to maximize the likelihood of success and to minimize the likelihood of additional airway injury.

Smoke inhalation can present on a spectrum from mild exposure to complete airway obstruction and death. The initial assessment is designed to identify the presence or absence of high-risk historical features (e.g., closed space fire) and physical findings (e.g., singed nasal hairs, perinasal or perioral soot, carbon deposits on the tongue, hoarse voice, and carbonaceous sputum). When evidence of significant smoke inhalation is present, direct examination of the airway, often with intubation, is important. This is best done with flexible endoscopy, which permits evaluation of the airway and immediate progression to intubation, if indicated. Supraglottic edema is an indication for intubation, even if the edema is mild, because progression can be both rapid and occult. Observation in lieu of airway examination can be hazardous because the airway edema can worsen significantly without any external evidence, and by the time the severity of the situation is apparent, intubation is both immediately required and extremely difficult or impossible. If examination of the upper airway identifies that the injury is confined to the mouth and nose, and the supraglottic area is spared (normal), then intubation safely can be deferred, with subsequent examination at the discretion of the operator. If it is unclear whether edema is present, it is useful to periodically perform a repeated upper airway examination (e.g., 30 to 60 minutes), even if symptoms or signs do not develop or worsen.

B—Traumatic Brain Injury

In the NEAR studies, head injury is the most common indication for emergency department trauma airway management. Traumatic brain injury (TBI) is the number one cause of injury-related death worldwide. The principles of management of the patient with TBI and elevated intracranial pressure are discussed in more detail in Chapter 32.

When neurologic status is altered, whether by traumatic brain injury, spinal injury, or both, a rapid, but thorough neurologic examination is important before intubation is undertaken, so that baseline neurologic status is documented to guide subsequent assessments and therapeutic decisions. Airway management decisions in the patient with severe TBI are centered around the prevention of secondary injury, that is, minimizing the magnitude and duration of hypoxia or hypotension. Secondary injury is the term applied when the insult to the injured brain is worsened by hypoxia, hypotension, or both.

Concrete steps can be taken to reduce the risk of secondary injury before, during, and after airway management:

First—Bring the principles of secondary brain injury prevention to the field. EMS providers should be educated and equipped to begin neuroresuscitation before the patient arrives in the ED. Maintenance of adequate perfusion pressure (mean arterial blood pressure) and oxyhemoglobin saturation are the keys.

Second—Optimize brain perfusion before intubation, if possible. Appropriate volume replacement with normal saline solution may mitigate or prevent hypotension caused by RSI drugs or positive-pressure ventilation.

Third—Don't delay. Often, fentanyl and lidocaine are given as pretreatment agents for patients with elevated intracranial pressure (see Chapters 19, 20, and 32). If the patient is hypoxic because of hypoventilation or lung injury, intubation should not be delayed for administration of these pretreatment drugs. Similarly, if respirations are depressed, fentanyl should be avoided. Often, despite the presence of known or suspected elevated intracranial pressure, conflicting clinical considerations argue for a simple approach, such as rapid RSI using etomidate and succinylcholine. However, it is precisely the brain injured patient who has the most to gain by mitigating the adverse physiologic responses to intubation, especially the very young who are endowed with the greatest potential for recovery.

Fourth—Select induction agents and doses carefully. Etomidate, because of its balance of preservation of hemodynamics and modest cerebroprotective properties, is frequently the agent of choice. The dose should be reduced from 0.3 mg per kg to 0.15 to "0.2" mg per kg in the face of compensated or decompensated hypovolemic shock. If the patient is severely compromised, ketamine, if available, is the agent of choice. The dose of ketamine is reduced to 0.5 mg per kg if the patient is in shock. The historical dogma that ketamine causes a clinically meaningful rise in intracranial pressure (ICP) is not evidence based. However, ketamine may raise the systemic blood pressure, so it probably should be avoided in head injured patients who are hypertensive.

Fifth—Avoid hyperventilation. Once felt to be a basic tool in the management of severe TBI, the use of hyperventilation is now known to lead to poorer outcomes. There is no question that hyperventilation transiently reduces intracranial pressure (ICP). It does so, however, by reducing CNS perfusion, violating the central tenant of secondary injury prevention.

C—Cervical spine injury

Severely injured blunt trauma patients are assumed to have cervical spine injury until proven otherwise, and require in-line stabilization during airway management. Although in-line stabilization is believed to help protect against spinal cord injury during intubation, it can create several problems as well. Intoxicated or head injured patients typically become agitated and difficult to control when strapped down on a backboard. Physical and chemical restraint may be required. Aspiration is a significant risk in the supine patient with traumatic brain injury or if they are vomiting. In the supine position, ventilation may be impaired, particularly for obese patients, and chest injury may make matters even worse. High-flow oxygen should be provided to all patients, and suction must be immediately available.

If urgent airway management is needed, no purpose is served by obtaining a crosstable-lateral cervical spine X-ray before intubation. This single view, even if technically perfect, with a sensitivity of <80% is inadequate to exclude injury. Additionally, delaying intubation for the X-ray expends precious time, only to provide the operator with a false sense of security if "normal." The intubation itself is performed as gently as possible, ideally using a video laryngoscope, and with in-line cervical stabilization by a second provider. Use of the BURP maneuver will improve visualization of the glottis during direct laryngoscopy (DL) without compromising spine stabilization. Both the preintubation neurologic status of the patient and the fact that in-line stabilization was used should be clearly documented in the medical record.

There is growing evidence that video laryngoscopy is superior to standard laryngoscopy when airway management is performed with the neck held in-line. Better views of the glottis are achieved in less time, and intubation success rates are higher. Traditional flexible endoscopic intubation remains a valuable tool in the patient with cervical spine trauma. Recent flouroscopic studies comparing cervical motion during standard laryngoscopy, video laryngoscopy, and flexible fiberoptic intubation demonstrate that the flexible endoscopic approach is associated with the least amount of cervical displacement. Translating this information into clinical practice, video laryngoscopy appears to be the best approach for the majority of at-risk blunt trauma patients requiring cervical immobilization. Flexible endoscopic intubation should be considered in patients with known or strongly suspected unstable cervical spine fractures, or those with coexisting anterior neck injuries with distorted anatomy, provided sufficient time, and appropriate equipment and expertise are available.

C—Chest trauma

Blunt and penetrating chest trauma produce injuries that are extremely relevant to the airway management process. Pneumothorax, hemothorax, flail chest, pulmonary contusion, or open chest wounds all impair ventilation and oxygenation. Preoxygenation may be difficult or impossible, and rapid desaturation following paralysis is the rule. The postintubation delivery of positive-pressure ventilation may convert a simple pneumothorax to a tension pneumothorax. When a pneumothorax is known or suspected, needle decompression should be performed before intubation when feasible.

Penetrating chest wounds with the potential to cause cardiac injury deserve special mention. Acute traumatic pericardial tamponade is a rapidly progressive and highly lethal condition. In the setting of tamponade physiology, cardiac output becomes preload dependent. For this reason, cardiovascular collapse can occur following administration of induction agents or use of positive-pressure ventilation. If available, a bedside ultrasound should be performed early in the resuscitation. If pericardial tamponade is detected, it should be relieved before the intubation or immediately following intubation whenever possible. If urgent intubation is required and a cardiac wound is known or suspected, volume infusion is important to increase cardiac preload. The dose of induction agent (ketamine or etomidate) ought to be substantially reduced in this setting (e.g., 50%) or perhaps opting for "amnesia over anesthesia" (midazolam or ketamine), particularly for the patient in extremis.

S—Shock

Shock in the multiple injured patient can be broadly classified as hemorrhagic or nonhemorrhagic (e.g., tension pneumothorax, pericardial tamponade, myocardial contusion, and spinal shock). A targeted physical examination and selective bedside testing (chest X-ray, pelvic X-ray, and e-FAST) will help identify the cause(s). As the causes of shock are elucidated and addressed, airway management decisions must consider the erosion of hemodynamic reserve in these patients. Common decisions include the following:

- Should the patient be intubated now, or is more resuscitation advisable?
- How does the patient's hemodynamic status influence the choice and dose of the induction agent?

Although there is no simple answer to these fundamental questions, the central tenet here is: the more hemodynamically unstable, the more important it is to resuscitate before intubation to mitigate the potential adverse hemodynamic effects of RSI drugs.

Patients in "compensated shock" can appear deceptively stable. The presence or absence of shock should never be simplistically equated with the presence or absence of a blood pressure reading of <90 mm Hg. Because of adaptive postinjury responses, relatively normal blood pressure is often maintained despite significant hypoperfusion. Hypotension is typically a late finding indicative of significant decompensation. The operator must select the induction agent (and its dose) and determine the rate, timing, and quantity of resuscitative crystalloid solution in the context of the patient's overall circulatory status and response to resuscitation, rather than be guided only by a systolic blood pressure.

Table 31-2 provides summary guidance on how to anticipate and manage changes in physiology during airway management.

TABLE 31-2
Anticipating Changes in Physiology during Trauma Airway Management

Clinical scenario	Challenge	Considerations
Airway injury		
• Facial/neck trauma	Will intubation be difficult?	• RSI vs. an awake technique? • Identify rescue device(s) • Prepare for surgical airway
• Smoke inhalation	Will intubation be difficult? Will there be airway edema? Will lung injury limit reserve?	• RSI vs. an awake technique? • Supraglottic rescue device may not work • Prepare for surgical airway • Have smaller ETT ready • Anticipate rapid desaturation
Brain injury		
• Isolated brain injury	Will laryngoscopy cause a rise in ICP?	• Pretreat with lidocaine and fentanyl if time and conditions permit • Etomidate induction
• Brain injury and multisystem trauma with hemodynamic compromise	Will BP (and CNS perfusion) fall further during induction?	• Optimize preload • Reduce dose of etomidate or ketamine • Avoid other induction agents
Cervical spine	Is there a risk of spinal cord injury during intubation?	• Blunt trauma patients are presumed to have this risk until proven otherwise • Maintain in-line stabilization • Use video laryngoscopy or flexible endoscopy if available
	Will in-line stabilization impair visualization of the airway?	• Use the BURP maneuver during DL • Video laryngoscopy is superior to DL
Chest injury		
• Blunt	Is there a pneumothorax or hemothorax? Will drugs or positive pressure ventilation precipitate cardiovascular collapse? Will chest injury limit reserve?	• Consider needle chest decompression • Optimize preload • Ketamine or reduced dose etomidate for induction • Anticipate rapid desaturation
• Penetrating	Is there a pneumothorax or pericardial tamponade? Will drugs or positive-pressure ventilation precipitate cardiovascular collapse? Will chest injury limit reserve?	• Consider needle chest decompression • Optimize preload • Ketamine or reduced dose etomidate for induction • Anticipate rapid desaturation
Shock	Will drugs or positive-pressure ventilation precipitate cardiovascular collapse?	• Optimize preload • Ketamine or reduced dose etomidate for induction

TECHNIQUE

Paralysis versus Rapid Tranquilization of the Combative Trauma Patient

The combative trauma patient presents a series of conflicting problems. The causes of combative behavior in the trauma patient are numerous and include head injury, drug or ethanol intoxication, preexisting medical conditions (e.g., diabetes), hypoxemia, shock, anxiety, personality disorder, and others. The priority is to rapidly control the patient so that potentially life-threatening causes can be identified and corrected. Controversy exists as to whether such patients ought to undergo rapid tranquilization with a neuroleptic agent or sedative, or whether immediate intubation with neuromuscular blockade is appropriate. Rapid tranquilization using haloperidol is well established as a safe and effective means for gaining control of the combative trauma patient who cannot be settled by other means. Haloperidol can be used intravenously in 5- to 10-mg increments every 5 minutes until a sufficient clinical response is achieved. There is extensive literature supporting the safety of this approach. The decision to use rapid tranquilization rather than RSI with neuromuscular blockade depends on the nature of the patient's presentation and injuries. If intubation is required based on the patient's injuries, independent of the combative behavior, then immediate intubation is indicated. If, however, the patient is presenting primarily with control problems and does not appear to have injuries that would mandate intubation, then rapid tranquilization is appropriate. In many situations, the decision will not be clear-cut, and judgment will be required. Control of the patient is an essential step in overall management.

Rapid Sequence Intubation of the Trauma Patient

Except when consideration of the patient's injuries argues otherwise, rapid sequence intubation (RSI) is the preferred method of airway management for the majority of injured patients. The potential for difficulty or failure is inherent in trauma airway management and formulation of a back up (rescue) plan is a key part of preparing for the airway interventions.

As in other critically ill patients, the universal, difficult, and failed airway algorithms will guide the clinician in navigating the multitude of unique clinical scenarios that may arise in the injured patient (see Chapter 3). Familiarity with the algorithms and with the drugs and techniques of RSI, and alternative airway techniques will maximize the likelihood of a positive outcome.

Choice of Pretreatment Agents

Pretreatment agents potentially can mitigate some of the detrimental side effects of upper airway stimulation during intubation. Pretreatment agents, when used, ideally are given 3 minutes before the paralysis step of RSI. In highly unstable patients or in other circumstances in which it appears necessary to secure the airway without delay, a simple intubation using only an induction agent and neuromuscular blocking agent may be preferable. Lidocaine, in a dose of 1.5 mg per kg, blunts the reflex rise in ICP during laryngeal manipulation and mitigates increased airway resistance in susceptible patients. Although controversy exists about the exact mechanism and magnitude of the effect on ICP, we recommend the use of lidocaine for patients suspected to have elevated ICP, when possible.

Fentanyl is indicated when the catecholamine surge, which accompanies intubation, is undesirable, such as in traumatic cerebral hemorrhage or brain injury with elevated ICP. In the trauma patient, increased sympathetic tone often is essential to preserve blood pressure in the face of blood loss. Administration of fentanyl, which reduces sympathetic tone may not be in the patient's best interest. In cases of isolated head injury with stable hemodynamics, fentanyl is indicated, as is lidocaine.

Choice of Neuromuscular Blocking Agent

Succinylcholine (SCh) is the NMBA of choice for RSI in the trauma patient because of its rapid, reliable onset and brief duration of action. Although patients with spinal cord injury, extensive burns, or severe crush injuries are at risk for SCh-induced hyperkalemia, the receptor upregulation that can lead to hyperkalemia takes several days to develop and is not a clinical concern in the acute setting. SCh is contraindicated in these patients beginning 5 days postinjury, and extending for 6 months or until the burns are healed. In these patients, rocuronium is a suitable replacement.

Suspected elevation of ICP is not a contraindication to SCh. SCh-induced fasciculations have been implicated in producing elevation of ICP in the patient with traumatic brain injury, and in the past using a defasciculating dose of a nondepolarizer was recommended. This rise in ICP is not felt to be clinically significant and defasciculation is not needed.

Choice of Induction Agent

In most circumstances, etomidate is the drug of choice for patients with trauma, because of its rapid onset, hemodynamic stability, favorable effect on cerebral metabolic oxygen demand and extensive experience with its use. Despite its reputation for hemodynamic stability, etomidate can aggravate hemodynamic status in susceptible patients leading to the recommendation to reduce the induction dose to 0.2 mg per kg in these patients. The transient depression of steroid synthesis by etomidate has not been shown to adversely affect outcome in patients with hemodynamic shock (see Chapters 21 and 35).

Ketamine may be the best induction agent for patients in compensated or decompensated shock. However, because ketamine may increase blood pressure in normotensive or hypertensive patients, such as patients with isolated severe head injury, etomidate is probably the preferable agent in these patients. Induction agent selection is summarized in Table 31-3.

THE FAILED AIRWAY

The failed airway is managed according to the failed airway algorithm. The LEMON, MOANS, RODS, and SMART guided evaluations during the preintubation assessment are intended to minimize the risk of encountering a failed airway. Cricothyrotomy equipment should always be readily available.

TIPS AND PEARLS

1. Airway management of the multiple injured patient follows the same general principles as any other patient. The primary challenge for the intubator is to resist distraction by the patient's

TABLE 31-3
RSI Sedative Induction Agent Selection in the Trauma Patient

Clinical scenario	First choice	Alternatives
No brain injury		
Hemodynamically stable	Etomidate	Propofol, thiopental, midazolam
Shock	Ketamine	Etomidate[a]
Brain injury		
Hemodynamically stable	Etomidate	Thiopental, propofol
Shock	Etomidate[a]	Ketamine[a,b]
Profound shock	Ketamine[a]	None

[a]In the presence of shock, reduce the dose by 25%–50%.
[b]Hemodynamic considerations outweigh intracranial pressure controversy.

external injuries, combative behavior, or the anxiety that accompanies care of the severely injured trauma victim.

2. Resist the temptation to observe the patient with upper airway injury or smoke inhalation. Delay can lead to disaster. Examine the upper airway periodically with a flexible endoscope passed nasally.

3. Consider early intubation for patients to be moved out of the ED for investigations or transport to another facility.

4. There is substantial and increasing evidence that video laryngoscopy is superior to DL for trauma airway management in the ED. Give serious consideration to incorporating video laryngoscopy into your practice.

5. The hemodynamically compromised trauma patient may be much more severely injured than is apparent. Young patients, in particular, can preserve a reasonably "normal" blood pressure in the face of significant hemorrhage. Occult instability may be suddenly unmasked by the administration of sedative agents or positive-pressure ventilation.

EVIDENCE

- **Are there large studies of intubated trauma patients?** Dunham et al.[1] performed a comprehensive evidence-based literature overview (demographics, airway management techniques, and success rates) of trauma patients requiring emergency airway management. Although most of these patients were critically ill, the degree of injury were highly variable; the mean injury severity score was 29 (range 17 to 54), and the mean Glasgow Coma Scale was 6.5 (range 3 to 15). On average, 41% of patients died (range 2% to 100%). In the recently published report from the NEAR, 26% of patients were victims of injury. Cricothyrotomy is required in approximately 1.7% of all trauma patients. It is almost always used as a rescue technique and when performed has a high success rate and low rate of adverse events.[2]

- **Has inadequate or inappropriate airway management been linked to preventable death?** In 1995, a panel of physicians and prehospital providers reviewed 629 trauma deaths in the state of Montana to determine the rate and cause of preventable mortality and "inappropriate" care. The overall preventable death rate was judged to be 13%. The most common cause of inappropriate care was inadequate airway management in either the prehospital setting (6.8% of cases) or emergency department (5.4% of cases).[3] A more recent study evaluating 51 preventable deaths at a large regional trauma center in Los Angeles found that only one death (1.9%) was directly attributable to failure to manage the airway in the ED.[4] Although this improvement is encouraging, it should not diminish the appreciation that trauma airways are high-risk and that developing and maintaining skills necessary for trauma airway management is a priority.[5,6]

- **Does hyperventilation worsen outcomes in patients with severe TBI?** Davis et al.[7] examined the impact of prehospital ventilation strategies on outcomes in 890 intubated head injury patients in San Diego County. By protocol, arterial blood gases were obtained upon ED arrival. Hyperventilation was defined as a PCO_2 <30 mm Hg, and hypoventilation as a PCO_2 >49 mm Hg. Patients with a PCO_2 of 30 to 49 mm Hg had a lower mortality and a better neurologic outcomes. Warner et al.[8] conducted a similar prospective assessment of 576 intubated TBI patients in Seattle. These authors defined severe hypocapnea as an arrival PCO_2 <30 mm Hg, severe hypercapnea as an arrival PCO_2 >45 mm Hg. Targeted ventilation was defined as an arrival PCO_2 between 30 and 35 mm Hg. The rate of severe hypocapnea (i.e., hyperventilation) was 18%. Patients in the targeted ventilation range were less likely to die than those who were hyperventilated (odds ratio, 0.57; 95% confidence intervals, 0.33 to 0.99). The most recent guidelines published by the Brain Trauma Foundation[9] discourage "routine" hyperventilation and restrict use to a very narrow segment of patients with unequivocal evidence of herniation (i.e., blown pupil or motor posturing) for whom mannitol therapy has failed (see Chapter 32).

- **Is video laryngoscopy superior to DL in trauma patients requiring in-line stabilization for those at risk for cervical injury?** In a prospective study of 198 NEAR patients, 26% of which were injured, Brown et al.[10] demonstrated superior visualization of the glottis using a Storz Video Macintosh Laryngoscope compared with standard laryngoscopy. In a simulation study assessing intubation success rates with in-line stabilization, Takahashi et al.[11] demonstrated that intubation with the Airway Scope (AWS) was more effective than DL (success rates 100% AWS; 93% DL). Three recent studies[12–14] have compared cervical motion with DL, video laryngoscopy, and flexible endoscopic intubation in healthy human volunteers. Cervical motion was examined using flouroscopy. The results demonstrated more cervical motion with DL than with video laryngoscopy, and the least amount of cervical motion with flexible endoscopic intubation.
- **Is pretreatment with lidocaine safe in patients with TBI?** Simply stated, there is no direct, evidence-based answer to this question, particularly in the TBI or blunt head injured patient. A 2007 review[15,16] revealed that much of the evidence in support of and against the use of intravenous lidocaine as a pretreatment agent is largely inferential. Frequently cited concerns regarding potential for dosing error or delay in RSI are arguably valid. Lidocaine is generally considered safe and possibly beneficial, but use of lidocaine should be carefully and appropriately timed, and not delay airway management (see Chapter 32).
- **Is etomidate safe in trauma patients?** In a single-center study, Hildreth et al.[17] confirmed transient suppression of the adrenal response to exogenous ACTH, and questioned the safety of etomidate in trauma patients, claiming such outcomes increased ventilator time, hospital length-of-stay, ICU days, and the requirement for blood products. The study was poorly designed failing to control for key clinical variables among many other fatal flaws. There is no credible evidence that use of etomidate in trauma patients, including those in shock, is risky. To the contrary, etomidate's ability to preserve hemodynamic status make it an excellent agent for use in trauma.
- **Is ketamine safe in patients with TBI?** A 2006 review of this topic by Sehdev et al.,[18] questioned the historical bias against the use of ketamine in patients with TBI as not evidence based. Ketamine is an attractive alternative in the hemodynamically unstable trauma patient that has been largely ignored because of the concern of increasing ICP. Although the use of ketamine has not, to date, been extensively studied in TBI patients, there is increasing evidence[19] that ketamine is safe to be used in trauma patients and that the use of ketamine may actually decrease ICP.

REFERENCES

1. Dunham MC, Barraco RD, Clark DE, et al. Guidelines for emergency tracheal intubation immediately after traumatic injury. *J Trauma*. 2003;55:162–179.

2. Walls RM, Brown CA, Bair AE, et al. Emergency airway management: a multi-center report of 8937 emergency department intubations. *J Emerg Med*. 2011;41:347–354.

3. Esposito TJ, Sanddal ND, Hansen JD, et al. Analysis of preventable deaths and inappropriate trauma care in a rural state. *J Trauma*. 1995;39:955–962.

4. Teixeira PGR, Inaba K, Hadijizacharia P, et al. Preventable or potentially preventable mortality at a mature trauma center. *J Trauma*. 2007;63:1338–1347.

5. Kortbeek JB, Turki SA, Ali J, et al. Advanced trauma life support, 8th edition, the evidence for change. *J Trauma*. 2008;64:1638–1650.

6. Chesnut RM, Marshall LF, Klauber MR, et al. The role of secondary brain injury in determining outcome from severe brain injury. *J Trauma*. 1993;34:216–222.

7. Davis DP, Idris AH, Sise MJ, et al. Early ventilation and outcomes in patients with moderate to severe traumatic brain injury. *Crit Care Med*. 2006;34:1202–1208.

8. Warner KJ, Cushieri J, Copass M, et al. The impact of prehospital ventilation on outcome after severe traumatic brain injury. *J Trauma*. 2007;62:1330–1338.

9. Brain Trauma Foundation, American Association of Neurological Surgeons. Guidelines for the management of severe traumatic brain injury. I. Blood pressure and oxygenation. *J Neurotrauma*. 2007;24(suppl):S7–S13.

10. Brown CA, Bair AE, Pallin DJ, et al. Improved glottis exposure with the video Macintosh laryngoscope in adult emergency department tracheal intubations. *Ann Emerg Med*. 2010;56:83–88.

11. Takahashi K, Morimura N, Sakamoto T, et al. Comparison of the Airway Scope and Macintosh laryngoscope with in-line cervical stabilization by the semisolid neck collar: manikin study. *J Trauma*. 2010;68:363–366.

12. Hirabayashi Y, Fujita A, Seo N, et al. Cervical spine movement during laryngoscopy using the Airway Scope compared with the Macintosh laryngoscope. *Anaesthesia*. 2007;62:1050–1055.

13. Maruyama K, Yamada T, Kawakami R, et al. Upper cervical spine movement during intubation: flouroscopic comparison of the Airway Scope, McCoy laryngoscope, and Macintosh laryngoscope. *Br J Anaesth*. 2008;100:120–124.

14. Wong DM, Prabhu A, Chakraborty S, et al. Cervical motion during flexible bronchoscopy compared with the Lo-Pro Glidescope. *Br J Anaesth*. 2009;102:424–430.

15. Salhi B, Stettner E. In defense of the use of lidocaine in rapid sequence intubation. *Ann Emerg Med*. 2007;49:84–86.

16. Vaillancourt C, Kapur AK. Opposition to the use of lidocaine in rapid sequence intubation. *Ann Emerg Med*. 2007;49:86–87.

17. Hildreth AN, Meija VA, Maxwell RA, et al. Adrenal suppression following a single dose of etomidate for rapid sequence induction: a prospective randomized study. *J Trauma*. 2008;65:573–579.

18. Sehdev RS, Symmons DAD, Kindl K. Ketamine for rapid sequence induction in patients with head injury in the emergency department. *Emerg Med Australas*. 2006;18:37–44.

19. Bar-Joseph G, Guliburd Y, Tamir A, et al. Effectiveness of ketamine in decreasing intracranial pressure in children with intracranial hypertension. *J Neurosurg Pediatr*. 2009;4:40–46.

32

Elevated Intracranial Pressure

Andy S. Jagoda • Bret P. Nelson

THE CLINICAL CHALLENGE

Elevated intracranial pressure (ICP) poses a direct threat to the viability and function of the brain. In head trauma, elevated ICP has been clearly associated with worse outcomes. The problems associated with elevated ICP may be compounded by many of the techniques and drugs used in airway management because they may cause further elevations of ICP. In addition, victims of multiple traumas may present with hypotension, thus limiting the choice of agents and techniques available. This chapter provides the basis for an understanding of the problems of increased ICP and the optimal methods of airway management in this patient group.

When increased ICP occurs as a result of an injury or medical catastrophe, the brain's ability to regulate blood flow (autoregulation) over a range of blood pressures is often lost. In general, ICP is maintained through a mean arterial pressure (MAP) range of 80 to 180 mm Hg. Elevation in ICP often is a sign that autoregulation has been lost. In this setting, excessively high or excessively low blood pressure could aggravate brain injury by promoting cerebral edema or ischemia. Hypotension, even for a very brief period, is especially harmful, and, along with hypoxia, has been shown to be an independent predictor of mortality and morbidity in patients with traumatic brain injury (TBI).

Cerebral perfusion pressure (CPP) is the driving force for blood flow to the brain. It is measured by the difference between MAP and ICP, expressed as the formula:

$$CPP = MAP - ICP$$

It is clear from this formula that excessive decreases in MAP, as might occur during rapid sequence intubation (RSI), would decrease CPP and contribute to cerebral ischemia. Conversely, increases in MAP, if not accompanied by equivalent increases in ICP, may be beneficial because of the increase in the driving pressure for oxygenation of brain tissue. It is generally recommended that the ICP be maintained <20 mm Hg, the MAP between 100 and 110 mm Hg, and the CPP near 70 mm Hg. There are a number of confounding elements that may increase ICP during airway management.

Reflex Sympathetic Response to Laryngoscopy

The reflex sympathetic response to laryngoscopy (RSRL) is stimulated by the rich sensory innervation of the supraglottic larynx. Use of the laryngoscope, and particularly the attempted placement of an endotracheal tube, results in a significant afferent discharge that increases sympathetic activity to the cardiovascular system mediated through direct neuronal activity and release of catecholamines. More prolonged or aggressive attempts at laryngoscopy and intubation result in greater sympathetic nervous system stimulation. This catecholamine surge leads to increased heart rate and blood pressure, which significantly enhances cerebral blood flow (CBF) at the apparent expense of the systemic circulation through redistribution. These hemodynamic changes may contribute to increased ICP, particularly if autoregulation is impaired; therefore, it is desirable to mitigate this RSRL. Gentle intubation techniques that minimize airway stimulation and pharmacologic adjuncts (e.g., β-blockade, lidocaine, and synthetic opioids) have been studied to accomplish this mitigation.

Evidence is mixed regarding the use of lidocaine to blunt the hemodynamic response to laryngoscopy. Studies in patients without cardiovascular disease have failed to show effect. Other studies have shown variable results with respect to hemodynamic protection, with some appearing to demonstrate benefit and others showing none. As a result, lidocaine cannot be recommended at the present time for mitigation of the RSRL associated with emergency intubation. However, it is useful as a premedication agent, as discussed in the evidence section of this chapter and in chapters 19 and 20.

The short-acting β-blocker esmolol, in contrast, has consistently demonstrated the ability to control both heart rate and blood pressure responses to intubation. A dose of 2 mg per kg given 3 minutes before intubation has been shown to be effective. Unfortunately, administration of β-blocking agents in emergency situations may be problematic for several reasons. Even a short-acting agent, such as esmolol, may exacerbate hypotension in a trauma patient, or confound interpretation of a decrease in the blood pressure immediately following intubation. For these reasons, although esmolol is consistent and reliable for mitigation of RSRL in elective anesthesia, it is generally not used for this purpose for emergency intubation.

Fentanyl at doses of 3 to 5 μg per kg has also been shown to attenuate the RSRL associated with intubation. Although a full sympathetic blocking dose of fentanyl is 9 to 13 μg per kg, the recommended pretreatment dose of fentanyl for emergency RSI is 3 μg per kg and should be administered as a single pretreatment dose over 60 seconds. This technique permits effective mitigation of the RSRL, with greatly reduced chances of apnea or hypoventilation before sedation and paralysis (see Chapter 20).

Several studies have investigated the potential advantages of flexible endoscopic intubation over direct laryngoscopy, working on the premise that these techniques minimize tracheal stimulation and thus the RSRL. Results of these studies are mixed and do not permit any conclusions recommending one technique over the other. In a controlled operating room setting, the insertion of the endotracheal tube into the trachea is more stimulating than a routine laryngoscopy.

At present, based on the best available evidence, it seems advisable to administer 3 μg per kg of fentanyl intravenously (IV) as a pretreatment agent 3 minutes before administration of the induction and neuromuscular blocking agents to mitigate the RSRL. Fentanyl should not be administered to patients with incipient or actual hypotension or to those who are dependent on sympathetic drive to maintain an adequate blood pressure for cerebral perfusion. In such cases, the ensuing hypotension may cause further central nervous system injury. In addition to pharmacologic maneuvers to reduce RSRL, intubation should be performed in the gentlest manner possible, limiting both the time and intensity of laryngoscopy.

Reflex ICP Response to Laryngoscopy

Laryngoscopy may also increase the ICP by a direct reflex mechanism not mediated by sympathetic stimulation of the blood pressure or heart rate. The details of this reflex are poorly elucidated. Insertion of the laryngoscope or endotracheal tube may, therefore, further elevate ICP, even if the RSRL is blunted. It would seem desirable to blunt this ICP response to laryngoscopy in patients at risk for having elevated ICP. The literature related to the use of lidocaine to blunt ICP response to laryngoscopy and intubation is discussed in Chapter 20. In patients with elevated ICP, lidocaine should be administered as a pretreatment drug in the dose of 1.5 mg per kg IV 3 minutes before the induction agent and succinylcholine (SCh) to mitigate the ICP response to laryngoscopy and intubation.

ICP Response to SCh

SCh itself may be capable of causing a mild and transient increase in ICP. Studies have shown that this increase is temporally related to the presence of fasciculations in the patient, but is not the result of synchronized muscular activity leading to increased venous pressure. Rather, there appears to be a complex reflex mechanism originating in the muscle spindle and ultimately resulting in an elevation of ICP. One recent study challenged the claim that SCh causes an elevation of ICP, and SCh remains the drug of choice for management of patients with elevated ICP because of its rapid onset and short duration. Although we recommended in early editions of this manual the routine use of a defasciculating agent when SCh is administered to a patient with elevated ICP, we no longer advocate this practice. There is insufficient evidence to support the use of a defasciculating agent, and it adds unnecessary complexity.

Choice of Induction Agent

When managing the patient with potential brain injury, it is important to choose an induction agent that will not adversely affect CPP. Ideally, one would like to choose an induction agent that is capable of improving or maintaining CPP and providing some cerebral protective effect. Sodium thiopental is an ultra–short-acting barbiturate induction agent. Historically, sodium thiopental often was the drug of choice for patients with elevated ICP. Thiopental confers some cerebro-protective effect because it decreases the basal metabolic rate of oxygen utilization of the brain ($CMRO_2$). This effect can be likened to decreasing myocardial oxygen demand in the ischemic heart. In addition, sodium thiopental decreases CBF, thus decreasing ICP. This combination of characteristics, the decrease in ICP and the decrease in $CMRO_2$, make thiopental a desirable agent for use in patients with elevated ICP and a normal or high blood pressure. However, thiopental is a potent venodilator and negative inotrope. Therefore, it has a tendency to cause significant hypotension and thus reduce CPP, even in relatively hemodynamically stable patients. In the hemodynamically unstable patient, this hypotensive effect can be profound. A single episode of hypotension significantly increases mortality in acute, severe head injury. Therefore, although thiopental has some desirable attributes for management of patients with elevated ICP, its hemodynamic instability relegates it to an alternative role, with etomidate being the agent of choice. Thiopental generally is difficult to obtain in North America and likely will fall out of use altogether.

Etomidate is a short-acting imidazole derivative that has a similar profile of activity to thiopental, but without the tendency to cause hemodynamic compromise. In fact, etomidate is the most hemodynamically stable of all commonly used induction agents except ketamine (see Chapter 21). Its ability to decrease $CMRO_2$ and ICP in a manner analogous to that of sodium thiopental and its remarkable hemodynamic stability make it the drug of choice for patients with elevated ICP. The use of etomidate in patients with elevated ICP has been challenged on the basis of evidence from a few animal studies. This preliminary evidence, which is addressed in Chapter 21, does not justify avoidance of etomidate, with its excellent hemodynamic profile, in patients with elevated ICP.

Ketamine, in general, has been avoided in patients with known elevations in ICP because of the belief that it may elevate the ICP further. The evidence regarding this phenomenon is mixed, however, and is discussed in Chapter 21. In patients with elevated ICP and hypotension, ketamine's superior hemodynamic stability, on balance, argue for its use. In the normotensive or hypertensive patient, etomidate is preferred.

APPROACH TO THE AIRWAY

RSI is the preferred method for patients with suspected elevated ICP because it provides protection against the reflex responses to laryngoscopy and rises in ICP. The presence of coma should not be interpreted as an indication to proceed without pharmacologic agents or to administer only a neuromuscular blocking agent without a sedative induction drug. Although the patient may seem unresponsive, laryngoscopy and intubation will provoke the reflexes described previously, if appropriate pretreatment and induction agents are not used. Following appropriate assessment and preparation, as described in chapter 2 and 19, the sequence in Box 32-1 is recommended for patients with elevated ICP.

INITIATING MECHANICAL VENTILATION

Mechanical ventilation in the patient with elevated ICP should be predicated on three principles: (1) optimal oxygenation, (2) normocapnia, and (3) avoidance of ventilation mechanics (e.g., positive end-expiratory pressure, high peak inspiratory pressure) that would increase venous congestion in the brain.

Although there never was a scientific basis for the use of "therapeutic" hyperventilation, it was widely and enthusiastically adopted, and, surprisingly, still is used in some centers today despite solid evidence that it promotes worse outcomes rather than better. The Brain Trauma Foundation Guidelines for the Management of Severe TBI recommend that prophylactic hyperventilation should be avoided and that patients with severe TBI be ventilated in such a way as to target the lower limits of normocapnia ($PaCO_2$ of 35 to 40 mm Hg). A similar approach seems prudent in patients with medical causes of elevations of ICP (e.g., cerebral hemorrhage).

Box 32-1. Doses for lidocaine, succinylcholine, and etomidate are mg not mcg.

Time	Action
Zero minus 10 min	Preparation
Zero minus 5 min	Preoxygenation
Zero minus 3 min	Pretreatment:
	Lidocaine 1.5 mg per kg IV
	Then on its own line,
	Fentanyl 3 mcg/kg (over 1 minute)
Zero	Paralysis with induction:
	Etomidate 0.3 mg per kg IV
	SCh 1.5 mg per kg IV
Zero plus 30 s	Positioning
Zero plus 45 s	Placement with proof: intubate, confirm placement
Zero plus 60 s	Postintubation management

Although there is no outcome evidence supporting its use or demonstrating any benefit, hyperventilation to a $PaCO_2$ of 30 mm Hg still may have a limited role as a temporizing measure in patients demonstrating definite clinical signs of herniation (blown pupil or decerebrate posturing) unresponsive to appropriate intervention using osmotic agents, cerebrospinal fluid drainage, or both. This should be initiated only with continuous capnography to guide ventilation efforts and avoid harmful sequelae of excessive hypocapnia. Normal initial physiologic ventilation parameters are described in Chapter 7. Initial inspired fraction of oxygen (FiO_2) should be 1.0 (100%). FiO_2 can later be decreased according to pulse oximetry, as long as 100% oxygen saturation is maintained. Carbon dioxide tension can be followed with arterial blood gases or, preferably, continuous capnography, the first assessment of which should occur approximately 10 minutes after initiation of steady-state mechanical ventilation. To permit early and frequent neurologic examinations (e.g., by a neurosurgeon to decide whether there is sufficient persisting neurologic functioning to warrant an attempt at surgical evacuation of a massive subdural hematoma), long-term sedation is best accomplished by using a propofol infusion, which can be terminated as needed with prompt patient recovery. Deep sedation is desired, however, to permit effective controlled mechanical ventilation and other necessary interventions, while mitigating the stimulating effects of the tube in the trachea and eliminating any possibility of the patient coughing or bucking. Propofol is not an analgesic, and an opioid analgesic, such as fentanyl, is used to improve endotracheal tube tolerance and reduce stimulation and responsiveness.

TIPS AND PEARLS

- RSI clearly is the desired method for tracheal intubation in patients with suspected elevation of ICP. The technique allows control of various adverse effects and optimal control of ventilation after intubation. However, the use of neuromuscular blockade in patients with potential neurologic deficit carries the responsibility of performing a detailed neurologic evaluation on the patient before initiation of neuromuscular blockade. The patient's ability to interact with the surroundings, spontaneous motor movement, response to deep pain, response to voice, localization, pupillary reflexes, and other pertinent neurologic details must be assessed carefully before administration of neuromuscular blockade. The careful recording of these findings will be invaluable for the ongoing evaluation of the patient.

- If the patient's ventilatory status is severely compromised by the head injury or by concomitant injuries, positive-pressure ventilation with bag and mask may be required throughout the intubation sequence. In such circumstances, one is trading off the increased risk of aspiration against the hazard of inadequate oxygenation and rising $PaCO_2$ during the intubation sequence. When such a tradeoff arises, it should be resolved in favor of oxygenation over the risk of aspiration.

EVIDENCE

Evidence-based recommendations depend on a careful analysis of the methodology used in the studies reviewed and an understanding of the outcome measure, which must be sound to make the study clinically relevant. In this light, it becomes challenging to make evidence-based recommendations regarding airway management in the patient with a brain injury, as is the case in many other areas of airway management. Regarding methodology, most of the studies of the effect of interventions discussed in this chapter were performed on stable patients in the operating room setting; others were performed on deeply anesthetized patients in the intensive care unit during tracheal suctioning. It is difficult to extrapolate the findings in these patient groups to critical patients undergoing emergency intubation. In addition, the timing and dosing of pharmacologic interventions varied significantly, making it difficult to compare one study with another. For example, in one study lidocaine was found effective when given 3 minutes before intubation and ineffective if given at 4, 2, or 1 minute before.[1] There is only one randomized double-blind interventional study identified that was performed in the ED on patients with head injury.[2] This prospective double-blind study found that esmolol and lidocaine had similar efficacy in attenuating the hemodynamic response to intubation of patients with isolated head injury.

Regarding outcome, there is no study in the literature that compares airway interventions with a functional outcome measure, that is, disability or death. Rises in heart rate, blood pressure, and ICP are the commonly measured parameters comparing one technique or pharmacologic intervention with the other because these affect CPP. However, there is no evidence that these are valid surrogates for more meaningful outcome measures such as disability, nor is there evidence that transient rises in any of the previously mentioned measures have any meaningful impact on morbidity or mortality. That said, there is no evidence that the interventions presented in this chapter do harm, and pending more direct evidence, it does seem intuitive that minimizing adverse changes in ICP, blood pressure, and heart rate can only contribute to maximizing good outcomes.

- **Is premedication indicated for patients with elevated ICP?** The choices of RSI premedications for patients with elevated ICP include lidocaine, fentanyl, esmolol, and a defasciculating dose of a nondepolarizing agent. Evidence for the use of lidocaine, 1.5 mg per kg IV, and fentanyl, 3 mg per kg IV, 3 minutes before induction, is discussed in Chapter 20. In summary, there is insufficient evidence that lidocaine can mitigate the RSRL, but it appears somewhat effective in limiting the intracranial response to upper airway stimulation, which is not mediated by catecholamines. Fentanyl, however, is known to blunt the reflex sympathetic response to upper airway manipulation, mitigating the extent of catecholamine release and, therefore, rise in MAP (see Chapter 20).

    Esmolol has been studied as a premedication to blunt the RSRL through its β-blocking properties. In one randomized double-blind, placebo-controlled study, esmolol, 2 to 3 mg per kg IV, provided better control of heart rate and blood pressure than either lidocaine or fentanyl.[3] Of note, fixed doses of drugs were used, and the lidocaine and fentanyl were given only 2 minutes before intubation. Similar results were reported in another randomized double-blind study using 1.4 mg per kg and 2 mg per kg.[4,5] In a randomized double-blind study comparing the hemodynamic response of esmolol and lidocaine, both were found equally effective.[2]

There is some controversy, but no evidence, whether the increase in ICP caused by SCh is clinically significant, and whether a defasciculating dose of a competitive neuromuscular blocking agent is capable of mitigating this response. On balance, we no longer recommend the use of a defasciculating dose (one-tenth of the paralyzing dose) of a competitive neuromuscular blocking agent such as vecuronium (0.01 mg per kg) or rocuronium (0.06 mg per kg) 3 minutes before SCh is given. Based on the best evidence available at this time, the following recommendations can be made regarding the pharmacologic mitigation of exacerbations of elevated ICP during emergency intubation:

- Administer lidocaine, 1.5 mg per kg, 3 minutes before airway manipulation to mitigate increases in ICP related to laryngoscopy.
- In patients without compensated or decompensated shock, administer fentanyl, $3\,\mu g$ per kg, 3 minutes before airway manipulation in order to mitigate increases in ICP from RSRL.
- When patients with elevated ICP are paralyzed with SCh, use of a defasciculating dose of a nondepolarizing paralytic agent is no longer recommended.
- Esmolol is an effective agent in mitigating rises in ICP from RSRL; however, because of its potential to cause or aggravate hypotension, especially in patients with hypovolemia, it is not recommended for routine use in emergency intubation.

- **Is hyperventilation (ETCO$_2$ 30 to 35 mm Hg) recommended in the management of the TBI patient with suspected elevated ICP?** Hyperventilation can be defined as a PaCO$_2$ <35 or an ETCO$_2$ <30 to 35; the correlation between the two measures is generally good in patients who are normotensive.[6] It causes vasoconstriction and thus reduces ICP.[7] Unfortunately, hyperventilation will also cause a reduction in CBF. Because CBF is reduced by almost 50% in the first days after TBI, hyperventilation poses a risk of exacerbating ischemia.[8] In a randomized, controlled trial, Muizelaar et al.[9] found that patients with an initial Glasgow Coma Scale score of 4 to 5 who were hyperventilated to a PaCO$_2$ of 25 mm Hg during the first days after head injury had significantly worse outcomes than patients kept at a PaCO$_2$ of 35 mm Hg.

  Despite observations that hyperventilation reverses the clinical signs of herniation, there is no evidence that hyperventilation improves outcomes.[10] In an observational study, 59 adult severe TBI patients who required RSI for intubation were matched to 177 historical nonintubated controls.[11,12] The study used ETCO$_2$ monitoring and found an association between hypocapnia and mortality, and a statistically significant association between ventilatory rate and ETCO$_2$. Both the lowest and final ETCO$_2$ readings were associated with increased mortality versus matched controls. Another retrospective study of 65 brain trauma patients with a Glasgow Coma Scale of ≤8 found that patients who were normocarbic on initial assessment had an in-hospital mortality of 15%.[13] In contrast, patients with hypercarbia had a mortality of 61% and hypocarbia was associated with a mortality of 77%. These studies contribute to the growing body of evidence arguing against hyperventilation under any circumstance in TBI patients, and this is likely analogous to patients with medically caused elevated ICP.

  Based on the best available evidence, the following recommendations can be made:

- Hyperventilation (ETCO$_2$ <30 to 35) should be carefully avoided in patients with medical intracranial catastrophe or TBI who do not demonstrate signs of increased ICP ("blown pupil" or extensor posturing) that is refractory to osmotic agents, CSF drainage, or both. Even in this circumstance, there is no solid evidence to support its use, so operator judgment prevails.
- There is no evidence that hyperventilation improves outcome in patients with elevated ICP, and there is some evidence that it causes harm. If hyperventilation is considered, it should only be used briefly, as a temporizing measure, in the management of patients exhibiting signs of increased ICP who have failed to respond to osmotic agents.

- Intubated patients with TBI should have continuous $ETCO_2$ monitoring in order to avoid inadvertent hypocapnia ($ETCO_2$ <35).

There is a clear need for a well-controlled comparative study using a meaningful outcome measure to determine which, if any, of these interventions will decrease morbidity or mortality in patients with elevated ICP undergoing emergency RSI. Pending such a study, which will likely never be done because of logistical challenges, the approach outlined in Box 32-1 seems rational. Management of the patient at risk for elevated ICP should ensure cerebral perfusion and oxygenation. When intubation is indicated, pretreatment should be provided using lidocaine 1.5 mg per kg and fentanyl 3 μg per kg. There is insufficient evidence to support the use of a defasciculating agent. Once the patient is intubated, continuous $ETCO_2$ should be provided to safeguard against inadvertent hypocapnia and its associated increase in mortality.

REFERENCES

1. Abou-Madi MN, Keszler H, Yacoub JM. Cardiovascular reactions to laryngoscopy and tracheal intubation following small and large intravenous doses of lidocaine. *Can Anaesth Soc J*. 1977;24:12–19.

2. Levitt M, Dresden G. The efficacy of esmolol versus lidocaine to attenuate the hemodynamic response to intubation in isolated head trauma patients. *Acad Emerg Med*. 2001;8:19–24.

3. Helfman SM, Gold MI, DeLisser EA, et al. Which drug prevents tachycardia and hypertension associated with tracheal intubation: lidocaine, fentanyl, or esmolol? *Anesth Analg*. 1991;72:482–486.

4. Singh H, Vichitvejpaisal P. Comparative effects of lidocaine, esmolol, and nitroglycerin in modifying the hemodynamic response to laryngoscopy and intubation. *J Clin Anesth*. 1995;7:5–8.

5. Feng CK, Chan KH, Liu KN, et al. A comparison of lidocaine, fentanyl, and esmolol for attenuation of cardiovascular response to laryngoscopy and tracheal intubation. *Acta Anaesthesiol Sin*. 1996;34:61–67.

6. Yosefy C, Hay E, Nasri Y, et al. End tidal carbon dioxide as a predictor of the arterial Pco_2 in the emergency department setting. *Emerg Med J*. 2004;21:557–559.

7. Raichle M, Plum F. Hyperventilation and cerebral blood flow. *Stroke*. 1972;3:566–575.

8. Marion D, Darby J, Yonas H. Acute regional cerebral blood flow changes caused by severe head injuries. *J Neurosurg*. 1991;74:407–414.

9. Muizelaar J, Marmarou A, Ward J, et al. Adverse effects of prolonged hyperventilation in patients with severe head injury: a randomized clinical trial. *J Neurosurg*. 1991;75:731–739.

10. Brain Trauma Foundation. Guidelines for the management of severe traumatic brain injury, third edition. *J Neurotrauma*. 2007;24(suppl 1):S1–S108.

11. Davis DP, Dunford JV, Poste JC, et al. The impact of hypoxia and hyperventilation on outcome after paramedic rapid sequence intubation of severely head-injured patients. *J Trauma*. 2004;57:1–10.

12. Davis DP, Dunford JV, Ochs M, et al. The use of quantitative end-tidal capnometry to avoid inadvertent severe hyperventilation in patients with head injury after paramedic rapid sequence intubation. *J Trauma*. 2004;56:808–814.

13. Dumont TM, Agostino JV, Rughani AI, et al. Inappropriate prehospital ventilation in severe traumatic brain injury increases in-hospital mortality. *J Neurotrauma*. 2010;27:1233–1241.

33

Reactive Airways Disease

Bret P. Nelson • Andy S. Jagoda

THE CLINICAL CHALLENGE

There are a number of confounders that make airway management of the patient with asthma or chronic obstructive pulmonary disease (COPD) challenging. These patients are often hypoxic, desaturate quickly, and can be hemodynamically unstable. Unlike many other clinical conditions, intubation itself does not resolve the primary problem, which is obstruction of the small, distal airways. The actual intubation may be the easiest part of the resuscitative sequence because postintubation ventilation may be extremely difficult with persistent or worsening respiratory acidosis, barotrauma, or worsening hypotension caused by high-intrathoracic pressures with diminished venous return. Thus, the decision to intubate must be made carefully, and the appropriate technique must be chosen to facilitate the best possible outcome.

Severe asthma often presents one of the most difficult airway management cases encountered in the emergency department. Diaphoresis is a particularly ominous sign, and the diaphoretic asthmatic patient who cannot speak full sentences, appears anxious, or is sitting upright and leaning forward to augment the inspiratory effort must not be left unattended until stabilized.

Standard initial management of acute severe asthma exacerbation includes reversal of dynamic bronchospasm using continuous β_2-agonist nebulization therapy (Albuterol 10–15 mg per hour) and anticholinergic nebulization therapy (ipratropium bromide 0.5 mg every 20 minutes for three doses). In addition, oral or intravenous (IV) steroids are indicated for the treatment of the inflammatory component. If the patient is severely bronchospastic and cannot comply with a nebulized treatment, subcutaneous epinephrine or terbutaline 0.3 to 0.5 mg may be of benefit. The use of IV terbutaline is controversial; and has no proven benefit in adults. However, if selected, it should be initiated in the child at 10 μg per kg over 30 minutes followed by a continuous infusion of 0.1–0.4 μg/kg/minute. For severe, refractory asthma, administration of IV magnesium sulfate 2 g in adults and 25-75 mg per kg (up to a maximum of 2 g) in children may be of benefit, although evidence supporting this is mixed. The addition of inhaled or IV anticholinergic agents (atropine or glycopyrrolate), titrated doses of IV ketamine, or inhalational helium/oxygen mixture is controversial but also may be considered in severe cases (Fig. 33-1).

In COPD, much of the obstruction is fixed, comorbidity (especially cardiovascular disease) plays a greater role, and the prognosis (even with short-term mechanical ventilation) is worse. In the patient with COPD, anticholinergic therapy may be as important as β_2-agonist therapy. Steroids are again important to attenuate underlying inflammation. As is the case for many asthma patients, it is progression of fatigue, not worsening bronchospasm that leads to respiratory failure and arrest. The intubated COPD patient may have a prolonged, difficult course, and weaning from the ventilator is not assured. Therefore, unless the patient's condition forces early or immediate intubation, a trial of noninvasive ventilation is recommended. Noninvasive ventilation (bi-level positive airway pressure [BL-PAP] or continuous positive airway pressure) is of proven value in certain COPD patients and may help avoid intubation (see Chapter 6). As for the asthmatic patient, mechanical ventilation after intubation in COPD is notoriously difficult to manage. Ventilation pressures often are high, and breath stacking (automatic positive end-expiratory pressure [auto-PEEP]) is common, even with excellent ventilator management. Increased intrathoracic pressures induced by mechanical ventilation, combined with volume depletion from the patient's work of breathing before intubation, coexisting cardiovascular disease, and hemodynamic changes related to decreased sympathetic tone after intubation makes the peri-intubation period highly dynamic and unstable. Ventilator management is discussed below. There is no role for IV aminophylline in the management of either acute severe asthma or acute severe COPD exacerbation, before or after intubation.

APPROACH TO THE AIRWAY

Despite this vast array of noninvasive treatment modalities, 1% to 3% of acute severe asthma exacerbations will require intubation. These patients are usually fatigued and have reduced functional residual capacity, so it is difficult (if not impossible) to preoxygenate them optimally, and rapid desaturation

Initial Assessment (auscultation, accessory muscle use, vital signs, PEF, FEV$_1$)

Severe (<40% PEF or FEV$_1$)

- Oxygen to maintain SaO2 >90%
- High dose inhaled beta agonist plus ipratropium every 20 minutes or continuously for 1 hour
- Oral systemic corticosteroids

Impending respiratory arrest

- Intubation and mechanical ventilation
- Nebulized beta agonist and ipratropium
- IV corticosteroids
- Consider adjunct therapies
- Admission to intensive care unit

Repeat Assessment (symptoms, physical examination, PEF)

Good response (No distress, >70% PEF or FEV$_1$)	Incomplete Response (Mild–moderate symptoms, 40-69% PEF or FEV$_1$)	Poor Response (Severe symptoms; drowsy, confused, <40% PEF or FEV$_1$)
• Discharge home • Continue oral corticosteroid • Consider starting inhaled corticosteroid • Review medicine use, action plan, followup	• Consider admission to ward • Inhaled beta agonist • Systemic corticosteroids • Consider adjunct therapies	• Consider admission to intensive care • Inhaled beta agonist • Systemic corticosteroids • Consider adjunct therapies • Possible intubation, mechanical ventilation

Figure 33-1 ● Approach to the Patient with Severe Asthma Exacerbation. (Adapted from National Heart, Lung, and Blood Institute, National Institutes of Health, National Asthma Education and Prevention Program. *Expert Panel Report 3 (EPR-3): Guidelines for the Diagnosis and Management of Asthma—Summary Report 2007.* NIH publication 08-5846. http://www.nhlbi.nih.gov/guidelines/asthma/asthsumm.pdf. Accessed May 15, 2011.)

must be anticipated. Because most of these patients have been struggling to breathe against severe resistance, usually for hours, they have little if any residual physical reserve, and mechanical ventilation will be required. In fact, the need for mechanical ventilation is the indication for tracheal intubation; the airway itself is almost invariably patent and protected. This fact argues strongly for rapid sequence intubation (RSI), which often is the preferred method even if a difficult airway is identified on preintubation assessment (the "forced to act" scenario; see Chapters 2 and 3). If the patient has a difficult airway, the operator might plan intubation even earlier than for the nondifficult patient, in an attempt to have the best conditions and greatest amount of time possible for an awake technique.

Technique

The single most important tenet in managing the status asthmaticus patient who requires intubation is to take total control of the airway as expeditiously as possible. Patients typically adopt an upright posture as their respiratory status worsens; this position should be maintained as much as possible during the preintubation period. Preoxygenation should be achieved to the greatest extent possible (see Chapters 5 and 19). Noninvasive ventilation may be considered as a means of increasing FiO$_2$ during this phase while decreasing work of breathing. The RSI drugs chosen should be administered with the patient in their position of comfort, often sitting upright. As the patient loses consciousness, place the patient supine, position the head and neck, and perform laryngoscopy and intubation, preferably with an 8.0- to 9.0-mm endotracheal tube to decrease resistance and facilitate pulmonary toilette. If bag-mask ventilation is required because of desaturation before intubation is achieved, Sellick maneuver may help prevent the passage of air down the esophagus, particularly in these patients, who have high pulmonary resistance to ventilation.

Drug Dosing and Administration

If time permits, patients with reactive airways disease or obstructive lung disease should be pretreated with 1.5 mg per kg of IV lidocaine 3 minutes before induction to attenuate the reflexive bronchospasm in response to airway manipulation. Ketamine is the induction agent of choice in the asthmatic patient because it stimulates the release of catecholamines and also has a direct bronchial smooth muscle relaxing effect that may be important in this clinical setting. Ketamine 1.5 mg per kg IV is given immediately before the administration of 1.5 mg per kg of succinylcholine or 1.0 mg per kg of rocuronium. If ketamine is not available, any of the other commonly used induction agents (propofol, etomidate, and midazolam) may be used, but the barbiturates should be avoided as they release histamine. For COPD patients, who often have concomitant cardiovascular disease, etomidate may be preferred to avoid the catecholamine stimulation of ketamine.

POSTINTUBATION MANAGEMENT

After the patient is successfully intubated and proper tube position has been confirmed, sedation and analgesia are titrated according to a sedation scale (see Chapter 19). Neuromuscular blockade may be required during the first few hours of mechanical ventilation to prevent asynchronous respirations, promote total relaxation of fatigued respiratory muscles, decrease the production of carbon dioxide, and allow optimal ventilator settings. Often, though, these same goals are achieved using a proper balance of sedation and analgesia. Prolonged neuromuscular blockade is not required and may worsen the patient's overall course of management. Meticulous ventilator management is critical in achieving the best patient outcome. Additional ketamine, as well as continuous in-line albuterol and other pharmacologic adjuncts, may also be given.

Mechanical Ventilation

All asthmatic patients have obstructed small airways and dynamic alveolar hyperinflation with varying amounts of end-expiratory residual intra-alveolar gas and pressure (auto-PEEP or intrinsic PEEP). Elevations in auto-PEEP increase the risk for baro/volutrauma. Reversal of airflow obstruction and decompression of end-expiratory filled alveoli are the primary goals of early mechanical ventilation in the asthmatic patient. The former requires prompt administration of IV steroids and continuous in-line nebulization with β_2-agonists until reversal is objectively measured (decrease in peak and plateau airway pressures) or unacceptable side effects are produced. Safe, uncomplicated alveolar decompression requires prolonged expiratory time (inspiration/expiration [I/E] ratio of 1:4 to 1:5), which is achieved by using smaller tidal volumes than usual, with a high-inspiratory flow (IF) rate to shorten the inspiratory cycle time, permitting a longer expiratory phase. A general discussion of ventilation parameters can be found in Chapter 7.

The initial goal of ventilator therapy in the asthmatic patient is to improve arterial oxygen tension to adequate levels without inflicting barotrauma on the lungs or increasing auto-PEEP. Initial tidal volume should be reduced to 6 to 8 ml per kg to avoid barotrauma and air trapping. The speed at which a mechanical breath is delivered in liters per minute, typically 60 L per minute, is called the inspiratory flow rate (IFR). In asthma, the initial IFR should be increased to 80 to 100 L per minute with a decelerating flow pattern. Pressure control is preferred to volume control because of the lower risk of barotrauma. If volume control is used, the operator should select the flow waveform to use ramp (decelerating) instead of square (constant). The ventilation rate should be determined in conjunction with the tidal volume. An initial rate of 8 to 10 breaths per minute (bpm) with a high IFR promotes a prolonged expiratory phase that allows sufficient time for alveolar decompression. It is acceptable to permit the maintenance or gradual development of hypercapnia through reduced minute ventilation (the product of tidal volume and ventilatory rate) in the asthma or COPD patient because this approach reduces peak inspiratory pressure (PIP) and thus minimizes the potential for barotrauma. High intrathoracic pressure may compromise cardiac output and produce hypotension; therefore, it is to be avoided.

The highest measured pressure at peak inspiration is the PIP. The patient's lungs, chest wall, endotracheal tube, ventilatory circuit, ventilator, and mucus plugs all contribute to the PIP. This reading has an inconsistent predictive value for baro/volutrauma, but ideally should be kept under 50 cm H_2O. A sudden rise in PIP should be interpreted as indicating tube blockage, mucous plugging, or pneumothorax until proven otherwise. A sudden, dramatic fall in PIP may indicate extubation.

The measured intra-alveolar pressure during a 0.2- to 0.4-second end-inspiratory pause is referred to as the *plateau pressure* (P_{plat}). Values <30 cm H_2O are best and are not usually associated with baro/volutrauma. Measurement and trending of P_{plat} is an excellent objective tool to confirm optimal ventilator settings and the patient's response, as well as the reversal of airflow obstruction. If initial ventilator settings disclose a P_{plat} of more than 30 cm H_2O, consider lowering minute ventilation and increasing IF, both of which will prolong expiratory time and attenuate hyperinflation. If P_{plat} is unavailable, PIP may be used as a surrogate.

Most status asthmaticus patients who require intubation are hypercapnic. The concept of controlled hypoventilation (permissive hypercapnia) promotes *gradual* development (over 3 to 4 hours) and maintenance of hypercapnia (PCO_2 up to 90 mm Hg) and acidemia (pH as low as 7.2). This treatment is done primarily to decrease the risk of ventilator-related lung injury and prevent hemodynamic compromise as a result of increasing intrathoracic pressure from auto-PEEP or intrinsic PEEP. Permissive hypercapnia is usually accomplished by reducing minute ventilation, increasing IF rate to 80 to 120 L per minute. Optimal sedation and analgesia is required, with some patients also requiring neuromuscular blockade, to tolerate these settings. Permissive hypercapnia may be instrumental in promoting prolonged expiratory times and reducing auto-PEEP.

Summary for Initial Ventilator Settings

1. Determine the patient's ideal body weight.
2. Set a tidal volume of 6 to 8 ml per kg with FiO_2 of 1.0 (100% oxygen).
3. Set a respiratory rate of 8 to 10 bpm.
4. Set an I/E ratio of 1:4 to 1:5. Pressure control is preferred. If using pressure control, the I/E ratio is adjusted directly by the I/E ratio parameter or by adjusting the inspiratory time parameter. If using volume control, the I/E ratio can be adjusted by increasing the peak flow rate, and the ramp inspiratory waveform should be selected. Peak IF can be as high as 80 to 100 L per minute.
5. Measure and maintain the plateau pressure at <30 cm H_2O; try to keep PIP at <50 cm H_2O.
6. Focus on the oxygenation and pulmonary pressures initially. If necessary, allow maintenance or gradual development of hypercapnia to avoid high plateau pressures and increasing auto-PEEP.
7. Ensure continuous sedation and analgesia with a benzodiazepine and a nonhistamine-releasing opioid, such as fentanyl, and consider paralysis with a nondepolarizing muscle relaxant if it is difficult to achieve ventilation goals.
8. Continue in-line β_2-agonist therapy and additional pharmacologic adjunctive treatment based on the severity of the patient's illness and objective response to treatment.

Complications of Mechanical Ventilation

Two of the more common complications seen in mechanically ventilated asthmatic patients are lung injury (baro/volutrauma) and hypotension. Lung injury is exemplified by tension pneumothorax. In those patients without tension pneumothorax, hypotension is usually related to either absolute volume depletion or relative hypovolemia caused by decreased venous return from increasing auto-PEEP and intrathoracic pressure. The inherent risks of developing either one of these complications are directly related to the degree of pulmonary hyperinflation. Of the two, hypotension occurs much more frequently than tension pneumothorax. Most asthmatic patients will have intravascular volume depletion because of the increased work of breathing, decreased oral intake following the onset of asthma exacerbation, and generalized increased metabolic state. It is appropriate for these reasons to infuse empirically 1 to 2 L of normal saline (NS) either before the initiation of RSI or early during mechanical ventilation.

The differential diagnosis for hypotension in the mechanically ventilated patient is discussed in Chapter 19. Pneumothorax and volume depletion are two common and important conditions to consider. Pneumothorax can reliably be excluded with the aid of point-of-care ultrasound or chest X-ray. Alternatively, a trial of hypoventilation (apnea test) may be used to distinguish tension pneumothorax from volume depletion. The patient is disconnected from the ventilator and allowed to be apneic up to 1 minute as long as adequate oxygenation is ensured by pulse oximetry. In volume depletion, the mean intrathoracic pressure will decline quickly, blood pressure should begin to increase, pulse pressure will widen, and pulse rate will decline within 30 to 60 seconds. If auto-PEEP is high, reductions in tidal volume and increases in IF and I/E times will be required to reduce auto-PEEP. If auto-PEEP is not an issue, then an empiric volume infusion of 500 ml NS should be instituted and may be repeated based on the patient's response to the additional volume. With tension pneumothorax, cardiopulmonary stability will not correct during the apnea time. If physical examination fails to identify the culprit lung, immediate insertion of bilateral chest tubes is indicated. Reassessment of ventilatory pressure settings will be required thereafter. The initial ventilator settings and potential ventilator complications of the asthma patient are shared by the COPD patient.

EVIDENCE

- **Does lidocaine improve clinical outcomes when patients with status asthmaticus are intubated?** IV lidocaine has been recommended to attenuate airway reflexes during intubation in patients with reactive airways disease.[1,2] Stimulation of the airway in asthmatic patients is reported to result in bronchoconstriction, which is believed to be mediated through the vagus nerve.[3] The recommendation to use IV lidocaine in RSI protocols for the severe asthmatic patient is extrapolated from the results of studies using healthy volunteers with a history of bronchospastic disease.[4,5] In one double-blind, placebo-controlled randomized study, volunteers who had demonstrated a decrease in forced expiratory volume (FEV_1) in response to histamine inhalation were shown to have a significant attenuation of response when pretreated with IV lidocaine.[5] Another study demonstrated that a combination of lidocaine and albuterol was more effective than either drug alone, but that each drug also was more effective than placebo, in decreasing bronchospastic response to histamine.[6] Unfortunately, there also is evidence that IV lidocaine does not protect against intubation-induced bronchoconstriction in asthma. In a prospective randomized double-blind, placebo-controlled trial of 60 patients, lidocaine and placebo groups were not different in their transpulmonary pressure and airflow immediately after intubation and at 5-minute intervals.[7] The same study evaluated inhaled albuterol (four puffs from a metered dose inhaler 20 minutes before intubation), which showed significant mitigation of intubation-induced bronchospasm. There are no studies that have demonstrated that premedicating with IV lidocaine in RSI changes outcome; conversely, there is no evidence that premedication with IV lidocaine is harmful. Until better data are available, it seems reasonable to minimize the risk of intubation-induced bronchoconstriction by using lidocaine premedication in the asthmatic patients.
- **Do inhaled anticholinergics improve outcomes in acute reactive airways disease when compared with inhaled β-agonists alone?** The bronchodilatory effects of anticholinergic agents are well known, but there has been controversy over whether these agents act synergistically with β-agonists in the setting of acute bronchospasm. A recent meta-analysis of the role of ipratropium bromide in the emergency management of acute asthma exacerbation concluded that there is a modest benefit when it is used in conjunction with β-agonists.[8] Thirty-two randomized controlled trials enrolling 3,611 subjects were included. The use

of inhaled anticholinergics was associated with reduced hospital admissions in adults and children, as well as improved spirometric parameters within 2 hours of treatment. For severe asthma exacerbations, the number needed to treat to prevent one admission was 7 for adults and 14 for children. The meta-analysis recommended the use of inhaled ipratropium bromide because the benefit appears to outweigh any risks. In addition, pooled data suggest that multiple doses convey more benefit than single-dose regimens. A recent prospective, double-blind, randomized controlled trial examined the benefit of adding continuous nebulized ipratropium bromide to a continuous albuterol nebulization.[9] In this study, the addition of ipratropium bromide was not found to improve peak expiratory flow rate (PEFR) or admission rates compared with albuterol alone in a total of 62 enrolled patients. Theoretically, in status asthmaticus where inhaled agents have limited delivery, IV anticholinergic agents may have benefit.[10] However, other than case reports, there is no evidence at this time supporting their use. There is strong evidence for the long-term use of anticholinergic agents in the routine management of COPD.[11–14] Use in acute exacerbations has been less well studied; a Cochrane Database review summarized four studies comparing inhaled albuterol with ipratropium bromide in the setting of acute COPD exacerbation.[15] Pooled data from these studies (129 total patients) demonstrated no difference in FEV_1 at 1 hour or 24 hours between the albuterol and ipratropium bromide groups. The addition of ipratropium bromide to albuterol did not yield any benefit over albuterol alone. Despite this relative paucity of evidence, the American Thoracic Society and European Respiratory Society[16] and the Global Initiative for Chronic Obstructive Lung Disease[17] advocate the use of inhaled ipratropium in acute COPD exacerbations. Thus, based on available evidence, anticholinergic agents should be used in acute asthmatic patients as standard therapy and should be considered in the treatment of acute COPD exacerbations, especially when little improvement is seen with β-agonists alone.

- **Does the use of IV magnesium improve outcomes in patients with acute asthma?** Magnesium plays a role in smooth muscle relaxation, and recent research has focused on the role of this medication in alleviating bronchospasm. A meta-analysis of magnesium sulfate use in 1,669 patients demonstrated efficacy of IV magnesium (used in 15 studies) but not nebulized delivery (used in 9 studies).[18] In children, the impact of IV magnesium was improved pulmonary function and reduced hospital admission rates. For adults, IV magnesium was weakly associated with improved pulmonary function, but not with admission rates. There is no good evidence that magnesium decreases the need for intubation. Based on these data, IV magnesium therapy should be considered as adjunctive therapy for severe asthma or in patients unresponsive to initial therapy.

- **Are there any noninvasive ventilatory strategies that may improve respiratory status in acute asthma?** Noninvasive positive-pressure ventilation has demonstrated a bronchodilatory effect in methacholine-induced bronchospasm,[19,20] and it has been postulated that the addition of positive pressure may offset intrinsic PEEP and decrease work of breathing. However, few studies have examined the role of noninvasive positive-pressure ventilation in the setting of acute asthma. In a prospective, randomized cross-over study of 20 pediatric intensive care unit (ICU) admissions, BL-PAP use for 2 hours decreased respiratory rate, accessory muscle use, wheeze, and dyspnea.[21] A 2003 emergency department study randomized 15 adult patients to BL-PAP and 15 to standard therapy for a 3-hour treatment period.[22] The BL-PAP group demonstrated fewer hospital admissions, improved respiratory rate, and improved PEFR and FEV_1. There were no cases in either study of pneumothorax. Based on these limited data, it would be reasonable to consider BL-PAP for more severe cases of acute asthma, when immediate intubation does not appear to be required, or as a strategy to improve oxygenation in preparation for intubation.

- **Is there a role for heliox in the management of acute asthma or COPD exacerbations?** In obstructive lung disease with bronchospasm, increased turbulent flow through proximal airways decreases airflow and may contribute to increased work of breathing. Heliox, with a lower density than air–oxygen mixtures, has been believed to decrease turbulent flow and could increase carriage of nebulized medications to distal airways. A Cochrane review of 10 trials (including 544 asthma patients) concluded heliox may be beneficial in patients unresponsive to initial therapy.[23] Another systematic review examined controlled studies of acute asthma and COPD exacerbations.[24] For asthma, heliox-driven nebulizers improved PEFR in pooled data from two studies. No differences in admission rates were found. Heliox was found in a single study to improve PEFR when used as a breathing gas in intubated asthmatics. In COPD, heliox-driven nebulizers did not change PEFR compared with controls. When used in conjunction with noninvasive ventilation, heliox did not improve PCO_2, change intubation rates, or decrease length of stay in the ICU. There was a decreased overall hospital length of stay in the heliox group, however. In intubated COPD patients, heliox used as a breathing gas demonstrated a reduction in intrinsic PEEP of 2.2 cm H_2O compared with controls and improved work of breathing, but did not affect other outcomes. There is one case series of seven intubated patients with elevated airway pressures who had remarkable improvement with a 60 to 40 helium/oxygen mixture; however, this is a case series and thus suffers from inherent bias, precluding recommendations.[25] At this time, there is insufficient evidence of outcome benefit to justify the cost and complexity of heliox administration.

- **Is IV ketamine of benefit in severe asthma?** Theoretically, ketamine is a logical choice in managing the airway of the severe asthmatic because it increases circulating catecholamines, it is a direct smooth muscle dilator, it inhibits vagal outflow, and it does not cause histamine release.[26] However, there are no good controlled studies demonstrating the benefit of IV ketamine in the management of the nonintubated asthmatic patients. Case reports of dramatic improvement in pulmonary function with ketamine have driven its popularity,[27,28] but no randomized studies have been performed to demonstrate ketamine's superiority over other agents. In a case series, 19 of 22 actively wheezing asthmatics had a decrease in bronchospasm during ketamine-induced anesthesia.[29] In one prospective double-blind, placebo-controlled trial of 14 mechanically ventilated patients with bronchospasm, the 7 patients treated with ketamine (1 mg per kg) had a significant improvement in oxygenation but no improvement in PCO_2 or lung compliance. Outcome (discharge from the ICU) was the same in both groups. The study population was heterogeneous, making conclusions of the benefit of ketamine difficult at best.[30] A randomized double-blind, placebo-controlled trial of low-dose IV ketamine, 0.2 mg per kg bolus, followed by an infusion of 0.5 mg per kg/hour in nonintubated adult patients with acute asthma failed to demonstrate a benefit from IV ketamine compared with standard therapy.[31] The incidence of dysphoric reactions led the investigators to decrease the bolus to 0.1 mg per kg. Recently, a double-blind, placebo-controlled study randomized 33 pediatric asthma patients to ketamine infusion (0.2 mg per kg bolus, followed by 0.5 mg per hour for 2 hours) and 35 patients to placebo.[32] Each group also received albuterol, ipratropium bromide, and glucocorticoids. No significant difference in pulmonary index scores (consisting of respiratory rate, wheeze, I/E ratio, accessory muscle use, and oxygen saturation) were found between the two groups. No difference in hospitalization rate was noted. At the present time, based on its mechanism of action and safety profile, ketamine appears to be the best agent available for RSI in the asthmatic. In the absence of ketamine, other agents may be used. There is insufficient evidence to support the use of IV ketamine as adjunctive therapy in nonventilated patients.

REFERENCES

1. Walls RM. Lidocaine and rapid sequence intubation. *Ann Emerg Med*. 1996;27:528–529.

2. Gal T. Bronchial hyperresponsiveness and anesthesia: physiologic and therapeutic perspectives. *Anesth Analg*. 1994;78:559–573.

3. Gold M. Anesthesia, bronchospasm, and death. *Semin Anesth*. 1989;8:291–306.

4. Groeben H, Foster W, Brown R. Intravenous lidocaine and oral mexiletine block reflex bronchoconstriction in asthmatic subjects. *Am J Respir Crit Care Med*. 1997;156:1703–1704.

5. Groeben H, Silvanus M, Beste M, et al. Both intravenous and inhaled lidocaine attenuate reflex bronchoconstriction but at different plasma concentrations. *Am J Respir Crit Care Med*. 1999;159:530–535.

6. Groeben H, Silvanus MT, Beste M, et al. Combined intravenous lidocaine and inhaled salbutamol protect against bronchial hyperreactivity more effectively than lidocaine or salbutamol alone. *Anesthesiology*. 1998;89:862–868.

7. Maslow A, Regan M, Israel E, et al. Inhaled albuterol, but not intravenous lidocaine, protects against intubation-induced bronchoconstriction in asthma. *Anesthesiology*. 2000;93:1198–1204.

8. Rodrigo GJ, Castro-Rodriguez JA. Anticholinergics in the treatment of children and adults with acute asthma: a systematic review with meta-analysis. *Thorax*. 2005;60:740–746.

9. Salo D, Tuel M, Lavery R, et al. A randomized, clinical trial comparing the efficacy of continuous nebulized albuterol (15 mg) versus continuous nebulized albuterol (15 mg) plus ipratropium bromide (2 mg) for the treatment of asthma. *J Emerg Med*. 2006;31(4):371–376.

10. Slovis C, Daniels G, Wharton D. Intravenous use of glycopyrrolate in acute respiratory distress due to bronchospastic pulmonary disease. *Ann Emerg Med*. 1987;16:898–900.

11. Vincken W, van Noord JA, Greefhorst AP, et al. Improved health outcomes in patients with COPD during 1 yr's treatment with tiotropium. *Eur Respir J*. 2002;19:209–216.

12. Donohue JF, van Noord JA, Batemane ED, et al. A 6-month, placebo-controlled study comparing lung function and health status changes in COPD patients treated with tiotropium and salmeterol. *Chest*. 2002;122:47–55.

13. Donohue JF, Menojoge S, Kesten S. Tolerance to bronchodilating effects of salmeterol in COPD. *Respir Med*. 2003;97:1014–1020.

14. Ringback T, Viskum K. Is there any association between inhaled ipratropium and mortality in patients with COPD and asthma? *Respir Med*. 2003;97:264–272.

15. McCrory DC, Brown CD. Anticholinergic bronchodilators versus beta$_2$-sympathomimetic agents for acute exacerbations of chronic obstructive pulmonary disease. *Cochrane Database Syst Rev*. 2003;(1):CD003900.

16. Celli BR, MacNee W; ATS/ERS Task Force. Standards for the diagnosis and treatment of patients with COPD: a summary of the ATS/ERS position paper. *Eur Respir J*. 2004;23(6):932–946.

17. Global Initiative for Chronic Obstructive Lung Disease. Global strategy for diagnosis, management and prevention of COPD. http://www.goldcopd.com/download.asp?intId=617. Accessed May 15, 2011.

18. Mohammed S, Goodacre S. Intravenous and nebulised magnesium sulphate for acute asthma: systematic review and meta-analysis. *Emerg Med J*. 2007;24:823–830.

19. Wang CH, Lin HC, Huang TJ, et al. Differential effects of nasal continuous positive airway pressure on reversible or fixed upper and lower airway obstruction. *Eur Respir J*. 1996;9:952–959.

20. Lin HC, Wang CH, Yang CT, et al. Effect of nasal continuous positive airway pressure on methacholine-induced bronchoconstriction. *Respir Med*. 1995;89:121–128.

21. Thill PJ, McGuire JK, Baden HP, et al. Noninvasive positive-pressure ventilation in children with lower airway obstruction. *Pediatr Crit Care Med*. 2004;5(4):337–342.

22. Soroksky A, Stav D, Shpirer I. A pilot prospective, randomized, placebo-controlled trial of bilevel positive airway pressure in acute asthmatic attack. *Chest*. 2003;123:1018–1025.

23. Rodrigo G, Pollack C, Rodrigo C, et al. Heliox for nonintubated acute asthma patients. *Cochrane Database Syst Rev*. 2006;(4):CD002884.

24. Colebourn CL, Barber V, Young JD. Use of helium-oxygen mixture in adult patients presenting with exacerbations of asthma and chronic obstructive pulmonary disease: a systematic review. *Anaesthesia*. 2007;62:34–42.

25. Gluck E, Onorato D, Castriotta R. Helium-oxygen mixtures in intubated patients with status asthmaticus and respiratory acidosis. *Chest*. 1990;98:693–698.

26. Huber F, Reeves J, Gutierrez J, et al. Ketamine: its effect on airway resistance in man. *South Med J*. 1972;65:1176–1180.

27. Hommedieu C, Arens J. The use of ketamine for the emergency intubation of patients with status asthmaticus. *Ann Emerg Med*. 1987;16:568–571.

28. Rock M, de la Roca S, Hommedieu C, et al. Use of ketamine in asthmatic children to treat respiratory failure refractory to conventional therapy. *Crit Care Med*. 1986;14:514–516.

29. Corssen G, Gutierrez J, Reves J, et al. Ketamine in the anesthetic management of asthmatic patients. *Anesth Analg*. 1972;51:588–596.

30. Hemmingsen C, Nielsen P, Odorica J. Ketamine in the treatment of bronchospasm during mechanical ventilation. *Am J Emerg Med*. 1994;12:417–420.

31. Howton J, Rose J, Duffy S, et al. Randomized, double-blind, placebo-controlled trial of intravenous ketamine in acute asthma. *Ann Emerg Med*. 1996;27:170–175.

32. Allen JY, Macias CG. The efficacy of ketamine in pediatric emergency department patients who present with acute severe asthma. *Ann Emerg Med*. 2005;46(1):43–50.

34

Distorted Airways and Acute Upper Airway Obstruction

Michael F. Murphy • Richard D. Zane

THE CLINICAL CHALLENGE

Anatomically, the term *upper airway* refers to that portion of the anatomy that extends from the lips and nares to the first tracheal ring. Thus, the first portion of the upper airway is redundant: a nasal pathway and an oral pathway. However, at the level of the oropharynx, the two pathways merge and redundancy is lost. The most common, life-threatening causes of acute upper airway distortion and obstruction occur in the region of this common channel and are typically laryngeal. In addition, disorders of the base of the tongue and the pharynx can cause obstruction (Box 34-1). This chapter deals with problems that distort or obstruct the upper airway. Foreign bodies in the upper airway are addressed in Chapters 27 and 40.

APPROACH TO THE AIRWAY

The signs of upper airway distortion and obstruction may be occult or subtle. Life-threatening deterioration may occur suddenly and unexpectedly. Seemingly innocuous interventions, such as small doses of sedative hypnotic agents to alleviate anxiety or the use of topical local anesthetic agents, may precipitate sudden and total airway obstruction. Rescue devices may not be successful and may even be contraindicated in some circumstances. The goal in these patients is to proceed rapidly in a sensible, controlled manner to manage the airway before complete airway obstruction occurs.

When Should an Intervention Be Performed?

Chapter 1 deals with the important question of when to intubate. If airway obstruction is severe, progressive, or potentially imminent, then immediate action (often cricothyrotomy) is required without further consideration of moving the patient to another venue (e.g., the operating room or another hospital). Failing such an indication for an *immediate* cricothyrotomy, the question becomes more difficult: What is the expected clinical course?

    Penetrating wounds to the neck and airway are notoriously unpredictable (see Chapter 31). Some experts advocate securing the airway regardless of warning signs, whereas others advocate

---

Box 34-1. Causes of Upper Airway Obstruction

A. **Infectious**
   a. Viral and bacterial laryngotracheobronchitis (e.g., croup)
   b. Parapharyngeal and retropharyngeal abscesses
   c. Lingual tonsillitis (a lingual tonsil is a rare but real congenital anomaly and a well-recognized cause of failed intubation)
   d. Infections, hematomas, or abscesses of the tongue or floor of the mouth (e.g., Ludwig angina)
   e. Epiglottitis (also known as supraglottitis)
B. **Neoplastic**
   a. Laryngeal carcinomas
   b. Hypopharyngeal and lingual (tongue) carcinomas
C. **Physical and chemical agents**
   a. Foreign bodies
   b. Thermal injuries (heat and cold)
   c. Caustic injuries (acids and alkalis)
   d. Inhaled toxins
D. **Allergic/idiopathic:** including ACEI-induced angioedema
E. **Traumatic:** blunt and penetrating neck and upper airway trauma

expectant observation. There are substantial problems with the second strategy. The first is that the patient often remains relatively asymptomatic until they suddenly and unexpectedly develop total obstruction, resulting in an airway (and patient) that cannot be rescued. The second is that unless a flexible endoscope is used, the observer is only able to see the anterior portion of the airway and not the posterior and inferior parts where the obstruction likely will occur. In other words, when not using a flexible endoscope, one sees only "the tip of the iceberg."

The time course of the airway threat also is important. All other things being equal, a patient who presents with substantial airway swelling, such as angioedema, which has developed over 8 to 12 hours, is likely at substantially less risk for sudden obstruction than a similar patient where the same degree of swelling has developed over 30 minutes. Overall, for any condition in which the obstruction may be rapidly progressive, silent, and unobservable externally (e.g., angioedema, vascular injuries in the neck, and epiglottitis), acting earlier to secure the airway rather than later is the most prudent course.

There are four cardinal signs of acute upper airway obstruction:

- "Hot potato" voice: the muffled voice one often hears in patients with mononucleosis and very large tonsils
- Difficulty in swallowing secretions, either because of pain or obstruction; the patient is typically sitting up, leaning forward, and spitting or drooling secretions
- Stridor
- Dyspnea

The first two signs do not necessarily suggest that total upper airway obstruction is imminent; however, stridor and dyspnea do. The patient presenting with stridor has already lost at least 50% of the airway caliber and requires immediate intervention. In the case of children younger than 8 to 10 years with croup, medical therapy may suffice. In older children and adults, the presence of stridor typically mandates a surgical airway or, at the least, intubation using a double setup. This technique uses an awake attempt from above, ideally using a flexible endoscope, with the capability, prepared in advance, to rapidly move to a surgical airway if needed. Properly performed bag mask ventilation often will be successful in cases with soft tissue obstructions, including laryngospasm, but generally will not overcome a fixed obstruction, such as extrinsic compression of the airway by a hematoma, and, in any case cannot be counted on as more than a temporizing maneuver.

What Options Exist If the Airway Deteriorates or Obstruction Occurs?

The key considerations here are as follows:

- *Will rescue bag-mask ventilation (BMV) be possible?* Will a mask seal be possible to achieve, or is the lower face disrupted? Has a penetrating neck wound entered the airway rendering it incompetent to high airway pressures? As discussed in Chapter 9, the bag and mask devices most commonly used in resuscitation settings are capable of generating 50 to 100 cm of water pressure in the upper airway, provided that they do not have positive-pressure relief valves and that an adequate mask seal can be obtained. Pediatric and neonatal devices often incorporate positive-pressure relief valves that easily can be defeated if needed. This degree of positive pressure often is sufficient to overcome the moderate degree of upper airway obstruction caused by redundant tissue (e.g., the obese), edematous tissue (e.g., angioedema, croup, and epiglottitis), or laryngospasm. Lesions that are hard and fixed, such as hematomas, abscesses, cancers, and foreign bodies, produce an obstruction that cannot be reliably overcome with BMV, even with high upper airway pressures.
- *Where is the airway problem?* If the lesion is at the level of the face or oro/nasopharynx and orotracheal intubation is judged to be impossible (for whatever reason), but there is oral access, then a supralaryngeal rescue device, such as a laryngeal mask airway, King LT, or Combitube may be considered. If the lesion is at or immediately above the level of the glottis, a supraglottic airway will not work and intubation (if the obstruction can be bypassed) or cricothyrotomy

(if it cannot) are required. If the lesion is below the vocal cords, cricothyrotomy will not bypass the obstruction and an entirely different strategy is used (see Chapters 27 and 40).

What Are the Advantages and Risks of an Awake Technique?

In most instances, unless the patient is in crisis or deteriorating rapidly, awake examination using a flexible endoscope is the best approach. The endoscopic examination allows both assessment of the airway and, if indicated, intubation (see Chapters 15 and 23). Alternatively, awake laryngoscopy is performed using a video or conventional laryngoscope. If adequate glottic visualization is achieved by direct or video laryngoscopy, intubation is performed. If visualization is suboptimal, but the epiglottis can be seen and is in the midline, orotracheal intubation using rapid sequence intubation (RSI) is probably possible, especially when using a bougie, unless the working diagnosis is a primary laryngeal disorder. On rare occasions, however, the airway may be more difficult to visualize after induction and paralysis or may have deteriorated abruptly between the awake examination and administration of RSI drugs. For these reasons, RSI drugs should be drawn up before the awake laryngoscopy is performed, and intubation, if required, often is best done at the time of the initial examination, rather than withdrawing the laryngoscope to perform RSI. If the lesion is suspected to be at the laryngeal level, complete visualization of the larynx and, particularly the glottis, is important (e.g., flexible endoscopic visualization).

Is RSI Reasonable?

If one is confident that orotracheal intubation is possible and highly confident that the patient can be successfully ventilated using BMV or extraglottic device (EGD), then it is reasonable to proceed with RSI (e.g., early in the course of a penetrating neck injury). A double setup with readiness for an immediate surgical airway is advisable. The decision to proceed with RSI (using a double setup) versus an awake examination or primary cricothyrotomy is a matter of clinical judgment. A patient with early upper airway injury (e.g., inhalation of products of combustion) often is easily intubated orally (absent preexisting difficult airway markers) provided this is done before the injury and airway swelling are allowed to progress. The key determinant is the clinician's confidence that intubation likely will succeed, and, if not, that oxygenation through BMV or EGD, or by cricothyrotomy, will be timely and successful.

The challenges of patients presenting with upper airway obstruction underscore the importance of possessing alternative airway devices, such as the flexible endoscope and a video laryngoscope, in addition to a conventional laryngoscope and bougie. Patients with upper airway obstructions, such as severe angioedema, in whom direct laryngoscopy likely would be impossible, often are reasonably straightforward candidates for flexible endoscopic intubation; the device essentially transforming an impossible intubation into a challenging, but very achievable one.

TIPS AND PEARLS

- Be reluctant to transfer patients with suspected acute upper airway obstruction and unsecured airways, even short distances. With rare exception, it always is prudent to secure the airway of a patient with significant acute penetrating neck injury or blunt laryngeal trauma (examples of 'dynamic' upper airway obstruction) before transport.
- Angioedema of the upper airway is a potentially dangerous and unpredictable condition, particularly when it has occurred over a short period of time. External examination of the lips, tongue, and pharynx may tell you little of what is going on at the level of the airway. Intervention earlier rather than later is the most prudent course of action. Usually, flexible endoscopy will provide definitive information and serve as a conduit for intubation, if indicated.

- The patient with acute upper airway obstruction, a disrupted airway, or a distorted airway who *can* protect and maintain the airway and *can* maintain oxygenation and ventilation should always be considered a *difficult airway*, and the difficult airway algorithm should be used.
- The patient with upper airway obstruction, a disrupted airway, or a distorted airway who *cannot* maintain oxygenation or ventilation should be considered a *failed airway*, and the failed airway algorithm should be used.
- Blind techniques (e.g., blind nasotracheal intubation) of airway management in these situations are contraindicated and should not be attempted.
- BMV alone cannot be relied on to rescue the airway, particularly if the obstruction is caused by a fixed lesion.
- RSI is usually contraindicated unless the awake look proves otherwise or the operator judges that RSI is likely to be successful and a backup plan (double setup) is in place.
- Be prepared for a cricothyrotomy before performing an awake laryngoscopy, recognizing that manipulation of an irritated upper airway, administration of a sedative agent, or application of a topical anesthetic may precipitate total obstruction.
- Heliox may buy time. Helium is less dense than nitrogen, reducing turbulent flow and resistance through tight orifices, as is the case with some causes of upper airway obstruction. The commercial preparations are usually 80% helium and 20% oxygen, and provided lung function is adequate, this mix will produce acceptable oxygen saturations. Other concentrations may be prepared.

EVIDENCE

- **What evidence guides emergency management of patients with acute upper airway obstruction?** The evidence with respect to the emergency management of the patient with an airway that is potentially or actually disrupted, distorted, or obstructed is essentially anecdotal. Most of the information dealing with the topic comes either from the surgical or anesthesia literature: primarily small series or case reports. There are no controlled studies comparing intervention with expectant observation. In the surgical literature, cricothyrotomy, as might be expected, is typically overrecommended. In the anesthesia literature, intubation under deep inhalation anesthesia and spontaneous ventilation has been the standard and, as might be expected, cricothyrotomy is underrecommended. Despite the lack of scientifically sound studies, the following additional reading is recommended.[1–3]
- **How commonly does angiotensin-converting enzyme inhibitor (ACEI)–induced angioedema require intubation?** The clinical course of ACEI-induced angioedema is extremely unpredictable, and life-threatening presentations requiring airway interventions are reported in up to 20% of these patients.[4–6] According to the literature, 0% to 22.2% of patients with angioedema will require intubation.[7] Researchers from Boston retrospectively analyzed cases of ACEI-related angioedema and determined that increasing age and oral cavity/oropharyngeal involvement predicted the need for airway intervention. These predictors had a sensitivity of 65.2% and specificity of 83.7%.[7] The clinical course of angioedema, especially ACEI induced, is unpredictable. Patients not requiring intubation should be observed in the emergency department (ED), an ED Observation Unit, or an inpatient setting. The optimal duration of observation is not known, and recommendations vary. Patients presenting <12 hours after onset of angioedema probably should be observed until it is clear that the condition is not progressing. Generally, this requires observation for at least 6 hours, longer for more severe cases. Patients presenting more than 12 hours after onset should be observed until there is confidence that no further progression is occurring.
- **Is it true that application of topical anesthetic agents to a distorted airway can trigger total airway obstruction?** There are no studies related to this topic, but most experienced airway managers have seen it, and there are published case reports.[8–10] Although the mechanism by which this occurs is a matter of speculation, it is a real phenomenon, and caution should

be exercised in the setting of preexisting airway obstruction when topical anesthesia and instrumentation of the airway is contemplated. Rescue strategies should be planned in advance, and the examination should occur in a setting where rescue quickly can be executed if complete obstruction occurs.

REFERENCES

1. Crosby E, Reid D. Acute epiglottitis in the adult: is intubation mandatory? *Can J Anaesth*. 1991;38:914–918.

2. Halvorson DJ, Merritt RM, Mann C, et al. Management of subglottic foreign bodies. *Ann Otol Rhinol Laryngol*. 1996;105:541–544.

3. Tong MC, Chu MC, Leighton SE, et al. Adult croup. *Chest*. 1996;109:1659–1662.

4. Kaplan AP, Greaves MW. Angioedema. *J Am Acad Dermatol*. 2005;23:373–388.

5. Kostis JB, Kim HJ, Rasnak J, et al. Incidence and characteristics of angioedema associated with enalapril. *Arch Intern Med*. 2005;165:1637–1642.

6. Reid M. Angioedema. April 26, 2006. http://www.emedicine.com/med/topic135.htm.

7. Zirkle M, Bhattacharyya N. Predictors of airway intervention in angioedema of the head and neck. *Otolaryngol Head Neck Surg*. 2000;123:240–245.

8. Shaw IC, Welchew EA, Harrison BJ, et al. Complete airway obstruction during awake fibreoptic intubation. *Anaesthesia*. 1997;52:582–585.

9. McGuire G, el-Beheiry H. Complete upper airway obstruction during awake fibreoptic intubation in patients with unstable cervical spine fractures. *Can J Anaesth*. 1999;46:176–178.

10. Ho AM, Chung DC, To EW, et al. Total airway obstruction during local anesthesia in a non-sedated patient with a compromised airway. *Can J Anaesth*. 2004;51:838–841.

35

The Patient in Shock

Alan C. Heffner

THE CLINICAL CHALLENGE

Airway management and hemodynamic support are defining priorities of critical care. Intubation is among the most complicated emergency resuscitation procedures and both preintubation hypotension and postintubation hypotension (PIH) during emergency airway control are associated with increased risk of adverse events and death. A clear understanding of pertinent principles and priorities helps to minimize and rapidly manage shock in the peri-intubation period. In this chapter, we focus on the interplay between the shock state, intubation technique, medication selection, and postintubation management. Comprehensive discussions of shock resuscitation can be found in standard emergency medicine and critical care textbooks.

The Patient in Shock

Shock is the final common pathway for many life-threatening diseases. Unfortunately, shock recognition is not always straightforward. Shock is defined by inadequate tissue perfusion in which oxygen delivery is insufficient to meet metabolic needs. Contrary to popular use, the term is not synonymous with perfusion pressure. Systemic blood pressure is an unreliable indicator of adequate oxygen delivery and perfusion. Normal or even elevated blood pressure does not assure normal organ perfusion. Inadequate perfusion in the setting of normotension is termed *compensated shock*. The difficulty in identifying these patients has spawned the terms *occult hypoperfusion* and *cryptic shock* to describe hemodynamically stable patients with microvascular insufficiency. The majority of critically ill patients present in compensated shock with normal or near-normal blood pressure.

Uncompensated shock is characterized by hypotension, which is a late sign of hypoperfusion that develops when physiologic mechanisms to maintain normal perfusion pressure are overwhelmed or exhausted. Mean arterial pressure (MAP) <65 mm Hg, systolic blood pressure (SBP) <90 mm Hg or MAP >20 mm Hg below baseline should raise clinical concern even in the absence of overt clinical hypoperfusion. Both the degree and duration of hypotension are directly correlated with likelihood of adverse outcomes. Similarly, brief self-limited hypotension represents progressive failure of cardiovascular compensation and is a common first sign of uncompensated shock. This *transient hypotension* is an important clue, as it is a marker of adverse outcome and often heralds further hemodynamic deterioration in the absence of effective intervention.

AIRWAY MANAGEMENT OF THE PATIENT IN SHOCK

Airway management of the patient in cardiovascular crisis is a high-risk situation. Determining the need for, and timing of, intubation requires balancing respiratory and cardiovascular considerations in these fragile patients. The airway manager should optimize conditions to achieve first attempt intubation success as prolonged airway management, including the need for multiple laryngoscopy attempts, is associated with increased risk of clinical deterioration. Box 35-1 summarizes some important practical issues and modifications required for safe airway management of patients in shock.

Timing of Airway Management

Patients in shock exhibit the same primary indications for airway management as those without hemodynamic compromise. Failures of airway maintenance, airway protection, oxygenation, or ventilation are often related to the patient's primary disease. Concomitant shock simply adds complexity to the airway management plan of such cases. However, often the airway is maintained and protected and oxygenation and ventilation are (at least marginally)

Box 35-1. Implications of Shock during Airway Management

- Hemodynamic monitoring and optimizing preintubation status
  - Monitor for precipitous hemodynamic decline
  - Adequate IV access
  - Empiric fluid loading prior to airway management
  - When appropriate, delay intubation to improve hemodynamic status
  - Immediate availability and use of vasopressor support to avoid or treat hypotension
- Preoxygenation
  - Ineffective spontaneous breathing may limit preoxygenation
  - Limited preoxygenation resulting from high systemic oxygen extraction
  - Rapid desaturation limiting period of apneic normoxia for laryngoscopy
- RSI and drug use
  - Greater untoward cardiovascular effects of RSI drugs
  - Need for reduced dose sedative-hypnotic agent
  - Slower onset of action of RSI drugs
- Postintubation management
  - Attention to controlled, slow, low-tidal volume ventilation
  - Avoid dynamic hyperinflation and auto-PEEP
  - Low-dose titrated sedation

---

adequate. The primary indication for intubation in most cases derives from the anticipated clinical course, which is one of increasing metabolic debt, progressive patient fatigue, worsening hypoxemia, and respiratory failure. Prioritization of immediate airway management versus hemodynamic support is a common clinical dilemma. Four main considerations may assist with the decision:

- The severity of respiratory compromise

  Inadequate spontaneous ventilation and oxygenation are late-stage sequelae of shock. Respiratory failure, particularly sudden hypoventilation (especially bradypnea or apnea) often signifies impending cardiac arrest and requires immediate attention. Prompt intubation is indicated, and ideally, airway and cardiovascular support are coordinated. Less severely ill patients may benefit from supplemental oxygen or bag-valve-mask support to optimize preoxygenation, while critical minutes for improvement of cardiovascular status are gained through administration of crystalloid and vasopressor support.
- The risk of intubation at the patient's current cardiovascular state and the benefit of hemodynamic support

  Preintubation shock increases the likelihood of severe complications, including cardiac arrest, during or following intubation. Intubation and mechanical ventilation can have substantial negative impact on fragile cardiovascular status. Medications and positive-pressure ventilation may reduce cardiovascular performance and precipitate irreversible decompensation. Cardiac arrest rates as high as 15% are described during airway management of patients in hypotensive shock. If the patient is adequately oxygenated, fluid and catecholamine support is advised before initiating the intubation sequence.

  Cardiac tamponade represents an extreme example where the ABC priorities must be reordered to minimize the risk of precipitating cardiac arrest with intubation. In the absence of apnea or cardiac arrest, volume loading and support of spontaneous ventilation may provide sufficient time to perform pericardiocentesis or enable rapid transfer

to the operating room, for immediate surgical intervention, if needed, at the time of intubation.
- The anticipated clinical course of the patient with shock

Many critically ill patients demonstrate a biphasic early course wherein early resuscitation slows the spiral of hypotension, malperfusion, and organ dysfunction, only to have the patient deteriorate a few hours later. In most instances, hypotension and organ malperfusion are improved, but not entirely reversed by initial therapy. Interstitial edema from volume resuscitation, the progression of end-organ dysfunction (including acute lung injury), cumulative work of breathing, and metabolic debt combine with other factors to exhaust the patient's physiologic reserve leading to respiratory failure minutes or hours following initial "successful" resuscitation. Frequent reassessment is required, with particular attention to respiratory parameters. Declining oxygen saturation or increasing respiratory work or rate signals the diffusion compromise and decreasing lung compliance of acute lung injury. Hemodynamic status may also subtly, but progressively deteriorate, indicated by malperfusion or escalating vasopressor support. Intubation should occur early when this downward cycle is identified, and should not wait for overt cardiovascular or respiratory failure.

Preoxygenation

Optimizing preoxygenation is more difficult in patients with shock. Ineffective spontaneous ventilation, decreased pulmonary and systemic perfusion, and high systemic oxygen extraction all compromise preoxygenation. Although saturated hemoglobin accounts for the majority of blood oxygen content, systemic oxygenation is regulated (and limited) by cardiac performance. Even with optimal preoxygenation, the rate of desaturation is dependent on cardiovascular status. Thus, suboptimal preoxygenation is compounded by rapid desaturation during shock. The clinical repercussion is a marked reduction in the period of apneic normoxia to complete intubation. Hypercapnia during rapid sequence intubation (RSI) has the potential to exacerbate acidemia. Bag-mask ventilation may be required in the interval between induction and intubation if adequate systemic oxygen saturation (>90%) cannot be maintained, or if preexisting acidemia is severe (pH < 7.1).

Delayed peripheral blood distribution during shock causes cutaneous oximetry to lag central SaO_2. The delay is exacerbated by signal averaging of pulse oximetry (see Chapter 8). This can be disconcerting, as the pulse oximeter reading continues to fall, despite 100% oxygen being delivered through an endotracheal tube whose position has been confirmed in the trachea. The discrepancy is accentuated during hypoxia (i.e., starting at the inflection point of the oxyhemoglobin dissociation curve) and rapid desaturation. Forehead and ear probes are closer to the heart and respond more quickly than distal extremity probes. Forehead reflectance probes are often preferred in critically ill patients for this reason, and they provide more reliable signal detection during hypotension. Limited detection of cutaneous arterial pulsatility generally reduces accuracy of pulse oximetry with SBP <80 mm Hg.

Rapid Sequence Induction

By definition, patients in shock have exhausted cardiovascular reserve. RSI drugs are a double-edged sword in the critically ill. They facilitate intubation but can have severe adverse cardiovascular consequences including precipitation of irreversible shock and cardiac arrest. Patients with reduced physiologic reserve because of hypovolemia, vasodilation, or abnormal cardiac function are at higher risk of adverse event during airway management. Patients with hypotensive shock represent the extreme example. Most shock states are associated with high sympathetic tone, which serves a compensatory mechanism to maintain critical cardiac output.

Pretreatment and sedative-induction agents induce potent sympatholysis and attenuate reflex sympathetic discharge during laryngeal manipulation. Any drug that extinguishes these endogenous catecholamine responses, including sedative hypnotic agents, neuroleptics, and opioids can have deleterious impact. Reduction of endogenous sympathetic tone leads to venous and arterial vasodilation with decreased venous return and hypotension. Some anesthetic agents also induce direct myocardial depression.

RSI agents and doses must be carefully selected. Pretreatment opioids are contraindicated in patients with compromised cardiovascular status including compensated shock. Sedative induction drugs exhibit similar sympatholysis but are essential for facilitation of rapid sequence intubation. Adverse cardiovascular effects are both agent and dose dependent. Commonly recommended doses are based on patients with normal hemodynamics and cardiovascular reserve and therefore can be hazardous to critically ill patients. Frank hypotension or compensated shock requires dose reduction to half of normal or even lower. Although deep anesthesia may not be produced with half-dose induction, reasonable sedation and amnesia is assured with the recommended agents, particularly with proper management of sedation and analgesia in the immediate postintubation period.

Cardiovascular effects vary with sedative-hypnotic agent. Etomidate and ketamine are widely regarded as the most hemodynamically stable induction agents, especially compared with propofol, midazolam, and thiopental (see Chapter 21). However, despite their improved cardiovascular effects, both etomidate and ketamine require dose adjustment for administration to shocked patients (e.g., etomidate 0.1 to 0.15 mg per kg or ketamine 0.5 to 0.75 mg per kg). It is better to err on the side of too little rather than too much. Airway managers should anticipate delay in drug onset resulting from dose adjustment and the prolonged circulation time. Neuromuscular blocking agents pose little hemodynamic risk and should be dosed normally. Succinylcholine, vecuronium, and rocuronium are the most hemodynamically stable drugs in their respective classes. In patients with identified difficult airway attributes, awake intubation using a flexible endoscope, facilitated by topical anesthesia and limited (or no) sedation addresses the difficult airway and also avoids the potential hypotension of induction agents. Intubation with succinylcholine alone virtually never is indicated, but might be the best approach for the patient with severe cardiovascular decompensation who is felt unable to tolerate even a small dose of an induction agent. These patients typically have systemic SBP <70 mm Hg and markedly depressed mental status. Sedation and analgesia are judiciously titrated as soon as the tolerance to positive-pressure ventilation is determined. Intubation without any medications is reserved for arrested or moribund patients (see Chapter 3). However, neither of these situations obviates the need for attention to safe ventilation to minimize the negative cardiovascular impact of positive-pressure breathing.

Given the risk associated with intubation of patients in hemodynamic crisis, close hemodynamic monitoring is indicated. Continuous cardiac monitoring with frequent noninvasive blood pressure recording at least every 3 to 5 minutes is indicated in the peri-intubation period. Invasive arterial monitoring may be established during the preintubation period to facilitate monitoring of high-risk patients. Regardless of the measurement tool, blood pressure is not equivalent to blood flow (i.e., cardiac output and oxygen delivery). Progressive bradycardia not associated with hypoxia or laryngoscopy is a frequent sign of terminal shock and impending cardiac arrest.

Postintubation Management

Following intubation, positive-pressure ventilation should be initiated with caution. Positive intrathoracic pressure limits right heart venous return, which is accentuated during hypovolemia. Intentional or inadvertent hyperventilation may also lead to dynamic hyperinflation if expiratory time limits complete tidal volume (TV) elimination (see Chapter 7). Dynamic hyperinflation results in retained intra-thoracic volume which ultimately results in positive intrathoracic pressure known as auto-PEEP which impedes venous return. Although dynamic hyperinflation is worst in patients with obstructive lung disease, any patient can develop auto-PEEP during controlled positive-pressure breathing. Unrecognized auto-PEEP can lead to irreversible hypotension and cardiac arrest.

Slow, low-TV (10 to 12 breaths per minutes with TV 7 ml per kg) ventilation is used, regardless of whether ventilation is provided by manual resuscitation bag or by mechanical ventilator.

Hyperventilation with inappropriately high rate and TV is particularly common during manual bag ventilation immediately following endotracheal intubation. This is a vulnerable period given the simultaneous action of induction anesthesia. Recognize that most resuscitation bags have 1,500 ml reservoirs and require single-hand ventilation to provide TV approximating 500 ml. Similarly, rapid reexpansion of the bag following breath delivery is not a cue for the next breath, and a clock second hand, or counting cadence should be used to ensure that rate is not excessive. The airway manager needs to be particularly attentive to the risk of manual hyperventilation when other staff provide this support. Specific instruction is required regarding both volume (extent of bag squeeze) and rate (counting cadence, such as "1, 2, 3, 4, 5, breath, 1, 2, 3, 4, 5, breath…"). That sufficient time is allowed for complete expiration can be ascertained by simply listening to the patient's chest during ventilation. The chest should be quiet, representing completion of expiratory airflow, before initiation of the subsequent breath. Interrogation of the ventilator time-flow graphics to confirm return to zero flow at the completion of each breath cycle is a more sophisticated analysis of the same issue.

Vasopressor support should be immediately available to reverse life-threatening hypotension. Preintubation hypotension is more easily managed with catecholamine infusion initiated before intubation.

Postintubation sedation holds the same potential to induce sympatholysis related hypotension as induction agents. Although many prefer benzodiazepines (e.g., lorazepam and midazolam) to propofol because of perceived hypotension risk, appropriately titrated dose of the selected agent is likely most important. In the absence of painful invasive procedures, light sedation that maintains patient tolerance of endotracheal intubation is preferred over deeper sedation, which may worsen hypotension or increase vaso pressor requirements. Despite its favorable hemodynamic properties, etomidate should not be used for postintubation sedation due to risk for severe adrenal suppression.

POSTINTUBATION HYPOTENSION

Post-intubation hyptension (PIH) is a common clinical situation but should not be interpreted as an innocuous consequence of intubation. PIH occurs in one-quarter of normotensive patients undergoing emergency intubation and is severe (SBP <70 mm Hg) in up to 10% of cases. This is discussed in Chapter 19. Hemodynamic deterioration following emergency intubation of any shock patient stems from the mechanisms previously discussed but effects may be exaggerated, as hypotension is often multifactorial (Box 35-2). Even at reduced dose, sedative-hypnotic induction obliterates endogenous catecholamines with subsequent arterial and venous vasodilation. The reduced pressure gradient for venous return induced by systemic venodilation is compounded by positive intrathoracic pressure upon initiation of mechanical breathing. Pathologic states of tension pneumothorax and auto-PEEP exacerbate intrathoracic pressure and negative hemodynamic effects. Although most clinicians recognize the risk associated with tension pneumothorax, dynamic hyperinflation is much more common. The risk of dynamic hyperinflation in increased with obstructive lung disease but any patient can develop auto-PEEP under positive-pressure breathing.

Positive-pressure ventilation directly affects cardiac function. Positive intrathoracic pressure, including PEEP augmentation, reduces transmural cardiac pressure and thereby reduces left ventricular afterload. This impact may improve the performance of severe left ventricular dysfunction. In contrast, patients with normal or mildly reduced function suffer greater impact because of impedance of venous return. In contrast to the left heart, mechanical ventilation increases pulmonary vascular resistance which exacerbates pulmonary hypertension. This can be an important and life-threatening factor in managing patients with decompensated right heart failure.

Hypotension following emergency intubation is independently associated with increased risk of hospital death. Whether PIH directly contributes to worse outcome or merely represents a high-risk marker of severe disease is unclear. In either case, the risk associated with PIH warrants an early and organized hemodynamic resuscitation response similar to systemic hypotension (uncompensated shock) unrelated to airway management.

Box 35-2. Factors Contributing to Peri-intubation Hypotension

- Acute shock physiology
- Chronic underlying cardiac dysfunction
- RSI-related sympatholysis
- Prolonged or multiple intubation attempts
  - Hypoxemia
  - Bradycardia
- Metabolic factors
  - Hypoxemia
  - Severe acidosis
  - Hyperkalemia
- Initiation of positive-pressure ventilation
  - Positive intrathoracic pressure reduces venous return
  - Exacerbation of pulmonary hypertension worsening right heart dysfunction
  - Dynamic hyperinflation and auto-PEEP
  - Tension pneumothorax
- Postintubation factors
  - Postintubation sedation
  - Hypercarbia resolution

SUMMARY

Shock is a dynamic state, in which most, or all, of the patient's physiologic reserve mechanisms are depleted. Intubation is an essential part of the resuscitation of a patient with acute shock, but the intubation technique, medications, and postintubation mechanical ventilation all can exacerbate the shock state, often heralding a worse outcome for the patient. Coordinated shock resuscitation and peri-intubation management seeks to optimize patient outcome.

EVIDENCE

- **Who is at risk for PIH?** PIH is a common complication of emergency intubation that impacts roughly 25% of patients.[1–3] Severe PIH occurs in >10% of patients.[4,5] PIH may occur in any patient undergoing emergency intubation. In the normotensive range, serial vital signs do not appear to discriminate those at risk. Clinical factors including intubation for acute respiratory failure, COPD, hypercapnea, and sepsis are independently associated with PIH. Multiple intubation attempts and reintubation following self-extubation are also associated with increased complications including hemodynamic deterioration.[4,5]
- **Is there any evidence supporting use of an "intubation bundle" for patients with shock?** One important multicenter prospective study incorporated use of an intubation management bundle and showed important reduction in life-threatening complications including severe hypoxia and hypotension.[6] Critical bundle interventions focused on hemodynamic support included preintubation empiric fluid loading (minimum 500 ml isotonic fluid), use of cardiostable induction agents (etomidate or ketamine), early norepinephrine infusion for hypotension, and low-TV mechanical ventilation.

REFERENCES

1. Lin CC, Chen KF, Shih CP, et al. The prognostic factors of hypotension after rapid sequence intubation. *Am J Emerg Med.* 2008;26(8):845–851.

2. Jaber S, Amraoui J, Lefrant JY, et al. Clinical practice and risk factors for immediate complications of endotracheal intubation in the intensive care unit: a prospective, multiple-center study. *Crit Care Med.* 2006;34(9):2355–2361.

3. Franklin C, Samuel J, Hu TC. Life-threatening hypotension associated with emergency intubation and the initiation of mechanical ventilation. *Am J Emerg Med.* 1994;12(4):425–428.

4. Griesdale DE, Bosma TL, Kurth T, et al. Complications of endotracheal intubation in the critically ill. *Intensive Care Med.* 2008;34(10):1835–1842.

5. Mort TC. Unplanned tracheal extubation outside the operating room: a quality improvement audit of hemodynamic and tracheal airway complications associated with emergency tracheal reintubation. *Anesth Analg.* 1998;86(6):1171–1176.

6. Jaber S, Jung B, Corne P, et al. An intervention to decrease complications related to endotracheal intubation in the intensive care unit: a prospective, multiple-center study. *Intensive Care Med.* 2010;36(2):248–255.

36

The Pregnant Patient

Valerie A. Dobiesz • Richard D. Zane

THE CLINICAL CHALLENGE

The physiologic and anatomic changes associated with pregnancy may pose challenges to all facets of airway management including oxygenation, ventilation, and securing the airway. Along with many physiologic changes, late-term pregnancy also present unique difficulties related to the airway. In fact, complications related to airway management in the parturient patient are the most significant cause of anesthetic-related maternal mortality. Pregnancy changes the patient's anatomy and physiology in a variety of distinct ways:

- Oxygen reserve and depletion: There is an approximately 20% reduction in expiratory reserve volume, residual volume, and functional residual capacity (FRC), and an increased maternal basal metabolic rate and oxygen demand by the fetal unit. These changes lead to more rapid desaturation of the fully preoxygenated pregnant woman during apnea (approximately 3 minutes compared to 8 for the normal non-pregnant adult).
- Physiologic hyperventilation: Progesterone increases the ventilatory drive and leads to hyperventilation. Maternal minute ventilation increases early in pregnancy largely because of an increase in tidal volume. This results in alteration of "normal" blood gas parameters, which must be considered when managing mechanical ventilation. Maternal $PaCO_2$ falls to approximately 32 mm Hg, which is associated with a compensatory decrease in bicarbonate from 26 to 22 mEq per L in order to maintain a normal maternal pH. Mechanical ventilation must provide some degree of hyperventilation in order to maintain maternal pH. A reasonable approach is to increase the minute ventilation by approximately 20% for the pregnant woman in the first trimester, increasing to 40% by term.
- Cardiopulmonary compromise in late pregnancy: In the late stages of pregnancy when the patient is placed supine, the effects of the gravid uterus on the diaphragm and, occasionally, increased breast size on the chest wall, further decrease the FRC. In addition to decreasing FRC, supine positioning in the late second and third trimester of pregnancy can result in aortocaval compression by the gravid uterus. This significantly reduces blood return to the heart, impairing maternal and fetal perfusion. This can be mitigated to a certain degree by placing the patient in the left lateral decubitus position.
- Effects on laryngoscopy and bag-mask ventilation (BMV): Pregnancy also can affect laryngoscopy and BMV. Weight gain, greater resistance to chest expansion by abdominal contents, and increased breast size may make BMV difficult in a manner analogous to that seen with an obese patient. The effects of estrogen and increased blood volume contribute to mucosal edema of the nasal passages and pharynx causing airway tissues to become redundant, friable, and more prone to bleeding, especially with airway manipulation. This mucosal edema can also lead to distortion of the airway structures, leading to difficulty both in identifying structures and in passing the endotracheal tube through the upper airway to the glottis. This upper airway distortion can be worsened by preeclampsia, active labor with pushing, and the infusion of large volumes of crystalloid fluids. Vascular engorgement also leads to a decrease in luminal size in the trachea requiring a smaller than expected endotracheal tube (6.5 to 7.0 on average). The engorged upper airway tissues also can make BMV more difficult.
- Increased propensity for aspiration: As pregnancy progresses, gastric acid secretion increases, causing a decrease in maternal gastric pH as well as an increase in gastrin levels, a reduction in gastric activity, and an increase in gastric emptying time that can result in an increase in resting gastric volume. Gastroesophageal sphincter tone is also reduced in pregnancy. Enlargement of the uterus increases the pressure exerted on the stomach, which combined with a reduction in gastroesophageal sphincter tone, increases the risk of reflux. A "full stomach" should always be a concern in these patients. Administration of neuromuscular blockade will exacerbate this further by causing a loss of supporting abdominal muscle tone. These normal changes in gastrointestinal physiology start early in the second trimester but become most problematic in the mid to late second and third trimesters.

- Effects on neuromuscular blocking agents: Maternal plasma cholinesterase activity is reduced by 25%; however, this does not result in any significant effects on elimination, half-life, or duration of effect of succinylcholine. Pregnancy, however, does result in enhanced sensitivity to the aminosteroid muscle relaxants such as vecuronium and rocuronium which may prolong their effect.

APPROACH TO THE AIRWAY

In early pregnancy, fluid and FRC changes predominate, but the airway itself is unchanged. As pregnancy progresses, difficulty in both intubation and BMV should be anticipated. Nevertheless, the approach to airway management in the pregnant patient is no different from that of any other emergent intubation, except for consideration of the unique features of pregnancy described in The Clinical Challenge Section, which may create airway difficulty beyond the sixth month of pregnancy.

Key issues to consider for airway management in these patients are as follows:

1. Anatomically, think of the third trimester pregnant patient as analogous to an obese patient, and use the difficult airway algorithm. If careful assessment using the LEMON, MOANS, RODS, and SMART mnemonics (see Chapter 2) indicates that rapid sequence intubation (RSI) is reasonable, have backup devices readily at hand, and anticipate more rapid oxyhemoglobin desaturation than for the nonpregnant patient.
2. If flexible endoscopic intubation is the chosen method, avoid the nasal route in favor of the oral. The mucosa may be engorged, edematous, and friable, and nasotracheal intubation is more likely to lead to mucosal damage and bleeding.
3. Preoxygenate carefully, using at least eight vital capacity breaths or 3 minutes of breathing 100% oxygen; as FRC is reduced, oxygen consumption is increased, and apnea leads to desaturation more rapidly. If possible, continue passive oxygenation during the apneic phase, using nasal cannula at 5 L per minute flow. Although this has not been studied in term pregnant women, it significantly delays desaturation in obese patients.
4. All opioids and induction agents may reduce maternal blood flow to the placenta and, therefore, blood flow to the fetus. These agents also cross the placental barrier. Because muscle relaxants are quaternary ammonium salts and are fully ionized, they do not readily cross the placenta. Antihypertensive agents such as metoprolol, labetalol, and esmolol cross the placenta and carry a risk of inducing fetal bradycardia. In the context of emergent airway management, however, maternal well-being supersedes the potential for fetal exposure. When these agents are administered and delivery of the fetus is imminent, the caregiver charged with the management of the neonate immediately after delivery should be fully briefed regarding the agents administered to the mother.
5. Although there is no hard evidence in support of I believe we have been using "Sellick maneuver" throughout as per LWW protocol maneuver, it is widely used and recommended in pregnant patients, in particular, because of the gastrointestinal changes described previously. We consider the maneuver optional, but if it is to be used, the person tasked with applying it should be trained and skilled in the application of cricoid pressure.
6. Although rescue airway devices, such as the laryngeal mask airway (LMA), intubating LMA, and the Combitube, may be used in the event of a failed intubation similar to the nonpregnant patient, the enhanced risk of aspiration in the nonfasted pregnant patient creates additional urgency for definitive airway control. The successful placement of one of these extraglottic rescue devices may achieve adequate gas exchange, giving the provider additional time to secure a definitive airway and avoid a surgical airway. Nonetheless, as the term pregnant patient may rapidly desaturate, cricothyrotomy should not be delayed

when intubation fails and adequate oxygenation cannot be maintained using a bag and mask or an extraglottic device (EGD).

Recommended Intubation Sequence

- *Preparation:* A detailed difficult airway examination, including LEMON, MOANS, RODS, and SMART, should always be performed before making a decision regarding the appropriateness of RSI. Even if other markers of difficult laryngoscopy are not present, obesity, enlarged breasts, and physiologic airway edema can nevertheless complicate the ability to successfully secure the airway of the pregnant patient. By default, even in the absence of typical predictors of a potentially difficult airway the difficult airway algorithm should be used for patients in late-term pregnancy. As with the nonpregnant patient, if the intubator does not have confidence that oxygenation (by BMV or EGD) and intubation will be successful, an awake, sedated, technique with topical anesthesia is used, such as flexible endoscopy, video laryngoscopy, or awake direct laryngoscopy.

  Assemble your airway equipment both for immediate management and for potential rescue of a failed airway. Be sure to include a selection of smaller-sized endotracheal tubes with stylets loaded; a bougie, short-handle laryngoscope if direct laryngoscopy will be attempted; and, if available, a rescue device with which you are familiar and equipment for a surgical airway.
- *Preoxygenation:* Preoxygenate fully using eight vital capacity breaths or 3 minutes with 100% oxygen (see Chapters 5, 19). Use left lateral decubitus positioning when in the supine position to avoid aortocaval compression; tilt the abdomen slightly to the left with a wedge or pillow under the right hip to displace the gravid uterus from the inferior vena cava.
- *Pretreatment:* Lidocaine and fentanyl are indicated as for the nonpregnant patient if time allows. Fentanyl should be used in the eclamptic or preeclamptic patient to mitigate hypertensive responses. Note the previously mentioned caveats regarding opioids and the fetus.
- *Paralysis with sedation:* Agent selection is as for the nonpregnant patient. Unless contraindicated, succinylcholine is recommended for paralysis in a dose of 1.5 mg per kg. If succinylcholine is contraindicated, a nondepolarizing agent, ideally rocuronium 1 mg per kg, should be administered, despite the risk of prolonged effect after administration. The choice of induction agent is dictated by maternal hemodynamic condition as in the nonpregnant patient. There is no evidence to support the use of one particular induction agent in pregnancy.
- *Positioning:* Intubation success can be significantly enhanced with proper positioning before administration of induction agents. For the obese parturient patient or one with excessive breast tissue, placing a roll, a pillow, or a liter bag of intravenous fluid vertically between the shoulder blades moves the glottic structures forward and assists in displacing the breasts away from the neck. Positioning of the occiput is equally important because too much extension of the neck can move the glottic structures anteriorly and impede visualization. Placing a pad or folded sheet under the patient's head to bring it into a neutral position may eliminate this. A head up position can help with ventilation both in the spontaneously breathing patient and when positive-pressure ventilation is required. Cricoid pressure intuitively may be more important in the pregnant patient, but evidence supporting its use is scant. If cricoid pressure is used and glottic visualization is difficult, release the glottic pressure to improve glottic view and allow the intubator to perform external laryngeal manipulation if desired.
- *Placement with proof:* As with the nonpregnant patient, tube placement must be confirmed by detection of end-tidal carbon dioxide in addition to physical examination no matter how certain the operator is that the trachea has been successfully intubated.

Management of the Failed Intubation

As with any patient for whom emergent intubation is required, unanticipated difficulty can be encountered despite a careful difficult airway assessment. In the pregnant patient, the approach needs to be modified slightly to accommodate the anticipated physiologic changes imposed by pregnancy. Primarily, this is driven by the rapidity with which the mother desaturates and the commonly encountered airway edema and friability. We recommend reducing the number of attempts at laryngoscopy before moving to the failed airway algorithm to two from three in the pregnant patient, unless success on the third attempt is believed to be highly likely. Even though maintaining oxygenation and ventilation is important for all patients, it is paramount in the pregnant patient, who has reduced physiologic reserve. In this circumstance, one should always choose a rescue device with which he or she is most facile and has the most experience. Properly performed, two-handed, two-person BMV may buy time to allow an alternative to cricothyrotomy. Nevertheless, one needs to be prepared to go to surgical airway if the rescue device is not able to provide adequate ventilation. Keep in mind that upper airway edema is a common cause of inability to both visualize the glottic structures and ventilate with BMV or supraglottic devices, making insertion of appropriately sized, or even oversized airways of even greater importance. Resistance to diaphragmatic excursion by the uterus and the weight of the gravid breast on the chest will further impede successful ventilation, which may be mitigated by placing the patient in a reverse Trendelenberg position to cause the abdominal contents to shift caudally.

Postintubation Management

Pregnancy is associated with an increased metabolic rate, which requires increasing minute ventilation as the pregnancy progresses. At term, this translates into a 30% to 50% increase in minute ventilation. Arterial blood gases or pulse oximetry and end-tidal carbon dioxide monitoring will aid in adjusting the ventilation parameters. Modest adjustments of both rate (start at 12 to 14 per minute) and tidal volume (start at 12 ml per kg) should meet the ventilatory need. If ventilation pressures are high, placing the patient in reverse Trendelenberg and left lateral decubitus position to move the abdominal contents down off the diaphragm may bring some improvement. In addition tidal volume can be reduced somewhat and the respiratory rate increased.

SUMMARY

Late-term pregnancy induces changes that affect almost every aspect of airway management. Classification of the late-term pregnant patient as a difficult airway, use of the difficult airway algorithm, and consideration of rapid oxyhemoglobin desaturation and the technical challenges of laryngoscopy and BMV will help the operator develop a cogent plan, including rescue from intubation failure.

TIPS AND PEARLS

- Proper positioning of the pregnant patient including placing the head slightly up with a roll between the shoulders and good support under the occiput before induction and attempting intubation may improve success.
- Supraglottic edema is a common cause for failure to secure the airway in the pregnant patient; therefore, a smaller (6.5 to 7.0 mm ID) endotracheal tube may be required.
- Although not specifically studied in the pregnant patient to date, it is likely that video laryngoscopy offers substantial advantages for glottic visualization and intubation when compared with direct laryngoscopy.
- As for the nonpregnant patient, cricoid pressure is optional. In the event of difficult laryngoscopy, or a failed airway requiring a rescue EGD, releasing cricoid pressure may improve success at placement.
- When choosing pharmacologic agents to facilitate intubation, the general rule of thumb is "if it benefits the mother in the acute setting, it will ultimately benefit the fetus."

EVIDENCE

- **Which extraglottic device is best for the pregnant patient?** There are no randomized studies comparing the various rescue airway devices in pregnant patients. There are, however, a number of case reports and case series detailing the use of the LMA Classic, LMA ProSeal, LMA Fastrach, laryngeal tube, and Combitube. Naturally, these reports largely focus on the positive outcomes when these devices are used, so the risks and benefits of each are difficult to discern. None of these devices provide complete protection against aspiration, which remains a significant concern in the airway management of the pregnant patient. The laryngeal tube modification with the second lumen for passing an oral gastric tube and the LMA ProSeal with a similar design may offer at least a conduit for stomach contents to exit if regurgitation occurs. The LMA ProSeal also has an airway cuff that seals at higher pressures than a classic LMA allowing for higher ventilatory pressures, a finding constant across a wide range of body mass index scores. Compared with a classic LMA, these features may be advantageous in the pregnant population. Both the Combitube and the laryngeal tube have a lumen/balloon that can provide some barrier to regurgitation; however, experience with both devices in obstetrics is limited.

  Although the LMA ProSeal, laryngeal tube, and Combitube may offer some advantage against the risk of aspiration, they cannot be used to secure definitive endotracheal intubation as can the intubating LMA. Currently, the intubating LMA is probably the best choice as a rescue device in the pregnant patient because it can be used as both a rescue device and an intubation device. Nonetheless, the choice of rescue device should be influenced by operator experience and device availability.[1-9]

- **What is the rate of failed intubations in obstetrics and has it improved with recent advances in difficult airway management?** There is variability and controversy regarding the exact rate of failed intubations in the pregnant patient reported in the Anesthesia literature but according to closed claim analysis it is 1 in 250 to 1 in 300.[10] Several studies have found this rate to be declining with the overall rate of general anesthesia in obstetrics decreasing over time. A cross-sectional study of obstetric complications extracted from the 1998 to 2005 Nationwide Inpatient Sample of Healthcare Cost and Utilization Project found a decrease of >40% in rates of severe complications of anesthesia including airway problems.[11,12] Several studies of obstetric anesthesia claims for injuries also found improved safety with a decrease in respiratory complications from 24% to 4% and a decrease in claims from inadequate oxygenation/ventilation or aspiration of gastric contents and esophageal intubations.[13,14] A third more recent study found the rate of difficult intubations in a 20-year cohort analysis of 2,633 patients to be 4.7% and failed intubations 0.8% and that these rates remained stable over the 20 years reviewed.[15] These studies suggest significant risks are associated with airway management in obstetrical patients and that these rates have been stable or declining in incidence. It is highly recommended to anticipate and recognize the difficult airway in pregnancy and to follow difficult airway algorithms with a few well-chosen devices considering the anatomic and physiologic changes occurring in pregnancy. It is also recommended to maintain ongoing training and education in this area.[16]

REFERENCES

1. Gaiser R. Physiologic changes of pregnancy. In: Chestnut DH, ed. *Obstetric Anesthesia: Principles and Practice*. 4th ed. Philadelphia, PA: Mosby; 2009:15–36.

2. Goldszmidt E. Principles and practices of obstetric airway management. *Anesthesiol Clin.* 2008;26(1):109–125.

3. Lewin SB, Cheek TG, Deutschman CS. Airway management in the obstetric patient. *Crit Care Clin.* 2000;16:505–513.

4. Minville V, N'guyen L, Coustet B, et al. Difficult airway in obstetrics using ILMA Fastrach. *Anesth Analg*. 2004;99:1873.

5. Munnur U, de Boisblanc B, Suresh M. Airway problems in pregnancy. *Crit Care Med*. 2005;33:S259–S268.

6. Vasdev GM, Harrison BA, Keegan MT, et al. Management of the difficult and failed airway in obstetric anesthesia. *J Anesth*. 2008;22(1):38–48.

7. Zand F, Amini A. Use of the laryngeal tube-S for airway management and prevention of aspiration after a failed tracheal intubation in a parturient. *Anesthesiology*. 2005;102:481–483.

8. Halaseh BK, Sukkar ZF, Hassan LH, et al. The use of ProSeal laryngeal mask airway in caesarean section—experience in 3000 cases. *Anaesth Intensive Care*. 2010;38(6):1023–1028.

9. Zamora JE, Saha TK. Combitube rescue for Cesarean delivery followed by ninth and twelfth cranial nerve dysfunction. *Can J Anaesth*. 2008;55(11):779–784.

10. McDonnell NJ, Paech MJ, Clavisi OM, et al; ANZCA Trials Group. Difficult and failed intubation in obstetric anaesthesia: an observational study of airway management and complications associated with general anaesthesia for caesarean section. *Int J Obstet Anesth*. 2008;17:292–297.

11. Kuklina EV, Meikle SF, Jamieson DJ, et al. Severe obstetric morbidity in the United States: 1998–2005. *Obstet Gynecol*. 2009;113:293–299.

12. Mhyre JM. What's new in obstetric anesthesia in 2009? An update on maternal patient safety. *Anesth Analg*. 2010;111:1480–1487.

13. Davies JM, Posner KL, Lee LA, et al. Liability associated with obstetric anesthesia: a closed claims analysis. *Anesthesiology*. 2009;110:131–139.

14. Kuczkowski KM, Reisner LS, Benumof JL. Airway problems and new solutions for the obstetric patient. *J Clin Anesth*. 2010;15:552–563.

15. McKeen DM, George RB, O'Connell CM, et al. Difficult and failed intubation: incident rates and maternal, obstetrical, and anesthetic predictors. *Can J Anaesth*. 2011;58:514–524.

16. Biro P. Difficult intubation in pregnancy. *Curr Opin Anaesthesiol*. 2011;24(3):249–254.

37

Prolonged Seizure Activity

Robert J. Vissers

THE CLINICAL CHALLENGE

A general discussion of the diagnosis and treatment of seizure disorder is beyond the scope of this book. This chapter focuses on the considerations of airway management in the seizure patient. In the simple, self-limited, generalized seizure, airway management is directed at termination of the seizure and prevention of hypoxia from airway obstruction. Paralysis and intubation should be considered when SpO_2 declines <90% or when typical first-line measures fail to terminate the seizure in a reasonable time. For the simple seizure, basic airway maneuvers, expectant observation (most seizures end spontaneously), supplemental high-flow oxygen, and vigilance are usually all that is necessary. Airway protection from aspiration is rarely required in the simple, self-limited seizure because the uncoordinated motor activity precludes coordinated expulsion of gastric contents.

Determining when to proceed from supportive measures to intubation is the main clinical challenge in the airway management of the seizing patient. *Status epilepticus* has been defined as continuous seizure activity for 30 minutes or multiple seizures without recovery of consciousness in between. The rationale for 30 minutes was that this is the minimum seizure duration that has been believed to produce neuronal injury. Recent literature questions the practical value of this, and it has been proposed that the "operational definition" of generalized convulsive status epilepticus in adults and children >5 years be modified to 5 minutes or more of continuous seizure activity. The intended implication of this change is that clinicians wait no longer than 5 minutes of continuous seizure activity before initiating therapy to terminate seizure activity. Any seizure lasting longer than 5 minutes is concerning because most single seizures are much shorter in duration than this. The brain's compensatory mechanisms to prevent neuronal damage rely on adequate oxygenation and cerebral blood flow, and brain compensation is often compromised before 30 minutes, particularly in patients with underlying illness. There is also evidence that with longer seizure duration, pharmacologic therapies become less effective. The mortality rate for status epilepticus is >20% and also increases with duration of seizure activity. Therefore, intubation should be undertaken early as a part of overall supportive therapy in cases where the seizure is not promptly terminated by anticonvulsant medications begun at a seizure duration of not >5 minutes. The absolute and relative indications for intubation in the seizing patient are listed in Box 37-1.

Box 37-1. Indications for Endotracheal Intubation for the Seizing Patient

Absolute indications
1. Hypoxemia (SpO_2 <90%) secondary to hypoventilation or airway obstruction
2. Treatment of underlying etiology (e.g., intracranial bleed with elevated ICP)
3. Prolonged seizure refractory to anticonvulsants (to prevent accumulating metabolic debt [acidosis and rhabdomyolysis])
4. Generalized convulsive status epilepticus

Relative indications
1. Prophylaxis for the respiratory depressant effect of large doses of anticonvulsants (e.g., benzodiazepines and barbiturates)
2. Termination of seizure activity to facilitate diagnostic workup (e.g., CT scanning)
3. Airway protection in prolonged seizures

APPROACH TO THE AIRWAY

Self-Limited Seizure

Most seizures terminate rapidly, either spontaneously or in response to medication, and require only supportive measures. Positioning the patient on his or her side, providing oxygen by face mask, suctioning secretions and blood carefully, and occasionally using the jaw thrust to relieve obstruction from the tongue are usually all that is necessary to prevent hypoxia and aspiration. Bite-blocks should not be placed in the mouths of seizing patients. They are not indicated and will only serve to increase the likelihood of injury. Attempts to ventilate during a seizure are usually ineffective and rarely necessary.

Prolonged Seizure Activity

Although most self-limited seizures do not require intubation, there are several indications for intubation in the prolonged seizure. Extensive generalized motor activity will eventually cause hypoxia, significant acidosis, rhabdomyolysis, hypotension, hypoglycemia, and hyperthermia. Respiratory depression may result from high doses or combinations of anticonvulsants. Oxygen saturation of <90%, despite supplemental high-flow oxygen, is an indication for immediate intubation.

There is no clear guideline that specifically defines the duration of seizure activity requiring intubation. A good rule of thumb is that patients with seizures lasting >5 minutes with evidence of hypoxemia (central cyanosis or pulse oximetry readings <90% despite supplemental oxygen and clearly inadequate respirations) or patients with seizures lasting >10 minutes despite appropriate anticonvulsant therapy should be considered for intubation. Generally, when first-line (benzodiazepine) anticonvulsants fail to terminate grand mal seizure activity, rapid sequence intubation (RSI) is indicated. Phosphenytoin, which has a relatively short loading time, may be initiated as a second-line agent before intubation, if time allows. Other second-line anticonvulsants (phenytoin and phenobarbital) require at least 20 minutes for a loading dose; therefore, at the time of initiation of such a load, intubation is advisable. The initiation of a propofol or phenobarbital infusion may also be an indication for intubation because of their respiratory depressant effects. Both agents also act synergistically with benzodiazepines, which increases the likelihood of apnea and the need for airway management.

TECHNIQUE

RSI is the method of choice in the seizing patient. In addition to its technical superiority, RSI ends all motor activity, allowing the body to begin to correct the metabolic debt. However, cessation of motor activity while the patient is paralyzed does not represent termination of the seizure, and effective loading doses of appropriate anticonvulsants (e.g., phenytoin) are required immediately after intubation. The recommended technique for the seizure patient is described in Box 37-2.

Standard RSI technique is appropriate in the seizing patient with the following modifications:

1. *Preoxyngenation*: Preoxygenation may be suboptimal because of uncoordinated respiratory effort; therefore, pulse oximetry is critical. After giving succinylcholine, the patient may desaturate to <90% before complete relaxation and thus may require oxygenation using a bag and mask before attempts at intubation or continuous passive oxygenation by nasal cannulae at 5 L per minute throughout the intubation sequence.
2. *Paralysis with induction:* Sodium thiopental shares anticonvulsant activity with other barbiturates and commonly was used for patients without hypotension. Propofol has also been used as an induction agent in this setting at a dose of 1.5 mg per kg. Little data exist on propofol as an induction agent in patients with seizures; however, there is evidence that it provides rapid suppression of seizure activity after a bolus and infusion and has been used in refractory status epilepticus. Midazolam is a reasonable alternative but dosage reduction is required in the hemodynamically compromised

---

Box 37-2. RSI for Patients with Prolonged Seizure Activity

Time	Action
Zero minus 10 min	Preparation
Zero minus 5 min	Preoxygenation
Zero minus 3 min	Pretreatment
	Continue anticonvulsant therapy
Zero	Paralysis with induction
	Sodium thiopental 3 mg/kg *or* midazolam 0.3 mg/kg *or*
	propofol 1.5–2 mg/kg *or* etomidate 0.3 mg/kg
	Succinylcholine 1.5 mg/kg
Zero plus 30 s	Protection and positioning
Zero plus 45 s	Placement with proof
Zero plus 60 s	Postintubation management
	Midazolam drip 0.05–0.2 mg/kg/h IV
	Or
	Propofol drip, 1–5 mg/kg/h IV
	Vecuronium 0.1 mg/kg IV (sedation preferable to paralysis)
	EEG monitoring if patient has ongoing paralysis
	Increased respiratory rate if significant acidosis present

patient, and midazolam functions poorly as an induction agent at lower doses. It is not known whether midazolam offers any additional anticonvulsant activity in a setting in which benzodiazepine seizure therapy has already been maximized. The full induction dose of midazolam is 0.3 mg per kg, but this often is reduced to 0.1 to 0.2 mg per kg for status epilepticus patients to prevent hemodynamic compromise, particularly because most patients have already received benzodiazepine therapy. Etomidate has an unclear effect on seizure activity but is the induction agent of choice if associated hypotension precludes the use of sodium thiopentothal, propofol, or midazolam. Although etomidate may raise the seizure threshold (and therefore inhibit seizure activity) in generalized seizures, it lowers the threshold in focal seizures. Either succinylcholine or rocuronium can be used for neuromuscular blockade in this setting. Succinylcholine offers a shorter duration of action, allowing early and frequent neurologic assessment, but this may be a moot point if sugammadex is approved and available for rapid reversal of rocuronium neuromuscular blockade.

3. *Postintubation management:* There are three additional considerations with respect to postintubation management.

- Prolonged, deep sedation with an agent that suppresses seizures is desirable for the first hour after intubation to facilitate investigations (e.g., CT scan) and to allow acidosis to correct with controlled ventilation. Propofol infusion permits rapid reversal of sedation, which allows repeated or on-going assessment of seizure activity and neurologic status, so often is used for this purpose.
- Long-term neuromuscular blockade should be avoided, if at all possible; however, if it is used, it should be accompanied by adequate doses of a sedation agent and continuous Electroencephalogram (EEG) monitoring, if available.

  Continuous bedside EEG monitoring is necessary in the paralyzed patient to assess for ongoing seizure activity. If this is not immediately available, motor paralysis should be allowed to wear off before repeat dosing, to evaluate the effectiveness of anticonvulsant therapy. Effective sedation with a convulsive suppressant such as a propofol or midazolam infusion is preferable to motor paralysis.
- If elevated intracranial pressure (ICP), head injury, known CNS pathology, or suspected meningitis is present, ICP intubation technique should be used (see Chapter 32).

Drugs and Dosages

1. Preintubation seizure management
   - Lorazepam 0.1 mg per kg intravenously (IV) up to 2 mg per minute

   or
   - Diazepam 0.1 to 0.3 mg per kg IV up to 5 mg per minute or 0.5 mg per kg per rectum

   or
   - Midazolam 0.1 to 0.3 mg per kg IV up to 5 mg per minute

   THEN
   - Phosphenytoin 20 mg per kg (as milligrams of phenytoin equivalent)

2. Induction agents
   - Sodium thiopental 3 mg per kg

   or
   - Propofol 1.5–2 mg per kg

   or
   - Midazolam 0.2–0.3 mg per kg

   or
   - Etomidate 0.3 mg per kg

3. Postintubation sedation and therapy
   - Midazolam 0.05 to 0.2 mg/kg/hour IV infusion, or
   - Propofol 1 to 5 mg/kg/hour IV infusion

TIPS AND PEARLS

1. Check early to ensure that hypoglycemia is not the cause of the seizure. Perform a bedside glucose measurement or administer IV dextrose solution in all cases. Similarly, check for hyponatremia.
2. Even in the difficult airway, RSI is generally preferred for airway management in the actively seizing patient because any technique without neuromuscular blockade is unlikely to succeed. Some difficult airway assessment components may be difficult (e.g., mouth opening for the 3-3-2 rule or the Mallampati assessment). Airway difficulty, therefore, often is a judgment call. If the airway is assessed to be difficult, a double setup may be desirable.
3. The paralyzed patient may continue to seize, possibly causing neurologic injury despite the lack of motor activity. Administer effective doses of long-acting anticonvulsants, and use benzodiazepines for long-term sedation. Avoid long-term paralysis, if possible. If a long-acting neuromuscular blocking agent is used, arrange continuous EEG monitoring, if possible, or allow motor recovery frequently (at least every hour) to assess response to therapy.
4. Prolonged seizure activity almost always represents a significant change in seizure pattern for the patient. A careful search for an underlying cause, including head CT scan, is indicated.

EVIDENCE

- **Which benzodiazepine is best?** The answer depends on the setting in which it is being used. In one multicenter study, 570 patients with status epilepticus were randomized to lorazepam (0.1 mg per kg), phenytoin (18 mg per kg), diazepam (0.15 mg per kg), and phenytoin or phenobarbital (15 mg per kg).[1] Lorazepam alone was most effective in terminating seizures within 20 minutes and maintaining a seizure-free state in the first 60 minutes after treatment. There was no difference in 30-day outcome or adverse events.[1] Lorazepam also performed better than diazepam or placebo in a double-blind prehospital study of 205 patients with status epilepticus, where termination of seizures occurred in 59% of patients versus 43% and 21%, respectively.[2] Diazepam remains a popular agent in the emergency setting because of its rapid onset (<20 seconds, compared to 1 minute for midazolam and 2 minutes for lorazepam).[3] Diazepam is stable at room temperature in a premixed form and is readily absorbed rectally; therefore, it is often the benzodiazepine of choice stocked on a resuscitation cart.

There are no data on the ideal benzodiazepine as an induction agent in status epilepticus; however, both propofol and midazolam are more familiar and available than thiopental to most providers, suggesting that one of these agents is the best choice.

- **Midazolam, propofol, or pentobarbital for postintubation therapy?** For postintubation care, the patient should be sedated using a drug that not only provides amnesia and anxiolysis, but also optimizes antiepileptic therapy. Benzodiazepines have all these properties and are readily available in the acute care setting. Midazolam is preferred over diazepam and lorazepam as a continuous IV infusion because of its shorter half-life, water solubility, hemodynamic stability, and greater clinical experience in refractory status epilepticus.[3,4]

Recent reports suggest midazolam or propofol being preferred as a first-line agent, and then pentobarbital as a second-line drug; however, no prospective randomized trial exists comparing these therapies directly.[5,6] A systematic review to evaluate the efficacy and outcomes of these three agents in refractory status epilepticus found 28 studies that described a total of 193 patients.[5] Pentobarbital was more effective at preventing breakthrough seizures; however, it was also associated with more episodes of hypotension, and there was no difference in outcomes between any of the agents. Pentobarbital is less desirable because it is rarely used in the emergency setting, making it less familiar or available.

Despite the popularity of propofol for refractory seizure management in the ICU setting, there is little experience in the emergency setting, and the ICU studies are too small to draw any conclusions.[7-10] The recommended dosing for propofol is 1 to 2 mg per kg IV bolus (or induction) followed by a 1 to 5 mg/kg/hour infusion.[11] Higher sustained doses have been associated with a propofol infusion syndrome.

REFERENCES

1. Abou Khaled KJ, Hirsch LJ. Advances in the management of seizures and status epilepticus in critically ill patients. *Crit Care Clin*. 2006;22(4):637–659.

2. Treiman DM, Meyers PD, Walton NY, et al. A comparison of four treatments for generalized convulsive status epilepticus. *N Engl J Med*. 1998;339(12):792–798.

3. Alldredge BK, Gelb AM, Isaacs SM, et al. A comparison of lorazepam, diazepam and placebo for the treatment of out-of-hospital status epilepticus. *N Engl J Med*. 2001;345(9):631–637.

4. Treiman DM. Pharmacokinetics and clinical use of benzodiazepines in the management of status epilepticus. *Epilepsia*. 1989;30:4–15.

5. Kumar A, Bleck TP. Intravenous midazolam for the treatment of refractory status epilepticus. *Crit Care Med*. 1992;20:483.

6. Claassen J, Hirsch LJ, Emerson RG, et al. Treatment of refractory status epilepticus with pentobarbital, propofol, or midazolam: a systematic review. *Epilepsia*. 2002;43(2):146–153.

7. Claassen J, Hirsch LJ, Emerson RG, et al. Continuous EEG monitoring and midazolam infusion for refractory nonconvulsive status epilepticus. *Neurology*. 2001;57:1036–1042.

8. Prassad A, Worrall BB, Bertam EH, et al. Propofol and midazolam in the treatment of refractory status epilepticus. *Epilepsia*. 2001;42:380–386.

9. Stecker MM, Kramer TH, Raps EC, et al. Treatment of refractory status epilepticus with propofol: clinical and pharmacokinetic findings. *Epilepsia*. 1998;39(1):18–26.

10. Shearer P, Riviello J. Generalized convulsive status epilepticus in adults and children: treatment guidelines and protocols. *Emerg Med Clin North Am*. 2011;29:51–64.

11. Rossetti AO, Reichhart MD, Schaller MD, et al. Propofol treatment of refractory status epilepticus: a study of 31 episodes. *Epilepsia*. 2004;45:757–763.

38

The Geriatric Patient

Patrick A. Nee • Diane M. Birnbaumer

THE CLINICAL CHALLENGE

Comorbid illnesses are common in the older population, and for any given illness or injury, older adults have a worse outcome. Aging causes progressive deterioration in physiologic reserve and these changes are exacerbated by preexisting chronic conditions, so the elderly are at increased risk of adverse responses to tracheal intubation.

Advanced age affects airway management decision making in three primary areas.

Decreased Cardio-Respiratory Reserve

Age-related changes in the lungs impair gas exchange, reducing oxygen tension at baseline. The normal PaO_2 falls by 4 mm Hg per decade after the age of 20. Total lung capacity does not change significantly, but functional residual capacity (FRC) and closing volume (CV) increase with age. CV increases more than FRC leading to atelectasis, especially in the supine position. Reduced sensitivity of central respiratory drive, weakened respiratory muscles, and altered chest wall mechanics impair the ability of the older adult to respond to hypoxia and hypercarbia. Consequently, oxygen saturation may fall rapidly in the face of a respiratory threat. Older patients also are at risk of pulmonary aspiration because of blunted airway reflexes, swallowing disorders, drug effects, and delayed gastric emptying.

The aging heart has reduced contractility and limited coronary blood flow, and dysrhythmias, such as atrial fibrillation, further impair the ability to increase cardiac output. This relatively fixed cardiac output impairs the physiologic response to the hypotensive effects of intubation drugs. Finally, the presence of cardiovascular or cerebrovascular disease reduces the patient's tolerance of hypoxemia or hypotension.

Increased Incidence of Difficult Airway

Advanced age, per se, is a marker for difficult bag-mask ventilation (BMV) (see Chapter 2). Older patients also have an increased incidence of difficult direct laryngoscopy, although this is not a factor of age itself, but rather a result of impairment of neck mobility and mouth opening. Similarly, changes associated with aging and the cumulative effects of disease cause difficulty with the insertion of extraglottic devices (EGDs) and provision of a surgical airway.

Ethical Considerations

In airway management, as in all other aspect of resuscitation, the patient's preferences regarding therapeutic interventions must be respected. Advanced age in and of itself is not a contraindication to advanced airway intervention. Poor outcomes relate more to functional limitation and comorbidities rather than chronologic age. In cases where life-sustaining interventions are either inappropriate or not desired, noninvasive ventilation can provide respiratory assistance and comfort.

APPROACH TO THE AIRWAY

As the elderly tolerate hypoxia poorly, intubation should be considered early in their management. A careful preintubation assessment will identify difficult airway predictors, such as poor mouth opening, absent teeth, stiff lungs and reduced cervical spine range of motion. Most often, the operator will be confident with respect to laryngoscopy, particularly if a video laryngoscope is used, and with respect to oxygenation using a bag and mask or EGD, so rapid sequence intubation (RSI) is usually the technique of choice.

Preoxygenation is particularly important as older patients may desaturate quickly because of age-associated changes in the heart and lungs and preexisting disease. For the same reasons, preoxygenation may not be as effective as in a younger, healthier patient. BMV may be required to maintain oxygen saturation >90% after the induction agent and neuromuscular blocking agent (NMBA) are given, particularly if more than one laryngoscopic attempt is required. Although not studied in the elderly patient, passive oxygenation during apnea by the provision of oxygen at 5 L per minute flow through nasal cannulae may retard the rate of oxyhemoglobin desaturation.

During bag-mask ventilation (BMV), mask seal may be problematic because of facial wasting and edentulousness, and a two-handed two-person technique, with a nasal or oral airway, is advisable. Well-fitting dentures should be left in place during BMV and removed for intubation. Loss of elastic tissues promotes collapse and partial obstruction of the upper airway. Older patients may have oropharyngeal obstruction because of hematoma or cancer of the head or neck. Reduced lung compliance and chest wall stiffness may make oxygenation using a bag and mask or EGD difficult, and this may be worsened by coexisting chronic obstructive pulmonary disease (COPD) or heart failure.

When preintubation assessment identifies a difficult airway, the operator should choose the best possible device (usually a video laryngoscope) and ensure optimal patient positioning to create the greatest likelihood of success. Alternative airway approaches, including awake flexible endoscopy, may be chosen over RSI, as guided by the difficult airway algorithm (Chapter 3).

Surgical cricothyrotomy is the appropriate choice in a "can't intubate, can't oxygenate" situation, but this procedure may be difficult in the elderly as they are more likely to have distortion of the tissues as a result of cancer or radiotherapy.

Drug Dosage and Administration

Pretreatment

The pretreatment agents considered for older adults are the same as for younger adult patients: lidocaine and fentanyl. In general, lidocaine is recommended for patients with elevated intracranial pressure or reactive airway disease and does not require dose adjustment. Its use in the elderly has not been specifically studied.

Fentanyl mitigates catecholamine response to laryngeal manipulation. Although senescence may blunt these autonomic responses, critically ill hypoxic and acidotic older patients requiring intubation are at risk of stroke, myocardial infarction, or other vascular events. Although premedication with fentanyl may attenuate these responses, its use is not without risk. Older patients are more sensitive to the respiratory depressant and hypotensive effects of opioids. Consequently, fentanyl should be given slowly (over more than 2 to 3 minutes) as the last of the pretreatment drugs. In frail patients, or those with significant comorbidities, including the use of antihypertensive medications, it may be advisable to reduce the fentanyl dose to 1 to 2 μg per kg, or avoid its use altogether.

Paralysis with induction

Etomidate is the preferred agent in older patients because of its superior hemodynamic stability, but it will not adequately blunt the pressor response to laryngoscopy (see "Pretreatment" section). Thiopental and propofol may cause significant hypotension in critically ill patients. With any induction agent, the elderly are more prone to drug-induced hypotension, which may be persistent. Ketamine causes less cardiovascular lability and is useful in reactive airways disease, however, its sympathomimetic properties can be a disadvantage in patients with ischemic heart disease, cerebrovascular disease, elevated intracranial pressure, or Parkinson's disease.

Succinylcholine is the paralytic agent of choice for RSI. Before using it in older patients, contraindications to succinylcholine should be sought by history from the patient or family members, physical examination (especially for neurologic disability), and review of clinical records, if possible. For example, a recent denervating stroke (3 days to 6 months) is associated with a high risk of drug-induced hyperkalemia. Where doubt exists, an alternative NMBA, ideally rocuronium, should be used. Chronic renal disease, including renal failure, is not a contraindication to succinylcholine use.

POSTINTUBATION MANAGEMENT

The principles of postintubation management, set out in Chapters 7 and 19, are appropriate to the aging adult. Anticipate greater sensitivity to both the sedative and hemodynamic effects of sedatives (e.g., midazolam and propofol) and analgesics (e.g., morphine, fentanyl, and alfentanil) and titrate accordingly. Neuromuscular blockade rarely is required. If used, the NMBA should also be given in reduced doses and with increased intervals between doses. Ventilator settings are not usually affected by age, but reduced compliance may increase ventilation pressures. In COPD, it is advisable to limit peak pressure and allow a prolonged expiratory phase, although severe respiratory acidosis should be avoided in ischemic heart disease. Positive-pressure ventilation, particularly with high levels of positive end-expiratory pressure, can cause hypotension, particularly if hypovolemia is present, and may exacerbate the hypotensive effects of sedative drugs. Pressure-controlled ventilation is the preferred mode.

TIPS AND PEARLS

- Older patients have an increased incidence of difficult airway management. These difficulties are identified and managed in generally the same fashion as for the younger patient. RSI usually is the procedure of choice.
- Elderly patients desaturate quickly, placing a premium on preoxygenation. Passive oxygenation during apnea (oxygen at 5 L per minute by nasal cannulae) may delay desaturation and BMV may be required after induction or between intubation attempts.
- Age-related cardiovascular changes, preexisting disease, and drug interactions enhance the hypotensive response to induction and reduced doses of sedatives and hypnotics should be used. Reduced cardiac output prolongs the arm–brain circulation time and a delayed onset of action should be anticipated for all intravenous drugs.

EVIDENCE

- **Is older age an independent predictor of difficult intubation or complications of intubation?** Airway morphology may be affected by age. Although one study showed Mallampati class, thyromental and sternomental distances, and cervical range of motion had the greatest reduction in patients aged 50 to 70 years,[1] another showed no relationship between mean age and Cormack and Lehane grade laryngoscopic view at intubation.[2] In two sizeable prehospital studies, age was not independently associated with intubation difficulty in either population.[3,4]

  Injury during tracheal intubation is more common in the elderly. In a comprehensive audit of airway management in the United Kingdom, patients older than 60 years accounted for one-third of major airway management complications in anesthesia cases and one-fifth of ED cases.[5,6] A North American group found an almost 3-fold increase in the risk of pharyngoesophageal perforation in patients older than 60 years.[7] The majority of 203 dental injuries reported over a 7-year period were sustained in patients aged 50 to 70 years.[8] Aspiration of gastric contents, a major complication of intubation, increases with advancing age and declining physical status.[9] Although most studies show the elderly at higher risk for intubation complications, a study of >3,000 emergency intubations showed age was not a risk factor.[10]
- **Which pretreatment drugs should be used in the elderly?** There is no literature addressing the use of lidocaine in older adults in the emergency setting.

  Fentanyl is the agent with which emergency physicians will be most familiar, and it is the sole pretreatment drug in most RSIs. Opioids onset more slowly in older subjects and their effects persist for longer, compared with younger age groups. The elderly are more sensitive to the respiratory and cardiovascular effects of these drugs and a 30% to 50% dose reduction is required.[11,12] Although there is literature addressing the pretreatment utility of fentanyl and alternative sedo-analgesic agents in the elderly, comparative studies of different agents in the emergency setting is lacking.

- **Which induction agent (and what dose) should be used in the elderly?** Etomidate is the intravenous induction agent of choice in older patients. A recent review of the literature on the use of etomidate in the ED setting concluded that the drug was effective and appropriate, even in hypovolemic patients and those with limited cardiac reserve.[13] Although dose reduction of etomidate in adults undergoing elective procedures has been described without loss of effect, evidence is lacking in the emergency situation and 0.3 mg per kg is the recommended dose.[14]

  Propofol or midazolam is a reasonable alternative to etomidate. Observational studies have shown that the plasma concentration required to induce the (desired and undesired) effects of these agents is up to 50% less in older subjects. Clinical effects take longer to become apparent and persist for longer. A 40% reduction in dose of propofol or midazolam is recommended in patients older than 65 years.[12,15] Midazolam may cause significantly more hypotension than etomidate, particularly in patients older than 70 years.[16] Similar advantage was found for etomidate compared with propofol when used for procedural sedation in the critically ill ED patients.[17]

- **Which muscle relaxant (and what dose) should be used in RSI in the elderly?** The advantages of succinylcholine in RSI are set out in Chapter 22. Many of the adverse effects are germane to the elderly patient and may prompt consideration of alternatives. The major adverse effect of SCh administration is hyperkalemia, which may occur in older subjects after a stroke.

  Although a reduced dose of SCh (0.6 mg per kg) produced *acceptable* intubating conditions in elective surgical patients with shortened neuromuscular recovery time,[18,19] data are lacking in respect of studies of RSI in elderly subjects in the emergency setting. The standard dose of 1.5 mg per kg is recommended in this age group.[14]

  Rocuronium in a standard dose of 1 mg per kg is as likely as SCh to produce *acceptable* intubating conditions but provides *excellent* conditions less often. When SCh is contraindicated, it is a reasonable alternative agent.[9] Prolonged neuromuscular blockade is a potential problem with this agent in older adults, and spontaneous breathing may not return for up to an hour. Sugammadex, a novel reversal drug that binds with rocuronium (and vecuronium) has been shown to reverse the block in this age group.[20]

REFERENCES

1. Turkan S, Ate Y, Cuhruk H, et al. Should we re-evaluate the variables for predicting the difficult airway in anesthesiology? *Anesth Analg*. 2002;94(5):1340–1344.

2. Reed M, Dunn MJG, McKeown DW. Can an airway assessment score predict difficulty at intubation in the emergency department? *Emerg Med J*. 2005;22:99–102.

3. Wang HE, Kupa DF, Paris PM, et al. Multivariate predictors of failed pre-hospital endotracheal intubation. *Acad Emerg Med*. 2003;10(7):717–724.

4. Combes X, Jabre P, Jbeili C, et al. Prehospital standardization of medical airway management: incidence and risk factors of difficult airway. *Acad Emerg Med*. 2006;13(8):828–834.

5. Cook TM, Woodall N, Frerk C; on behalf of the Fourth National Audit Project. Major complications of airway management in the UK: results of the Fourth National Audit Project of the Royal College of Anaesthetists and the Difficult Airway Society. Part 1: anaesthesia. *Br J Anaesth*. 2011;106:617–631. doi:10.1093/bja/aer058.

6. Cook TM, Woodall N, Harper J, et al; on behalf of the Fourth National Audit Project. Major complications of airway management in the UK: results of the Fourth National Audit Project of the Royal College of Anaesthetists and the Difficult Airway Society. Part 2: intensive care and emergency departments. *Br J Anaesth*. 2011;106:632–642. doi:10.1093/bja/aer059.

7. Domino KB, Posner KL, Caplan RA, et al. Airway injury during anesthesia: a closed claims analysis. *Anesthesiology*. 1999;91(6):1703–1711.

8. Givol N, Gershtansky Y, Halamish-Shani T, et al. Perianesthetic dental injuries: analysis of incident reports. *J Clin Anesth*. 2004;16(3):173–176.

9. Neilipovitz DT, Crosby ET. No evidence for decreased incidence of aspiration after rapid sequence induction. *Can J Anaesth*. 2007;54(9):748–764.

10. Martin L, Mhyre JM, Shanks AM, et al. 3,423 emergency tracheal intubations at a university hospital: airway outcomes and complications. *Anesthesiology*. 2011;114(1):42–48.

11. Vuyk J. Pharmacodynamics in the elderly. *Best Pract Res Clin Anaesthesiol*. 2003;17(2):207–218.

12. Martin G, Glass PSA, Breslin D, et al. A study of anesthetic drug utilization in different age groups. *J Clin Anesth*. 2003;15(3):194–200.

13. Oglesby AJ. Should etomidate be the induction agent of choice for rapid sequence intubation in the emergency department? *Emerg Med J*. 2004;21:655–659.

14. Reynolds SF, Heffner JH. Airway management of the critically ill patient. Rapid sequence intubation. *Chest*. 2005;127:1397–1412.

15. Schnider TW, Minto CF, Shafer SL, et al. The influence of age on propofol pharmacodynamics. *Anesthesiology*. 1999;90:1502–1516.

16. Choi YF, Wong TW, Lau CC. Midazolam is more likely to cause hypotension than etomidate in emergency department rapid sequence intubation. *Emerg Med J*. 2004;21:700–702.

17. Miner JR, Martel ML, Meyer M, et al. Procedural sedation of critically ill patients in the emergency department. *Acad Emerg Med*. 2005;12(2):124–128.

18. Naguib M, Samarkandi A, Riad W, et al. Optimal dose of succinylcholine revisited. *Anesthesiology*. 2003;99(5):1045–1049.

19. Mohammad I, El-Orbany M, Ninos JJ, et al. The neuromuscular effects and tracheal intubation conditions after small doses of succinylcholine. *Anesth Analg*. 2004;98:1680–1685.

20. McDonagh DL, Benedict PE, Kovac AL, et al. Efficacy, safety, and pharmacokinetics of sugammadex for the reversal of rocuronium-induced neuromuscular blockade in elderly patients. *Anesthesiology*. 2011;114(2):318–329.

39

The Morbidly Obese Patient

Richard D. Zane • Abbie L. Erickson

THE CLINICAL CHALLENGE

The World Health Organization and the National Institutes of Health define a person to be overweight when he or she has a body mass index (BMI) between 25 and 29.9 kg per m², and a person to be obese when BMI is ≥30 kg per m². Morbid obesity is variably defined as a BMI >35 or 40 kg per m². The National Health and Nutrition Examination Survey for 2003 to 2004 estimates that 66.2% of the adults in the United States between the age of 20 and 74 years are either overweight or obese (33.4% overweight, 32.9% obese) and early data from 2005 to 2006 show no significant change in the prevalence of obesity; however, the 2008 Behavioral Risk Factor Surveillance System, a state-based cross-sectional random survey of the adult population of United States, showed considerable differences in the prevalence of obesity across states.

APPROACH TO THE AIRWAY

As for all patients, managing the airway of obese patients requires a structured, methodical assessment to identify the specific predictors of difficult bag-mask ventilation (BMV), cricothyrotomy, extraglottic device (EGD) placement, and tracheal intubation. It is controversial whether obesity, per se, is a predictor of difficult laryngoscopy, or whether obese patients tend to have a higher incidence of other markers of difficult intubation. Patient attributes differ, and some obese patients may have multiple anatomical risk factors for difficult airway in addition to obesity, whereas others may not. Nevertheless, morbidly obese patients develop both physiologic and anatomic changes that can make airway management particularly challenging as morbidly obese patients not only have excess adipose tissue on the breast, neck, thoracic wall, and abdomen but also internally in the mouth and pharynx. When compared with lean patients, this excess tissue makes accessing the airway (intubation and tracheostomy) and maintaining patency (during sedation or mask ventilation) of the upper airway more difficult.

The degree of pathologic, physiologic, and anatomical changes correlate with the degree and extent of obesity and many comorbidities common with obese patients. The physiologic and anatomical changes associated with morbid obesity are listed in Box 39-1. The main effects of obesity on airway management are (1) rapid arterial desaturation, secondary to a decreased functional residual capacity (FRC) and increased oxygen consumption; (2) difficult airway management, specifically difficult BMV, resulting from increased risk of obstruction from excess pharyngeal adipose tissue and increased resistance resulting from the weight of the chest wall and the mass of abdominal contents limiting diaphragmatic excursion; and (3) difficult laryngoscopy, intubation, and cricothyrotomy.

Obesity affects almost every aspect of normal physiology, most notably the respiratory and cardiovascular systems. Obese patients often have baseline hypoxemia with a widened alveolar–arterial oxygen gradient, which is primarily because of ventilation–perfusion (V/Q) mismatching. Lung volumes develop a restrictive pattern with multiple disturbances, the most important of which is decreased FRC. Notably, these indices change exponentially with the degree of obesity. The decline in FRC has been ascribed to "mass loading" of the abdomen and splinting of the diaphragm. FRC may be reduced to the extent that it falls within the range of closing capacity, thus leading to small airway closure and V/Q mismatch. The FRC declines further when the individual assumes the supine position, resulting in worsening of the V/Q mismatch, right-to-left shunt, and arterial hypoxemia. Although the vital capacity, total lung capacity (TLC), and FRC may be maintained in mild obesity, they can be reduced by up to 30% in morbidly obese patients and up to 50% in severely obese patients. The decreased FRC causes rapid oxyhemoglobin desaturation during the apneic phase of rapid sequence intubation (RSI), even in the setting of adequate preoxygenation (see Chapter 19).

The work of breathing (WOB) is increased 30% to 400% in morbidly obese patients because of decreased chest wall compliance, increased airway resistance, and an abnormal diaphragmatic position. These changes limit the maximum ventilatory capacity (MVC). The obese patient has elevated oxygen consumption and carbon dioxide (CO_2) production because of the metabolic activity of the excess body mass.

Cardiovascular changes in obesity include increased extracellular volume, cardiac output, left ventricular end diastolic pressure, and left ventricular hypertrophy (LVH). The absolute total blood volume (BV) is increased, but it is relatively less on a volume/weight basis when compared with lean patients (50 vs. 75 ml per kg). Cardiac morbidity, including hypertension (HTN), ischemic heart disease, and cardiomyopathy, all correlate with progressive obesity.

Other changes include an increase in renal blood flow (RBF) and glomerular filtration rate (GFR), fatty infiltration of the liver, and a propensity for diabetes mellitus and obstructive sleep apnea (Box 39-1).

Box 39-1. Physiologic and Anatomical Changes Associated with Obesity

Physiologic changes associated with obesity according to system	Anatomical changes associated with obesity

Pulmonary:

- Increased intrathoracic pressure with a restrictive respiratory pattern: ↓FRC, ↓ERV, ↓TLC

- Increased WOB, decreased MVC

- V/Q mismatching (predisposes to hypoxemia)
- Risk of pulmonary HTN
- Obesity hypoventilation syndrome

Cardiac:

- Increased cardiac output
- Increased BV, SV
- HTN, LVH
- Increased metabolic rate: ↑VO_2, ↑CO_2 production

Renal:

- Increased RBF and GFR

Hepatic/gastrointestinal:

- Fatty infiltration of the liver
- Increased intraabdominal pressure
- Risk for hiatal hernia, GERD

Endocrine:

- Increased risk of diabetes
- Hyperlipidemia

Hematologic:

- Increased risk of DVT
- Polycythemia (with chronic hypoxemia)

Musculoskeletal:

- Degenerative joint disease
- Decubital changes

Anatomical changes associated with obesity

- Increased facial girth
- Increased tongue size
- Smaller pharyngeal area
- Redundant pharyngeal tissue (risk of obstructive sleep apnea)
- Increased neck circumference
- Increased chest girth
- Increased breast size

- Increased abdominal girth

ERV, expiratory reserve volume; SV, stroke volume; VO_2, oxygen consumption; GERD, gastroesophageal reflux; DVT, deep venous thrombosis.

Increased chest wall weight, increased facial girth, and redundant pharyngeal tissue all contribute to defining obesity as an independent risk factor for difficult BMV (see Chapter 2). Obese patients tend to have a smaller pharyngeal space because of deposition of adipose tissue into the tongue, tonsillar pillars, and aryepiglottic folds. Patients with obesity have an increased risk of having obstructive sleep apnea and facial hair (in men), which are also independent risk factors for difficult BMV. Difficult BMV should be anticipated in the obese patient, often requiring a two-person technique with both oral and nasopharyngeal airways in place. In severe or super-obese patients, BMV may simply be impossible as the mask seal pressure required to overcome the increased weight and resistance may be far in excess of that possible with a bag and mask. In addition, challenging BMV is associated with difficult intubation in 30% of the cases. Intubation difficulty is also associated with increased neck circumference and high Mallampati scores. Cricothyrotomy is more difficult because of the increase in neck circumference, the thickness of the subcutaneous tissues, anatomical distortions, and adipose tissue obscuring landmarks, often requiring deeper and longer incisions. EGDs may not be able to overcome the high resistance of the weighted chest wall and restricted diaphragms.

TECHNIQUE

Morbidly obese patients vary with respect to airway difficulty, and a methodical LEMON assessment is essential to anticipate and plan appropriately for intubation (see Chapter 2). When the airway appears particularly difficult, the difficult airway algorithm advocates for careful preparation and awake video or direct laryngoscopy or a flexible endoscopic approach with topical anesthesia and systemic sedation.

Proper positioning is essential in obese patients in order to ensure the best attempt at direct laryngoscopy and tracheal intubation. Ideally, the patient should be propped up on linens, or on a commercially available pillow, from the midpoint of the back to the shoulders and head for proper positioning, as shown in Figure 39-1. To confirm proper positioning, the patient should be viewed from the side, and an imaginary horizontal line should be able to be drawn from the external auditory meatus to the angle of Louis. This position facilitates intubation and both spontaneous and BMV, thus improving preoxygenation and prolonging the duration of time before arterial desaturation with apnea. Upright positioning improves the effectiveness of preoxygenation for obese patients. Similarly, continuous passive oxygenation, provided by nasal cannulae at 5 L per minute flow, delays oxyhemoglobin desaturation significantly in the obese patient.

To determine the best technique, the risks and benefits of managing the airway with the patient awake versus unconscious are weighed. When time and conditions permit, particularly in the morbidly obese patient, or the obese patient with additional markers of difficult laryngoscopy, awake flexible endoscopy is the preferred method. No matter which route is chosen, the proper airway equipment must be available and checked for proper functioning, and ideally help is readily available in the event intubation proves to be exceedingly difficult. Video laryngoscopy is preferred because it has a greater likelihood of providing an excellent view of the glottis. When performing direct laryngoscopy, a short-handled laryngoscope can be easier to insert because the chest prevents the longer handle from gaining blade access to the mouth. During ventilation by BMV or using an EGD, placing the patient in reverse Trendelenberg or a semi-upright position reduces upward pressure against the diaphragm by the abdominal contents and may also mitigate some of the "weight effect" of chest wall tissues, such as the breasts. Both the standard and the intubating laryngeal mask airway have been shown to be effective in providing ventilation, with the latter also serving as a conduit for tracheal intubation. Rigid fiberoptic intubating devices and video laryngoscopy have been shown to be successful in managing the airway of the obese patient as well. During direct laryngoscopy, the bougie may be helpful when only the arytenoids or the tip of the epiglottis is visible.

BMV often requires two providers using two-handed bilateral jaw thrust and mask seal, with oropharyngeal and nasopharyngeal airways in place and the airway pressure relief valve and mask seal set so that continuous positive airway pressure (5 to 15 cm H_2O) is delivered to the pharynx. Relaxation of the upper airway muscles during RSI will often cause collapse of the adipose-laden,

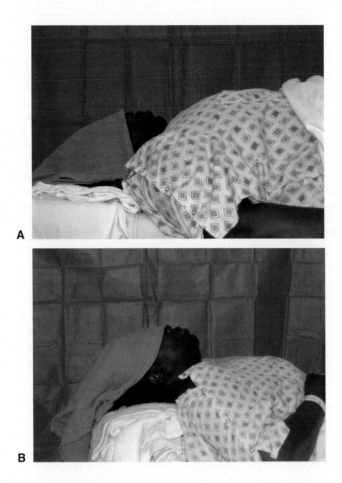

Figure 39-1 ● **A:** Patient is supine with the weight of the breast/chest obstructing access to the airway. **B:** Patient is propped on linens to establish better anatomical landmarks and remove the weight of the breasts/chest off the airway. Here it is possible to draw an imaginary horizontal line from the external auditory meatus to the angle of Louis.

soft-walled pharynx between the uvula and epiglottis, making BMV and tracheal intubation more difficult, and greatly reinforcing the need to use oral and nasal airways, augmented by positioning the patient semi-upright, as described above.

Cricothyrotomy may be extremely challenging in the severely obese patient because the chin may be directly contiguous with the chest wall, making identification of and access to anatomical landmarks difficult. In the moderately obese patient, care must be taken to ensure that landmarks are found. This step may require one or two assistants whose sole role is to hold or retract neck, facial, and chest fat folds. As in all patients, cricothyrotomy is a tactile procedure.

Drug Dosage and Administration

Obesity, along with any associated comorbidities, affects all aspects of the pharmacodynamic and pharmacokinetic properties of medications, including absorption, onset, volume of distribution (V_d), protein binding, metabolism, and clearance. In the obese patient, there is not only an increase in adipose tissue, but also an increase in lean body mass of approximately 30% of the total excess weight. The ratio of fat to lean mass increases, however causing a relative decrease in the percentage of lean mass and water in obese patients when compared to lean patients. In addition, there is an increase in BV and cardiac output. The V_d for a particular agent is affected by the combination of these obesity-associated factors, along with the specific lipophilicity of the drug. Protein binding is affected by an increased concentration of triglycerides, lipoproteins, cholesterol, and free fatty acids. These lipids limit the binding of some drugs, thus increasing the free plasma concentration. In contrast, increased α_1-glycoprotein may increase protein binding of other drugs, thus decreasing the free plasma concentration. For most agents that undergo hepatic metabolism, there is minimal change in effective half-life despite the high incidence of fatty infiltration of the liver. Agents handled by the kidney, however, have accelerated clearance because of increased GFR. These pharmacokinetic and pharmacodynamic changes can make the net effect of these agents somewhat unpredictable and dosage adjustment is required. Monitoring of clinical end points is important in addition to empirical drug dosing based on the available data.

In general, the lipophilicity of the agent can indicate the dosage requirement. Most anesthetic agents are lipophilic, thus an increase in V_d and dose of the drug is expected, but this is not consistently demonstrated in pharmacologic studies because of factors such as end-organ clearance or protein binding. Less lipophilic agents have little or no change in V_d and should therefore be dosed according to ideal body weight (IBW) or lean body weight (LBW). Unfortunately, few studies have investigated the effects of obesity on the disposition of anesthetic agents, so for many drugs, it is unclear if weight-related dosage adjustments should be made and whether these should be based on actual weight, ideal weight, or a percentage of the actual body weight. See Table 39-1 for specific recommendations.

Drug dosing for obese patients can be difficult to remember, given that some drugs are dosed using IBW, some using LBW, and some using total body weight (TBW). IBW must be estimated or looked up in a table or nomogram, based on the patient's height. TBW may be reported by the patient, or obtained using a bed scale. LBW can be thought of as IBW plus 30% of the difference between TBW and IBW. In other words, for every pound or kilogram the patient is overweight, about one-third of this contributes to lean body mass.

Succinylcholine is a TBW drug. This has been very well studied (see Chapter 22). The commonly used competitive neuromuscular blocking agents (rocuronium and vecuronium) are IBW drugs. Lidocaine also is an IBW drug. The induction agents and the opioid, fentanyl, generally are LBW drugs. Exceptions are midazolam and propofol, which generally are dosed according to IBW.

POSTINTUBATION MANAGEMENT

The changes in the anatomy and physiology of obese patients have important implications for ventilator management. The initial tidal volume should be calculated based on IBW and then adjusted according to airway pressures, with the success of oxygenation and ventilation indicated by pulse oximetry and capnography, or arterial blood gas monitoring. Generally, the use of at least 5 cm H_2O of positive end-expiratory pressure is recommended to prevent end-expiratory airway closure and atelectasis, particularly in the posterior lung regions. In severe obesity, it may be necessary to ventilate the patient in the semierect position to move the weight of the breasts, abdominal fat, or pannus off the chest wall.

Portable bedside radiographs are usually of poor quality in the obese patient, limiting their clinical value, although one can usually determine if the endotracheal tube (ETT) is in a mainstem bronchus.

When considering extubation of the obese patient, a conservative approach should be taken. Review documentation regarding the difficulty of BMV and tracheal intubation, and consider the possibility of the patient requiring emergent reintubation.

TIPS AND PEARLS

- The predicted difficulty in intubation combined with the decreased physiologic reserve in obese patients makes timely airway management important, and the decision to intubate cannot be delayed.

TABLE 39-1
Dosing Recommendations for Drugs Commonly Used in Airway Management

Drug	Dosing	Comments
Propofol	IBW	Lipophilic, systemic clearance and V_d at steady-state correlate well with TBW. High affinity for excess fat and other well-perfused organs. High hepatic extraction and conjugation relates to TBW. Cardiovascular depression limits dosage to IBW for use in induction. Maintenance dosing may be initiated at TBW but titrated to effect using sedation scales
Thiopental	LBW	Lipophilic, increased V_d, prolonged duration of action, cardiovascular depression limits dosage to LBW. Caution with reactive airway disease
Midazolam	IBW	Lipophilic, increased V_d, prolonged sedative effect due to accumulation in adipose tissue and inhibition of cytochrome P450 3A4 by other drugs or obesity itself
Succinylcholine	TBW	Hydrophilic, increased plasma cholinesterase activity increases in proportion to body weight
Atracurium	TBW	Hydrophilic, clearance, V_d, and elimination half-life is unchanged. No prolongation of recovery
Vecuronium	IBW	Hydrophilic, V_d increased and clearance decreased, significant delay in recovery if given according to TBW
Rocuronium	IBW	Hydrophilic, similar to vecuronium, prolonged duration of action if used with TBW
Fentanyl	LBW	Lipophilic, increased V_d and elimination half-life, distributes extensively in excess body mass. Respiratory depression limits dosing to LBW. Maintenance dosing is initiated at LBW but should be titrated using a sedation scale
Remifentanil	IBW	Lipophilic, decreased V_d, and clearance
Lidocaine	IBW	Increased V_d. Contraindicated with high-grade heart block
Etomidate	LBW	Increased V_d, dose may need to be decreased with liver disease

- For many obese patients, an awake technique, usually awake flexible endoscopy, is the preferred method of intubation. If RSI is performed, rescue strategy should be well laid out, and the necessary equipment immediately available.
- Most tracheostomy tubes will not be long enough for the morbidly obese patient; a 6-mm inner diameter ETT may be advanced through the cricothyrotomy incision.

EVIDENCE

- **Is obesity an independent risk factor for difficult intubation?** Classically, morbid obesity has been described as an independent predictor of difficult intubation although it has not been clear if obese patients have more commonly described predictors of difficult intubation or if obesity itself is an independent predictor. In 2008, Gonzalez et al.[1] compared the incidence of difficult intubation in obese and nonobese patients and found that neck circumference and increased BMI were independent predictors of difficult intubation. Obesity also proves to be a risk factor for difficult intubation in the prehospital environment. In 2011, Holmberg et al.[2] found obesity to be an independent risk factor for difficult intubation after reviewing >800 prehospital intubations.

- **What is the best position for preoxygenation and intubation of the obese patient?** Not only is intubation more difficult in obese patients but so is bag valve mask ventilation. In addition, obese patients desaturate more rapidly than nonobese patients, making preoxygenation challenging as well. Positioning with the head elevated anterior to the shoulders aligning the external auditory meatus with the sternal notch or angle (Fig. 39-1) has been shown to make both oxygenation and intubation easier. Dixon et al.[3] found that by elevating the head, obese patients were able to achieve 23% greater oxygen tension when compared with the supine position in obese patients undergoing elective bariatric surgery. Oxyhemoglobin desaturation was significantly delayed and fewer patients desaturated <90% when oxygen was continuously administered at 5 L per minute by nasal cannulae during the apneic phase of intubation.[4]

- **Are obese patients more difficult to ventilate with bag valve mask ventilation?** Obesity makes bag valve mask ventilation difficult for a number of reasons including difficulty in obtaining mask seal, deposition of intraglottic adipose tissue, and the increased weight of the breast and pannus requiring higher positive ventilation pressures often overcoming the mask seal. In 2009, Kheterpal et al.[5] demonstrated that obesity was an independent predictor of difficult bag valve mask ventilation after reviewing >50,000 patients requiring general anesthesia.

REFERENCES

1. Gonzalez H, Minville V, Delanoue K, et al. The importance of increased neck circumference to intubation difficulties in obese patients. *Anesth Analg*. 2008;106:1132–1136.

2. Holmberg TJ, Bowman SM, Warner KJ, et al. The association between obesity and difficult prehospital tracheal intubation. *Anesth Analg*. 2011;112:1132–1138.

3. Dixon BJ, Dixon JB, Carden JR, et al. Preoxygenation is more effective in the 25 degrees head-up position than in the supine position in severely obese patients: a randomized controlled study. *Anesthesiology*. 2005;102(6):1110–1115.

4. Ramachandran SK, Cosnowski A, Shanks A, et al. Apneic oxygenation during prolonged laryngoscopy in obese patients: a randomized, controlled trial of nasal oxygen administration. *J Clin Anesth*. 2010;22:164–168.

5. Kheterpal S, Martin L, Shanks AM, et al. Prediction and outcomes of impossible mask ventilation: a review of 50,000 anesthetics. *Anesthesiology*. 2009;110:891–897.

40

Foreign Body in the Adult Airway

Ron M. Walls

THE CLINICAL CHALLENGE

Many upper airway foreign bodies, such as a fish bone in the oropharynx, do not present any threat to the airway and simply are removed using one or a combination of techniques. This chapter deals with foreign bodies whose location or size presents an actual or potential threat of airway obstruction.

Airway obstruction caused by a foreign body presents a unique series of challenges to the practitioner. First, when incomplete obstruction is present, there exists the possibility that a particular action, or the failure to take specific action, could aggravate the situation by converting a partial obstruction to a complete obstruction. Second, when complete obstruction is present, instinctive interventions, such as bag-mask ventilation, have the potential to make the situation worse, for example, by causing a supraglottic obstruction to move below the cords, making retrieval more difficult (or impossible). Third, a common maneuver, like endotracheal intubation with bag ventilation, may meet with an unexpected result, such as the complete inability to move any air, defying the provider's attempts to find a solution to a problem perhaps never before encountered. Finally, the completely or partially obstructed airway is a unique clinical situation, unlike other airway threats, and requires a specific set of evaluations and interventions, often in a very compressed period of time.

The patient with a foreign body in the airway may present with signs of upper airway obstruction or may present comatose and apneic, with only the history of onset to provide clues as to the cause of the crisis. The obstruction may be complete, as in the patient who aspirates a food bolus, and is unable to move sufficient air to phonate. Although these situations usually arise in the out-of-hospital setting, they may occasionally present to the emergency department (ED), usually when an incomplete obstruction converts to a complete obstruction at the time of the patient's arrival. A partially obstructing foreign body will cause symptoms and signs of incomplete upper airway obstruction, specifically stridor, altered phonation, subjective difficulty breathing, and often a sense of fear or panic on the part of the patient. In many cases, there will be a preceding condition that has increased the risk of aspiration. Many patients who aspirate food are physically or mentally impaired, elderly, or intoxicated with drugs or alcohol.

APPROACH TO THE AIRWAY

Management of the suspected or known foreign body in the adult airway follows similar rationale to that used in the pediatric patient (see Chapter 27) and depends on the location of the foreign body and whether the obstruction is incomplete or complete. Location may be supraglottic, infraglottic, or distal to the carina. Because the precise location of the foreign body is usually not known, the following discussion focuses on the approach to the foreign body whose location is uncertain.

Incomplete Obstruction by a Foreign Body

When the patient presents with an incompletely obstructing foreign body, the objective is to reestablish a fully patent airway and prevent the conversion of a partial obstruction to a complete obstruction. If the patient is cooperative and breathing spontaneously and oxygen saturation is adequate (possibly with supplemental oxygen), then the best approach often is to have emergency airway equipment immediately accessible in case the patient deteriorates, but as part of a plan to rapidly mobilize the necessary providers for prompt removal in the operating room (OR). Some foreign bodies are obviously accessible and can be removed in the ED. There is risk, however, with an incompletely obstructing foreign body just proximal to the glottis, that attempts at removal in the ED might result in displacement of the foreign body into the trachea, where it is no longer amenable to removal with common ED instruments. If transfer to the OR is not an option, for example, because it would require transfer to another hospital, then a decision must be made as to whether the foreign body should be removed in the ED. If so, the best approach is to handle the airway much as one would handle awake laryngoscopy for a difficult intubation (see Chapter 23). The operator assembles the appropriate equipment, preoxygenates the patient, explains the procedure to the patient, and administers titrated sedation and topical anesthesia recognizing that either may trigger total obstruction. With the patient sedated, the operator carefully inserts the laryngoscope with the left hand, inspecting at each level of insertion before advancing to ensure that the foreign body is not pushed farther down by the tip of the laryngoscope. Either a conventional or a video laryngoscope may be used. The technique is one of "lift and look" followed by a small advance (perhaps 1 cm), and then another lift and look, and so on. It may be necessary to take a break to allow the patient to reoxygenate or to administer more sedation or anesthesia. When the foreign body is identified, the best instrument for removal (Magill forceps, tenaculum, and towel clip) is selected. Some foreign bodies, such as smooth-surfaced objects, cannot be grasped well with the Magill forceps. After the object is grasped and successfully removed, laryngoscopy is again performed to ensure that no additional foreign body remains in the airway. The patient should then be observed until fully recovered from the sedation and topical anesthesia to ensure that symptoms have resolved and there are no other issues. Some patients may require a longer period of observation or admission to hospital if the provider suspects additional small foreign bodies (small food items, such as peas) below the vocal cords, significant aspiration, symptoms of upper airway edema after removal of the foreign body, or if there is concern about the patient's comorbidities (e.g., chronic health issues and intoxication).

Upper airway foreign body causing incomplete obstruction should be considered a true emergency, and an early decision is required regarding the appropriateness of removal in the ED versus expedited transfer to the OR. If, at any point, the airway becomes completely obstructed, then the patient is managed as described in the following section.

Complete Obstruction of the Airway

When airway obstruction is complete, the patient is unable to breathe or phonate and may hold his or her neck with one or both hands, the so-called universal choking sign. The patient may appear terrified and will be making attempts at inspiration. In general, after complete obstruction of the airway with ensuing apnea, oxygen saturation will rapidly fall to levels incompatible with consciousness within seconds to a minute.

Initial management is dictated by whether the patient is conscious or unconscious. If the patient is conscious, the abdominal thrust maneuver should immediately and repeatedly be applied until either the foreign body is expelled or the patient loses consciousness (see algorithm, Fig. 40-1). Whether the maneuver is called the abdominal thrust maneuver or the Heimlich maneuver is of no importance; they are one and the same. There is no point in attempting instrumented removal of an upper airway foreign body while the patient is still conscious. If the abdominal thrust maneuver is successful in expelling the foreign body, and the patient can phonate and breathe normally, then observation for a few hours is sufficient, and it is not mandatory to visualize the airway if the patient remains asymptomatic. If the abdominal thrust maneuver is unsuccessful in removing the foreign body and the patient loses consciousness, a rapid series of chest thrusts (equivalent to those used during CPR) may be tried.

Thereafter, the first step is immediate direct or video laryngoscopy *before any attempts at bag-mask ventilation, which may cause the foreign body to move from a supraglottic to an infraglottic position.* Generally, the patient will be flaccid, and it will not be necessary to administer a neuro-muscular blocking agent. Time should not be lost waiting for an intravenous line to be established. Under direct or video laryngoscopy, a foreign body above the glottis is easily identifiable. Again, Magill forceps, a tenaculum, a towel clip, or any other suitable device can be used to remove the foreign body. After removal of the foreign body, the larynx is inspected through direct or video laryngoscopy to ensure that there is no residual foreign material. When the foreign body is removed, the patient may begin spontaneous ventilation immediately. If the patient does not begin to breathe spontaneously, immediate intubation and initiation of positive-pressure ventilation is indicated and can be performed during the same laryngoscopy (Fig. 40-1).

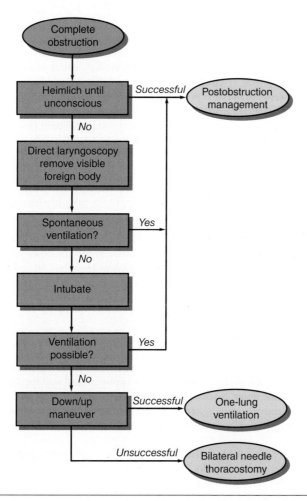

Figure 40-1 ● Management of Complete Obstruction by a Foreign Body.   See text for explanation.

If laryngoscopy does not identify a foreign body, and the glottis is clearly visualized, then either there is no foreign body or the foreign body is below the vocal cords. In this case, the patient should immediately be intubated and ventilated. If ventilation is successful, then resuscitation proceeds as for any other patient. If bag ventilation through the endotracheal tube meets with total resistance (no air movement, negative end-tidal carbon dioxide detection), then the trachea must be assumed to be completely obstructed. The stylet should immediately be replaced into the endotracheal tube, the cuff deflated, and the tube advanced all the way to its hilt in an attempt to push a tracheal foreign body into the right (or left) mainstem bronchus. If the foreign material is thought to be soft, then an attempt at ventilation can be made with the tube inserted to its deepest extent, on the basis that the tube may have passed through the obstruction. If ventilation is not successful, then the foreign body is assumed to be solid and to have been pushed into the mainstem bronchus ahead of the tube. The tube is withdrawn to its normal level and the cuff is reinflated, and then ventilation is attempted. The strategy here is to try to convert an obstructing tracheal foreign body (which will be lethal) to an obstructing mainstem bronchus foreign body (which can be removed in the OR). Thus, the patient can be kept alive by ventilating one lung while the other lung is obstructed.

If the down-then-up maneuver just described is not successful in establishing one-lung ventilation, there are two clinical possibilities. The only reversible situation is when the patient has one
obstructed mainstem bronchus and a tension pneumothorax on the other side. Pneumothorax can
occur in foreign body cases because of the abnormally high pressures generated both by the patient,
while conscious, and by the rescue maneuvers. Because the operator has no way of knowing into
which mainstem bronchus the foreign body was advanced (most commonly the right, but possibly
the left), bilateral needle thoracostomy should be performed, in the hope of identifying a tension
pneumothorax. If a pneumothorax is not identified, the second clinical possibility is complete bilateral mainstem obstruction, a condition from which survival is not possible, regardless of treatment.

POSTINTUBATION MANAGEMENT

Postintubation management depends on the clinical circumstances. If the foreign body has been
successfully removed and the patient remains obtunded, perhaps from posthypoxemic encepha-
lopathy, then ventilation and general management are as for any other postarrest patient. If the
foreign body has been pushed down into one mainstem bronchus, the other lung must be ventilated carefully at low rates with reduced tidal volumes to minimize the risk of pneumothorax
while waiting for the OR.

TIPS AND PEARLS

1. If the obstruction is incomplete, usually the best approach is to wait for definitive removal in the
   OR under a double setup. If you are forced to act, move cautiously and deliberately to ensure
   that you do not convert a supraglottic obstruction into an infraglottic obstruction.
2. If the obstructing foreign body is above the vocal cords and cannot be removed, cricothyrotomy
   is indicated.
3. If the obstructed foreign body is distal to the vocal cords and cannot be seen from above by direct
   laryngoscopy, it is extremely unlikely that cricothyrotomy will place an airway below the level
   of the obstruction, and therefore cricothyrotomy is not indicated.
5. A rapid series of abdominal thrust maneuvers is a reasonable first step in any case of complete
   obstruction and is the only maneuver that can be performed on a patient with a complete obstruction who is awake and responsive. In the unconscious patient, chest thrusts may help, but
   plan to proceed quickly to direct laryngoscopy.

EVIDENCE

- **When should I use abdominal thrust maneuvers versus back blows?** There are no completely
  sound studies comparing the effectiveness of various methods for expelling an obstructing
  foreign body. There is no clear evidence to establish the superiority of chest compressions
  over abdominal thrusts or vice versa. The American Heart Association (AHA), in its 2010
  guidelines for emergency cardiac care, recommends a progression of airway clearing maneuvers in the conscious patient, beginning with back blows and progressing to abdominal
  thrusts.[1] If the abdominal thrust maneuver is not successful despite repeated attempts, and
  the patient is unconscious, then chest thrusts can be tried, but there is no evidence that
  they will be more successful than abdominal thrusts. For obese patients or women late in
  pregnancy, chest thrusts are preferred. A cadaver study indicates that greater airway pressures can be developed using chest thrusts than with abdominal thrusts when the patient is
  unconscious, and this evidence is reflected in the AHA recommendations.[2]

REFERENCES

1. Berg RA, Hemphill R, Abella BS, et al. 2010 American Heart Association guidelines for cardiopulmonary resuscitation and emergency cardiovascular care. *Circulation*. 2010;122:S685–S705.

2. Langhelle A, Sunde K, Wik L, et al. Airway pressure with chest compressions versus Heimlich manoeuvre in recently dead adults with complete airway obstruction. *Resuscitation*. 2000;44:105–108.

INDEX

Note: Pages followed by f indicate figures; pages followed by t indicate tables; pages followed by b indicate boxes

The 'Gold Standard' in Airway Management Education

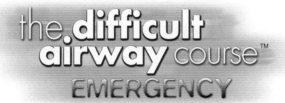

"One of the most important courses I have ever attended. The lectures, demos and hands-on workshops were all amazing."
Andrew C. Jones, MD, Florida

This 2 ½ day immersion experience in emergency airway management sets the standard for airway education. Evidence-based and comprehensive, this course is taught by a world-class faculty of airway experts who want you to succeed.

"Instructors were all phenomenal – smart, cutting-edge, super-approachable and friendly."
Michael Imperato, MD, New York

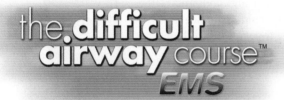

"This course is miles ahead of any other class I have taken. Being a medic for 24 years, I still learned new and better skills and approaches to my practice."
Karen Dougherty, MICP, NREMT-P

This intensive, two-day immersion program in EMS airway management will provide you with the knowledge and skills you need to confidently manage any airway situation.

"Excellent course! Great hands-on experience and very knowledgeable instructors!"
Ryan T. Koch, EMT-P, New York

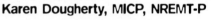

"This course was one of the most intensive and sophisticated courses I have ever attended in 30 years of anesthesia practice. The faculty was outstanding."
Robert Amrhein, MD, Massachusetts

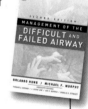

Taught by a world-renowned faculty of airway experts, this intensive, 2 ½ day course focuses exclusively on the difficult and failed airway. Even the most experienced anesthesia providers will take their airway practice to the next level with this course!

"Far and away the most useful educational adventure I've undertaken." **Sue Schulz, MD, Texas**

For Course Dates, Locations and Registration Information, visit www.theairwaysite.com.

Airway Management Resources

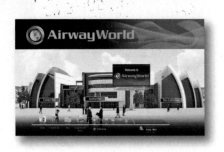

Airway World™ is the only multi-disciplinary virtual knowledge center dedicated to airway management. Join your colleagues in the Airway World community and gain access to live webinars, videos, moderated chats, research reports, airway literature, discussion groups and more! Register for Airway World at **www.AirwayWorld.com**. Registration is free (and easy)!

The Difficult Airway App™ is an essential tool for clinicians who manage emergency airways in any setting: the ED, ICU, in-patient unit or the many EMS practice environments. The app features easy, yet sophisticated, adult and pediatric drug dosing, decision-making support, rapid sequence intubation guidelines and educational resources including illustrations and videos.

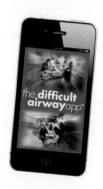

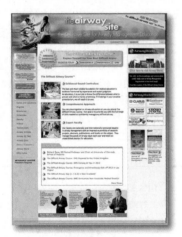

The Airway Site™ features the 'gold standard' airway management courses including: The Difficult Airway Course: Emergency™, The Difficult Airway Course: Anesthesia™, The Difficult Airway Course: EMS™ and Fundamentals of Airway Management™. Visit **www.theairwaysite.com** to register for these courses and link to other valuable airway resources.

The Airway Cards™ are the definitive pocket reference guides containing essential information including airway algorithms, mnemonics and drug dosing. *These include:* The Airway Card™, The Airway Card Anesthesia™, and The Airway Card EMS™.

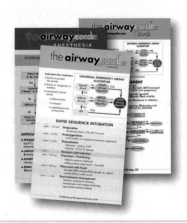